Smart Bodyweight Training

by Matt Schifferle

Text Copyright © 2018 Matthew J. Schifferle
All Rights Reserved

ISBN-13:978-1718906648
ISBN-10:1718906641

The information provided in this book is designed to provide helpful information on the subjects discussed. This book is not meant to be used, nor should it be used, to diagnose or treat any medical condition. For diagnosis or treatment of any medical problem, consult your own physician. The publisher and author are not responsible for any specific health or allergy needs that may require medical supervision and are not liable for any damages or negative consequences from any treatment, action, application or preparation, to any person reading or following the information in this book. References are provided for informational purposes only and do not constitute endorsement of any websites or other sources. Readers should be aware that the websites listed in this book may change.

Cover photo and design by Chris Clemens at http://www.thinkpilgrim.com

Dedicated to Grand Master Stephen Barrett.
Thank you for your endless patience while teaching me how to be a technician.

Table of Contents

Introduction	5
Chapter 1 Unfair Advantages of Bodyweight Training	7
Chapter 2 Smart Training Part I	15
Chapter 3 Smart Training Part II	19
Chapter 4 Smart Training Part III	29
Chapter 5 The Elements Of Progression	38
Chapter 6 Chain Training	53
Chapter 7 Extension Chain	63
Chapter 8 Squat Chain	82
Chapter 9 Pull Chain	106
Chapter 10 Push Chain	125
Chapter 11 Flexion Chain	151
Chapter 12 The Lateral Chain	167
Chapter 13 Weighted Calisthenics	174
Chapter 14 Calisthenics Cardio	178
Chapter 15 Principles of Programming	191
Chapter 16 Eating For Success	207
Bonus Chapter: DIY Tools Of The Trade	216

Introduction

The phrase "work smarter, not harder," has become so commonplace it's almost become a cliché but how many times do we take this advice to heart? These days, a busy schedule and an over-caffeinated lifestyle seem to be the norm. When was the last time you ran into someone who said they weren't busy, tired or stressed?

This idea of always working harder particularly applies to fitness and exercise. Our fitness culture loves to extol the virtues of blood, sweat, and tears. A quick scroll through social media makes it clear that hard work is what all the cool kids are doing while working easier or taking shortcuts is for wimps and sissies.

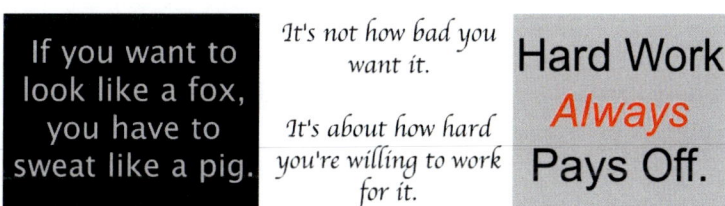

Motivation phrases like this are all over our fitness culture, but while Hard work is very important, it isn't everything.

It's easy to understand why hard work is put on a pedestal. In a world of scams, inflated hype, and empty promises, hard work is quickly becoming one of the few reliable ways to invest your time and energy. Sooner or later, everyone gives up the search for shortcuts and resolves to get results through brute force.

Hard work is incredibly important, but while this strategy can work for a little while, it's incredibly limiting and even dangerous. This is because hard work is extremely hard to scale. Eventually, everyone reaches the limit of how hard they can work.

Trying to succeed through brute force is like running at a wall as fast as you can. You'll make some initial progress but eventually, you'll have to stop moving forward. You may even crash and suffer burnout or injury. Once you reach that wall, your only options are to either quit and walk away, or you can continue to push against that wall in an attempt to maintain your results. Continuing to push your limits will prevent you from falling back, but you're now stuck working as hard as possible for the rest of your life just to stay where you are.

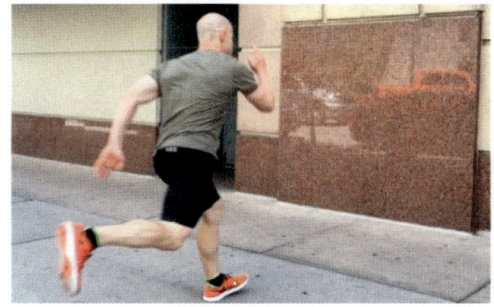 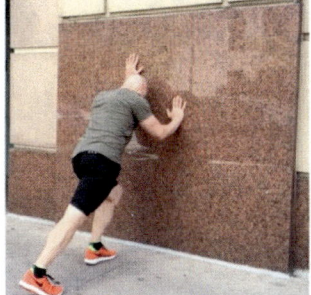

Hard work is like running at a wall. You make progress for a while, but eventually, you stop moving forward no matter how hard you keep pushing.

Working smarter gives you the opportunity to escape the exercise rat race. The more you learn about training intelligently, the better your results will be even if you're not putting in more effort than before.

Learning to train in a smarter way teaches you how to move around that wall so your efforts can continue to move your forward.

About the author

My name is Matt Schifferle and I've spent most of my life learning that hard work alone holds limited potential for success in fitness. I used to pride myself on how hard I could work with exhausting workouts, and punishing routines. This approach did bring me some progress, but it cost me a lot of time, money, and energy. It also beat my body and mind to a pulp by the time I was 30.

I almost gave up on fitness entirely, but as a last resort, I decided to give bodyweight training a try. Within a few months, every aspect of my fitness improved dramatically, plus my body and mind felt refreshed. The real shocking part was that I was making more progress while working less, not more.

Calisthenics taught me that even though I had spent most of my life working hard, I was also working dumb. I thought I would get results if I could work hard enough while using the right exercises, the right routine, or the right equipment. I eventually learned that none of that stuff works very well when I neglect to use them in a progressively smarter way. I've spent months, even years working as hard as I could without building any muscle or strength nor was I improving my performance in any of my hobbies. These seemingly endless plateaus came to an end once I realized that training smarter was a much easier to way to make progress than always trying to work harder.

What you'll learn from this book

The information in this book can potentially improve every exercise and workout you do for the rest of your life.

That's a bold statement, and I write it because I have absolute faith in what the information in this book can do for you. You see, this is not just a book about bodyweight training. It's a book about using calisthenics as a tool to consistently learn how to exercise in a smarter, and more productive, way no matter what style of exercise you practice.

I'll start out in the next chapter explaining why bodyweight training is a scientifically sound method for helping you reach your goals. In fact, it provides some massive advantages compared to more equipment based methods. The following chapters will show you the three things you must focus on to achieve success regardless of what exercise methods you use. After that, I'll teach you my unique approach towards progressive bodyweight training so you can build a custom program to perfectly fit your goals, your body, your fitness level and your lifestyle.

Who is this book for?

Maybe you're looking to break free from the shackles of a gym membership. Perhaps you want to add some new tools to an established workout routine. Or maybe you're tired of the iron game and want to explore a new way to get stronger. You may even be an experienced bodyweight practitioner and are just looking for some new ideas. No matter what you've done in your past, or what you hope to accomplish in the future, Smart Calisthenics can help you break free of the false hope of hard, yet dumb, work.
-Matt Schifferle Founder of the Red Delta Project 2017

Chapter 1 Unfair Advantages of Bodyweight Training

There was a time when I was very skeptical of bodyweight training. I used to believe it was impossible to get very far without a gym full of equipment. Over the years, my views have changed, and now I prefer bodyweight training over weights and machines by a mile and a half. It's not just because I enjoy practicing calisthenics; it's because of the practically unfair advantages it has for building muscle, burning fat and improving performance.

The biggest advantages have to do with helping you satisfy what I call the Delta Principles of Fitness. To quickly recap from my book, Fitness Independence, the five Delta Principles are the essential make-it-or-break-it principles in fitness. All of your potential depends upon your ability to fulfill all five of those principles. The more you satisfy them the better your results are. However, if just one of these principles is lacking, you have almost zero chance of getting what you want. Calisthenics makes it much easier to fulfill all five. Let's take a closer look at each one to find out why.

Delta Principle #1 Consistency

All exercise success comes from constantly adhering to beneficial habits for extended periods of time. When your training is here and there, you stand little chance of making any progress. Even if you do make progress, it will be next to impossible to maintain it with inconsistent habits.

Even the most dedicated equipment user will admit that bodyweight training is incredibly efficient. You can train anywhere at any time you like. You don't need a gym nor do you need to buy any fancy equipment. You're completely in control of your exercise fate. Even though many will admit that calisthenics is convenient, that convenience is usually considered to be a novelty at best. It's nice, but it's not that big of a deal. They are right, the simple nature of bodyweight training isn't a big deal. It's a supermassive black hole size deal. The reason is the more convenient and efficient your training is the easier it is to continue doing it on a consistent basis.

Evidence of this is in almost every trend, fad, and habit that's become more prolific in society. Everything from the popular use of the automobile to checking email has progressed because technology and innovation have made it cheaper and easier to use on a consistent basis.

Bodyweight training has always been one of the easiest and most efficient means of training. Maintaining that essential consistency is much easier than with any equipment based exercise, and this sets you up for long-term progress.

Delta Principle #2 Progression

Progression is the essence of what makes you stronger, leaner and more fit. It doesn't matter what your routine looks like. If your training stays the same, you stay the same. The moment you start to train better is the moment you start getting better results.

Progression is also the biggest stumbling block people face when it comes to bodyweight training. It's widely believed that basic moves, like push-ups and lunges, have a limited range of progression. I used to believe this myth myself, but now I know it's straight up nonsense. I would even argue there's more potential to progress in bodyweight training than with other methods.

Most equipment based training focuses on just two ways to advance, namely weight and reps. Bodyweight training uses these same two methods plus seven other ways to progress your training. That's right; there are nine ways you can progress any bodyweight exercise! This variety of progression gives you the flexibility to progress your training in a way that best suits your current fitness level and body type. Instead of trying to force yourself to conform to a limited range of progression, you can now create a custom progression plan that directly addresses the weaknesses and imbalances that are holding you back.

Delta Principle #3 Learning

Knowledge is power, and the more you know, the more you grow. If you fail to absorb new information, you'll fail to make progress. Naturally, learning is the key to training smarter rather than just harder.

Bodyweight training requires constant mental focus and attention to what you're doing. Every workout requires your mind to work just as hard as your body. As you'll discover in the next few chapters, your mental strength is the very essence of success.

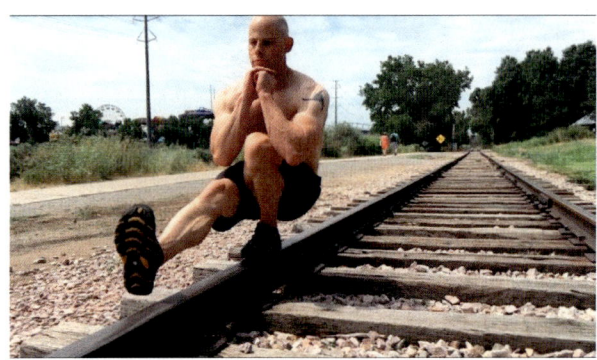

Your thoughts and focus are the key to keeping your training on track.

Many folks claim the advantage with lifting weights is it's easy to add resistance through just putting more weight on the bar. While just adding weight is easier, you can do it without achieving a deeper understanding of how to do the exercise. You can get under both a 100# bar and a 300# bar without learning a thing.

Calisthenics forces you to learn how to apply more resistance to your muscles. It's not as easy as sliding a plate onto a bar, and that's a good thing. You'll be able to apply plenty of resistance to your muscles once you understand how to use that resistance. The more you understand how your body works the more effective your training will be.

Delta Principle #4 Emotional Drive / Motivation

This is one of the biggest advantages of bodyweight training. Your mind and maybe even your very soul thrives on moving around. Just consider how active children are. There's just something about moving through space that's emotionally rewarding. Even exercising in place seems to lack that emotional stimulation.

Just consider the proliferation of electronic entertainment you see around gyms these days. Every stationary piece of equipment has a TV attached and people whip out their cell phones or tablets in between sets while using weight machines. The body is working, but the mind is bored and starving for distraction. The result is the person's attention is just as focused on the latest celebrity news or email as it is on their workout. Not only does this suck the life-is-good vibes out of your workout, it also severely compromises your progress.

There are no screens or distractions in bodyweight training. Whereas such things are a welcome distraction on a treadmill they become unwelcome disturbances once your body is moving around. Your mind needs to stay focused just to continue doing the exercise so not only is your training far more effective, but it's also a lot more enjoyable and rewarding.

Delta Principle #5 Plan of Action

Nothing great ever happens without a plan. Whether you're building a house or making a sandwich, having a plan ensures you make the appropriate choices to achieve your goals. The old saying that if you fail to plan then you plan to fail is truer than people know.

The most effective exercise plans are simple, easy to put into action and quickly adapt to your changing circumstances. It's difficult to maintain a consistent and progressive workout routine when your plan is complicated and difficult to use.

Bodyweight training uses the most basic and effective plan in all of fitness. In fact, it's so simple it can be summed up in a single word:

MOVE!

Yep, that's it, just move around. All other considerations are merely details. Even then, most workout plans and routines are very simple in nature. There aren't many fancy exercises to distract you from what's most important. Most routines only focus on a handful of exercises which use primal movements to work your whole body.

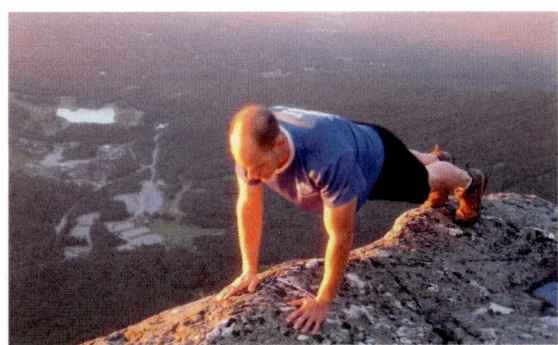

My Sunday workout plan: Step 1 hike up mountain. Step 2 do 50 push-ups. Step 3 walk down mountain.

So there you have it, the five Delta Principles for guaranteed success and every single one of them is easier to satisfy when you make calisthenics the cornerstone of your training. There's nothing special or magical about them and you probably won't find them trending on social media any time soon but that's a good thing. It's often the dull unpolished methods that produce the most exciting results.

But maybe you want something a little more than five principles to believe bodyweight training can produce the goods. Fair enough, let's look at some advantages of calisthenics concerning the three objectives covered in this book, fat loss, building muscle and performance.

Calisthenics Advantages For Fat Loss

Losing weight is not unlike having a tank full of gas in your car and your goal is to make the low fuel light come on. Imagine if I gave you a luxury car with the gas tank topped off and said if you could get the fuel light to come on you would win the car. The only catch is, you have to put some amount of gas back into the car every day. What would your strategy be?

I imagine your first step would be to monitor and regulate the gas you're putting in the car. That would be a good start, but it still wouldn't use any of the gas that's in the tank to begin with. You're going to have to proactively burn that fuel so how would you burn it off as quickly as possible?

Here's a common strategy; pay a monthly fee to drive the car at a race track. You also have to tow your car to a race track where you endlessly drive around in boring mind-numbing circles. Forget the thrill of speed, you don't want to wear out the car so you drive at a modest pace. After that, you tow the car back to your garage where it sits until you can find the motivation and/or time to do it again. All the while you're still required to go out and put at least some gas back in the car every day.

Now imagine I give you the same scenario but I tell you that you can drive the car anywhere you like, at any time without any restrictions whatsoever. How might your strategy change? You would drive it any chance you got! You would offer carpool for your whole office every day. Or you could drive the kids anywhere they wanted to go and take the long route to and from work. Forget evenings in front of the TV, nothing beats cruising the coastal highway every evening to watch the sunset.

Given the two scenarios, it's a wonder why anyone would pick the first option, but that's exactly what many people do. They have a full tank of gas so they spend money at a local gym, mostly to use the boring cardio equipment and take aerobic style classes like Spinning or kickboxing. Nothing is wrong with this strategy, but it's costly and very limited. Once you set your mind to burn calories on a piece of equipment you enclose your fat burning potential in a cage. You can only burn extra fuel at certain times, in a certain place while using equipment that doesn't do very much. Also, it's a good thing the modern equipment has "amenities" like satellite TV to keep you distracted. Heaven knows your mind needs something to do because you're not getting much else out of the activity.

When your body becomes your calorie burning machine the whole world is your gym. The sidewalk is your treadmill, your bicycle is a spinner, and the local hiking trails are your stair machine. All of this is readily available to you 24/7 and you're not confined to using it for a few hours each week. Best of all, it's all available at a low cost or even free. You may even find you save money by using your car less and your body more!

The biggest limiting factor in burning extra calories is time. You can burn more calories by working harder, but when your physical activity is infrequent it doesn't matter how hard you push yourself. You just can't burn very much energy in a single workout. On the other hand, if your physical activity is more frequent you don't have to throttle yourself with high-intensity exercise. All of those frequent moments of physical activity add up. This is why I always encourage people who are looking to lose weight to get their body moving in some sort of daily activity that's not necessarily a workout.

One of the best options is to have an active commute. Back when I lived in Japan, I rode my bike to and from school 40 minutes each way. I was doing nearly 90 minutes of activity every day just to get around Kyoto.

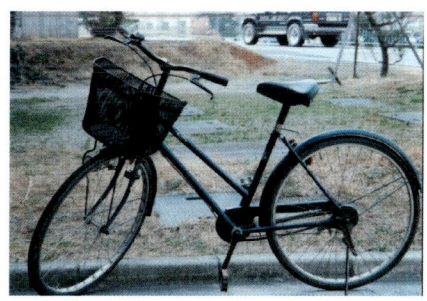

It may not look like much, but commuting on this bike, in Sonobe Japan, made me burn more calories in a week than most people burn in a month at the local gym.

If you're searching for employment, look for a job that involves a great deal of physical movement. If you can be active 8-9 hours a day landscaping, waiting tables or doing construction the caloric burn you'll receive along with your paycheck will blow away even the most serious gym rats. After all, what sounds better; being active 4 hours a week or 40?

Lastly, when you engage in bodyweight activity you're doing more than just moving your limbs in an effort to burn calories. You're actually doing something! Be it riding a bike with friends, hiking up a mountain or just taking a walk after dinner, you're doing something with a purpose beyond just burning calories.

The biggest lesson is that all calories count and it doesn't matter how you're burning them. Suffering boredom while watching the clock tick down on a treadmill doesn't make the exercise any more effective. In many cases, it's less so. When you get out and do something there's far less mental stress involved which makes it easier to start the activity and continue doing it for much longer periods of time. I can hike for hours, but even 30 minutes on a stair machine is more than enough for me thank you very much.

Calisthenics Advantages For Building Muscle

By far the most common question I'm asked about bodyweight training is if it's possible to build as much muscle with bodyweight training as with weights. To that, my answer is always a big fat NO. I firmly believe most folks will build MORE muscle and strength with bodyweight training than they would with weight training alone for the following reasons.

#1 Efficiency = consistency

Here's the honest truth about building muscle. If you want to have any hope of success you need to be able to stick to a regular training routine, every week, for years on end. Work can't stop you, school can't get too busy and family and friends can't convince you to skip a workout each week. In other words, life can't get in the way. The biggest reason why many people fail to build up their body is a lack of long-term consistency. Building muscle requires time and a whole lot of persistence in your training. I've never met anyone with a strong muscular physique who hasn't dedicated themselves to consistent training for years on end.

When I tell folks the need for such consistency I'm often met with skepticism and push back. "I can't make working out my life," they say. "You can't expect me to rearrange my priorities around going to the gym; I want a life!" I fully agree with these statements. Very few people can or will make training in a gym enough of a priority to make serious gains. Thankfully, you don't have to do that when your own body is your gym.

With calisthenics, there's no gym to drive to, and no complicated equipment to set up. Working out is as simple as laying down on the floor, jumping onto a pull-up bar or walking out the front door. Now, your workouts can bend to the whims of your life rather than the other way around. This means your chances of keeping to that consistent routine greatly increase along with your chances for success.

#2 Progression

The biggest progressive advantage of Bodyweight training is what many people consider its greatest weakness. When you use little more than your own bodyweight, there isn't a whole lot of adjustment you can make. No pads to move, or weights to change. This causes people to believe there is a limited progressive adjustment with bodyweight training.

The truth is, there is very little difference between progressive bodyweight training and training with adjustable equipment. Both methods are actually a form of strength training, and both methods use progressive resistance to further challenge your muscles over time. The only real difference is how you make adjustments to facilitate the progression. With equipment, you keep your technique relatively the same while adjusting the weight you lift. With bodyweight training, you keep your weight about the same and adjust your technique.

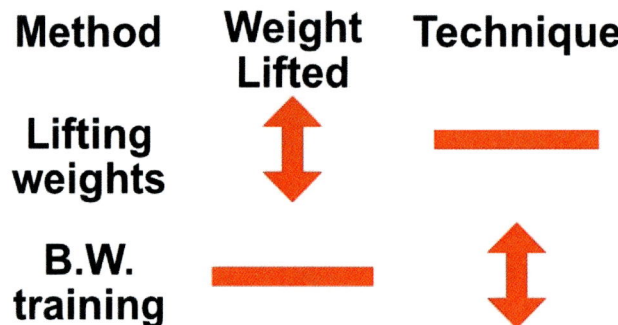

Both weightlifting and calisthenics use progressive resistance. The difference is in how you adjust that resistance.

Outside of that one difference, the actual process you use to build muscle is the same.
It's also a myth that adjustable equipment makes progress easier. In fact, it actually makes moving beyond the beginner stages of an exercise much more difficult. This is due to something I call functional fragmentation and functional integration.

Functional integration vs functional fragmentation

Functional integration refers to the way the human body uses multiple muscles and capabilities to perform an activity. Progressive leg training is a good example of this idea in action. When you do a lunge, you use every muscle in your lower body in an integrated way. Everything from the muscles in your feet to the prime movers, like your quads, play an important role.

You also integrate multiple physical abilities at the same time. Lunges require strength, balance, stability, coordination, flexibility, endurance, and mobility. So even if you're doing lunges to strengthen your legs, you'll still develop those other qualities at the same time.

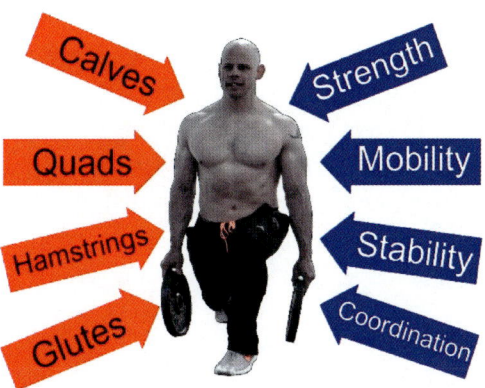

Progressive calisthenics integrates multiple muscles and functional elements into one basic movement to develop multiple benefits in one exercise.

In contrast, functional fragmentation breaks up your muscles and capabilities. This is usually done in an effort to focus on developing a specific muscle or capability and it's not always a bad thing to do. Physical therapists and trainers use functional fragmentation all the time to shore up a chronic weakness that's causing pain or holding back performance.

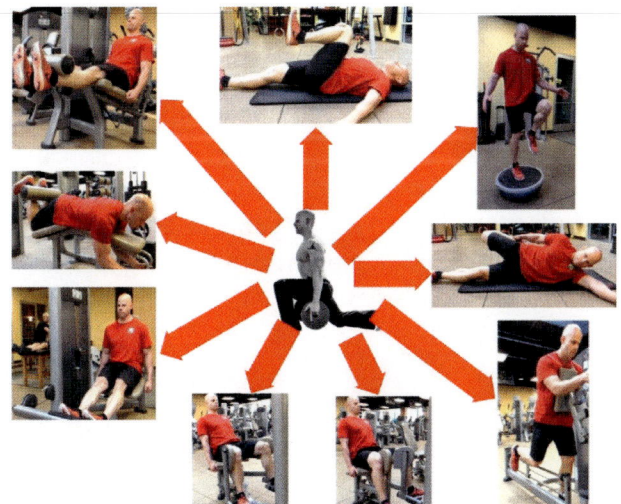

You can fragment many of the benefits of lunges into several exercises.

There are legitimate applications for functional fragmentation, but for the most part, you'll make better gains with less stress by embracing functional integration. It ensures that you won't work around any handicapping weaknesses and progressive calisthenics forces you to confront those weaknesses through holistic training. You may get away with unstable hips on a leg press, but lunges and single leg squats will expose such instability and make your hips rock-solid as a necessity.

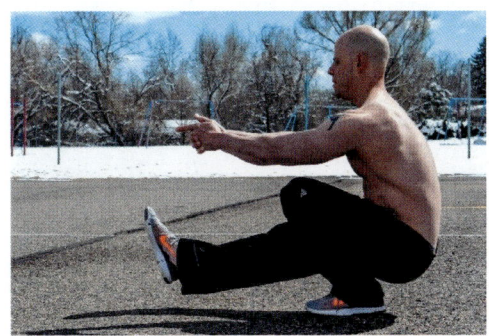

The basic pistol squat requires you to be strong in multiple ways, not just in how hard you can contract a few major muscles.

Believe it or not, your muscles want to grow. They're just sitting there waiting for you to tell them to do so. Once you give them a clear and consistent growth signal they will gladly grow without hesitation.

The biggest reason why people struggle to build muscle is that some sort of weakness is inhibiting that muscle building signal. Your body is smart, it knows imbalances and weaknesses can compromise your safety. A lack of hip stability can cause stress on your knees. Weak hamstrings can place stress on your lower back. Even weakness in your ankles can increase the risk of injury. Your body naturally holds back your strength and muscle development to prevent you from overloading yourself.

Progressive calisthenics will help you address any weaknesses that inhibit your muscle building potential. The more advanced your training becomes the stronger you will be as a whole which helps take the brakes off your muscle building potential.

Calisthenics Advantages for Health and Performance

As you'll discover in the next chapter, the ultimate goal of Smart Bodyweight Training isn't to build muscle, lose fat or get stronger. Those are merely side effects to the real true goal which is to learn how to use your body better. Learning how to use your body better will help you gain a massive amount of functional carry over toward almost any athletic activity. You'll also greatly improve your everyday functional strength. You'll climb stairs with more ease, get out of your car without strain and even standing for long periods of time won't be an issue at all.

While the exercises in this book are no replacement for your sports specific training, they will improve your ability to train for any sport or activity you enjoy. You may not improve your golf game by just doing pushups, but building more shoulder control will pay large dividends at the driving range.

I could go on about the benefits of bodyweight training, but I would rather let you experience them for yourself. Your journey starts with the next page.

Chapter 2 Smart Training Part I

As you can tell from the previous chapter, I just think the world of bodyweight training. With that said, I don't believe for a second that calisthenics exercises can make you leaner, stronger or more muscular on their own. It's entirely possible for you to do the best bodyweight exercises, and use them in the best routine and still make very little progress regardless of how hard you work.

I know that's not the message you usually come across in a fitness book. Most books tell you success depends on doing the right exercises with the right routine. While the routine and exercises you select are important, they are not truly responsible for the results you want. Instead, the exercises and routine you follow are like an alkaline battery you plug into an electronic device. It's not the physical battery, but the electrical juice within the battery that makes the device work. It doesn't matter if you use the right battery or install it in the correct way. If it's empty you won't have any power to get the result you want.

Your training success doesn't come from using the right exercises or routine. It comes from making sure those exercises and routines are filled with the electronic juice that makes them work. The next three chapters are going to cover the three essential elements of smart training that produce the electrical juice which powers your training.

Smart Element #1 Your Neural Code

It's easy to make the assumption that training is mostly a physical discipline. Sometimes exercise is even referred to as physical training when people talk about muscles, movement, and might. This focus on the physical can make it easy to forget that training is actually more of a mental discipline than a physical one.

Your body is like any other machine. It operates according to the instructions it receives from the central computer that is your brain. Every motion you do, from blinking your eyes to kicking your leg out, is the physical result of coded neurological instructions that are created in your mind.

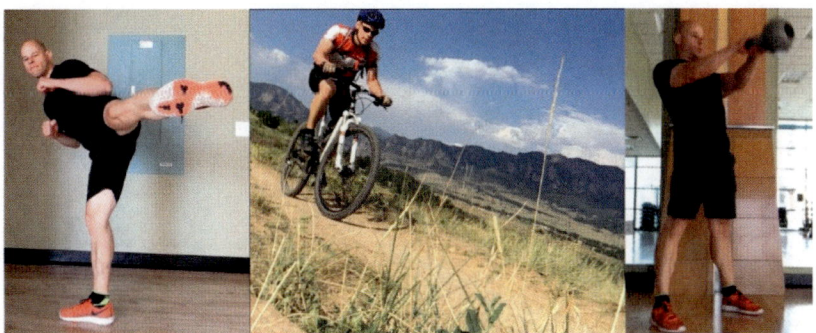
All forms of physical activity are the physical expression of what's going on in your mind.

When you want to do something with your body, your brain creates a coded signal that travels down your spinal cord and branches out through your peripheral nervous system.

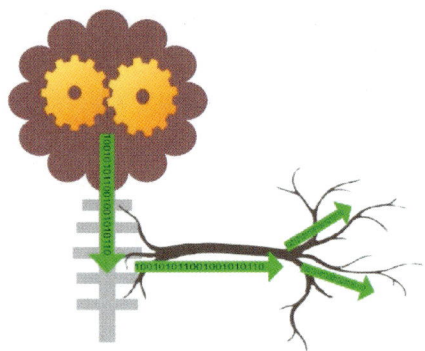

Physical activity occurs when your mind creates a signal that then travels down your spinal cord and is distributed through your nervous system.

This coded signal reaches a very specific number of muscular switches which are called motor units. A motor unit is a neuron with some muscle fibers attached to it. When that neuron receives that neurological signal, all of the muscle fibers it's associated with fully contract. When the neuron no longer receives that signal the muscle fibers relax.

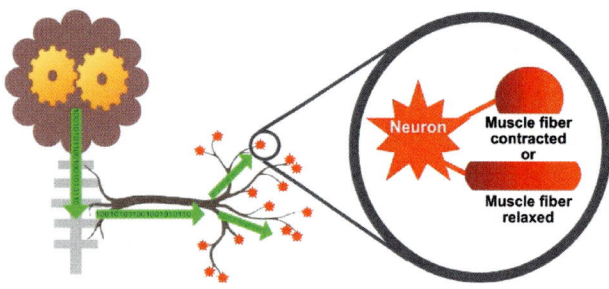

Your neurological signal is expressed through stimulating specific neurons telling them to contract their muscle fibers.

All of the physical activity you do is the result of the code you create in your brain to stimulate various motor units throughout your body. Just as all digital data is a binary stream of 1s and 0s, your neural code is also binary telling your motor units to turn on or off. This neural code is the source of all of your training success.

The creation and manipulation of this neural code is why this book is titled Smart Bodyweight Training. The word smart means to possess an essential element that produces the desired result. Going back to the analogy of the battery, you could say the battery is "smart" when it's fully charged. In the case of training, your thoughts are the essential element that makes your body move and work in an effective way.

The opposite of smart is dumb meaning to lack an essential element to make something work. You could say a battery is dumb once it's become drained and can no longer power on your device.

So smart training means you have the essential neurological code that makes your training effective. Even though a good routine or fancy equipment can be helpful, the real essence of effective training comes from what you think, not what you use.

Understanding that the origin of all training success comes from your mind brings some interesting lessons to light.

#1 Physical cultivation is psychological

If you want to get better results from your training, you need to use exercise methods that progress over time. The only way your training can progress is if your thoughts progress as well. If your mind never changes how it works, it will never progress your neural code. If your code doesn't change your physical abilities won't change. If your abilities don't change then your results will never progress. In other words, you can't get better results from your training until you progress your thoughts.

#2 Distractions are training poison

The success of your workout depends entirely on the signal your brain sends to your muscles. In light of this, anything that weakens this signal can jeopardize the quality of your training.

I know a TV or smartphone may seem like a siren call, especially when your mind is under stress, but they won't do you any favors. The more your mind is focused on things external to your workout, the less it can be focused on improving your training.

#3 Avoid unnecessary pain and discomfort

Pain is not weakness leaving the body, it's just the opposite actually. Your nervous system's natural reaction to a risky situation is to put on the brakes to prevent further damage. Just think of trying to run with a blister on your foot, or how strong you feel with a sore muscle. Even if you can fight through the pain, I guarantee you would have gotten more out of your effort if you didn't have that discomfort.

This principle also applies to situations where you feel uneasy or unsure of what to do. You cannot put as much power through your legs while walking on a frozen pond as you would on AstroTurf. Again, the reason is the same. Your mind perceives your situation as being a bit riskier and inhibits your neurological code.

Some pain and discomfort is a natural part of training so it's impractical and not necessary to avoid it at all costs. The key is to look for ways you can minimize unnecessary discomfort and uneasiness. Be sure to wear comfortable clothing when working out, drink enough water and prepare for the weather you'll be experiencing. Allowing your mind to be at ease will take off the mental brakes that are slowing down your progress.

#4 Stress alone doesn't stimulate change

I grew up with the belief that stress was what initiated change in the body. While stress does play an important role, it's time to recognize that the body won't always progress just because you exhaust yourself.

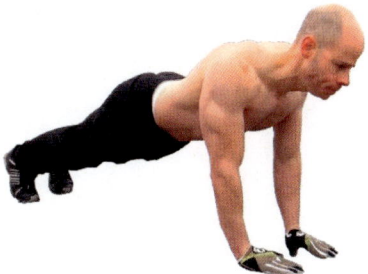

You can do push-ups until you collapse on the floor, but that won't get you very far if you're not thinking about how to do them better.

It's not stress that directs physical change, it's education. When your neural code changes you literally think differently about how to use your body. This directly carries over to how you use your body which then creates a cascade of change and adaptation.

#5 Habit will make or break your results

Your brain is a habit-forming machine. When you repeatedly do something you wear "neural groves" into the wiring of your brain making that action neurologically easier to do. Over time, this groove becomes the default neural code you use without even thinking about what you're doing.

This ability to form habits can work for you as well as against you. If you have a habit of using your hips when you walk or run, you'll strengthen those muscles without too much mental effort. On the other hand, if you've developed the habit of not using your hips you'll struggle to strengthen or tone them even through vigorous exercise.

The good news is you can condition any habit over time. Don't worry if you're struggling to turn on certain muscles, or move a certain way. With enough repetition, you'll create a neural code that will make even difficult activates easier over time.

#6 What are you thinking about?

The effectiveness of every workout you do boils down to one simple question:

What are you thinking about?

How you answer this question will determine the effectiveness of your training. Sadly, most people struggle to answer this simple question. Sometimes they tell me what they are planning, like what exercises they are doing or what muscles they are working. While these answers are certainly better than "I dunno", they still don't assure an effective workout.

So what should you think about in your training? That's the second part of smart training that I'll cover in the next chapter.

Chapter 3 Smart Training Part II

Successful training starts with the thoughts in your mind, but that doesn't mean you can become a world-class athlete by just thinking about exercise. As my Taekwon-do Instructor always told us "you can learn everything there is to know about ice skating and still fall on your butt the first time you step onto the ice."

The mental aspect of training is necessary, but it's only the first step towards training smarter. In this chapter, we'll explore the second part which deals with what you want to think about while training.

Smart Element #2 Tension Control

It makes sense that your mind controls your body, but how do you put that to practical use during your workouts?

The answer rests in how the neurological process of training is a two-way street between your mind and your muscle. When your mind sends a neurological code to your muscles, your muscles also send neurological feedback to your brain regarding what's going on. This feedback is the sensory perception of muscle tension.

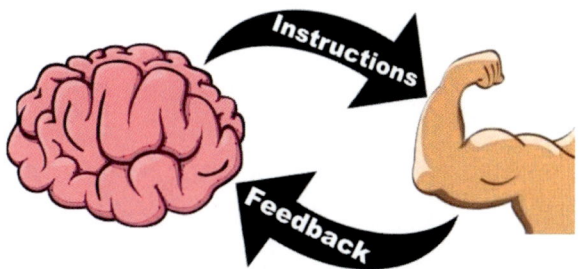

Your mind sends instructions to your muscles and your muscles return sensory feedback back to your mind so you can feel what's going on.

Tension isn't everything; it's the only thing

It doesn't matter what your goals are or what sort of exercise you're doing. The single purpose of your neurological code, and thus your training, is to create and control muscle tension.

Your muscle tension is the very essence of what creates the results you're hoping to achieve. As an athlete or exercise enthusiast, your primary job is to use tension just as a painter uses paint and a writer uses words. The better you use tension, the better your results will be. The thing is, what should you focus on while training to use tension more effectively? The answer to this can be found in the three qualities of muscle tension.

The Three Qualities Of Muscle Tension

You can manipulate muscle tension in an infinite number of ways, but all variations involve a particular combination of just three different variables.

Quality #1 Where you place tension throughout your body

Controlling where you send muscle tension can significantly improve the effectiveness of your training. Essentially, it's the skill of being able to engage a muscle on demand. Being able to actively put tension where you want it is the gateway towards muscle size and strength plus it can help prevent injury while enhancing performance.

Controlling the placement of muscle tension is an essential skill few people seek to cultivate. Part of the reason is the myth that tension is controlled by the equipment you use or the technique you perform. While the technique and equipment you use do influence what muscles are working, neither directly controls muscle tension.

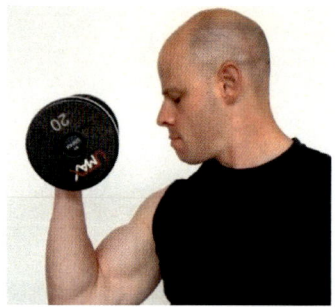 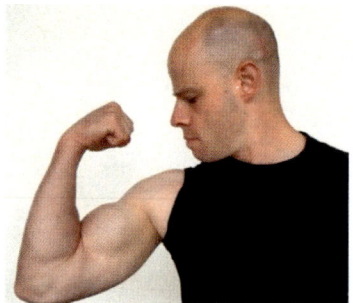

You can still place tension in a muscle even without a weight because the mind, not a weight or even a particular exercise controls where tension goes.

A bigger reason that many people are not aware they need to focus on tension control is that some experts claim it's not very important. I once read an article, by a prominent weightlifter, who stated that all you need to do is lift heavy weight with correct technique to get bigger and stronger. That's like saying the best way to drive a race car is to point the car down the track while mashing the accelerator to the floor.

Make no mistake, tension control is a vital part of your training, and it should be something you're always striving to improve. Personally, enhancing my tension skills has been the answer to every challenge I've ever faced in my training. Every injury and recurring pain have been because of poor tension control. Stubborn muscles that refused to grow were always the result of a weak mind-muscle connection. Every performance issue, from balance and stability to explosive power was solved by figuring out how to engage my muscles in a better way. Whatever you're struggling to achieve, improving tension control is an important part of the solution.

The modern plague of muscle amnesia

The neurological path between your brain and your muscles can become stronger or weaker just like the muscle fibers themselves. Also, just like your muscles, these pathways operate on the principle of "use it or lose it."

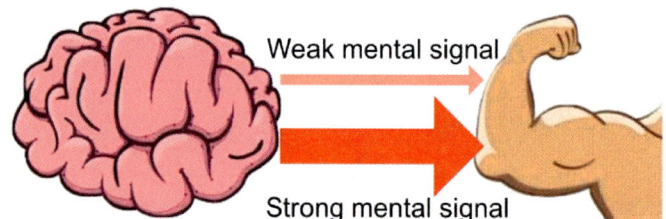

You can strengthen the neurological connection between your mind and muscle just as you strengthen the muscles themselves.

As I mentioned in the last chapter, repetition is the foundation for building and maintaining your tension control habits. It doesn't matter how your muscles are supposed to behave while you do an exercise, they're going to behave how you've used them through daily habit.

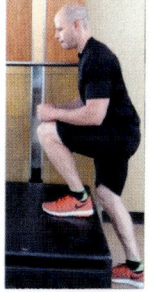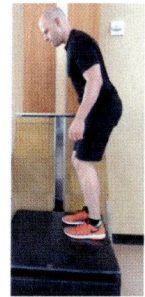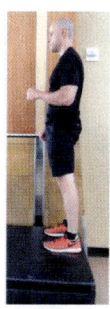

Stepping up on a box is a pretty simple exercise, but your glutes and hamstrings won't fully extend your hips to help you stand up straight if you're not in the habit of using those muscles outside your workout.

Even the most active individuals experience daily habits that condition poor tension control. Sitting is one of the most common culprits since it conditions the mind to shut down many of your muscles for hours at a time.

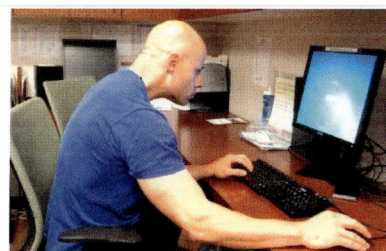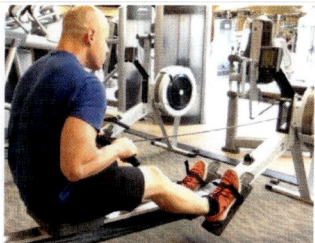

Even though a rowing machine is supposed to strengthen the back, you won't send much tension through those muscles when your mind is stuck in the habit of slouching forward.

Any activity can create a habitual neurological code that neglects to put tension in certain muscles. Ironically, many forms of exercise and recreation can be a big problem. Spending hours doing cardio can cause just as much muscle amnesia as sitting.

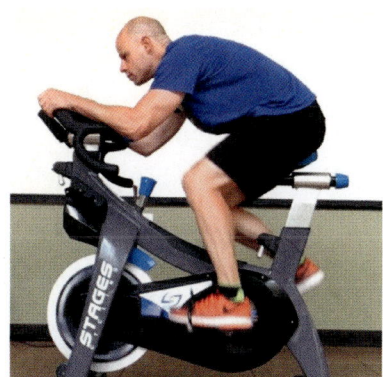

Pedaling an exercise bike may strengthen your legs and build endurance, but it can also create poor tension control in the back and hips.

Engaging in any activity long enough will put your mind at risk of forgetting how to send tension to various muscles. Just as you may not remember all of the foreign language lessons from high school, your mind will have trouble engaging certain muscles even if you're exercising for the sake of health and fitness.

The cure for muscle amnesia

Muscle amnesia is a serious threat to your health and fitness, but the solution is quite simple. All you need to do is practice sending tension to your muscles on a regular basis. You don't necessarily need to do taxing exercises or flex in awkward postures. Just tense up a muscle and hold the tension for a few seconds. Doing this will strengthen the neurological highway that your neural code travels through between your mind and your muscles.

I'll be including some simple ways you can practice turning on your muscles later on. I also highly recommend the book Muscle Control by the old-time strongman, Maxick. He was a pioneer in the health and strength field and firmly believed tension control was the key to developing his herculean capabilities. He proved his methods worked too. He went from a sick weakling to accomplishing feats of strength that would make strength athletes of today quiver in their lifting shoes.

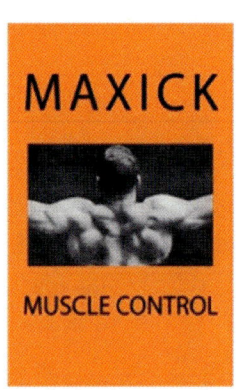 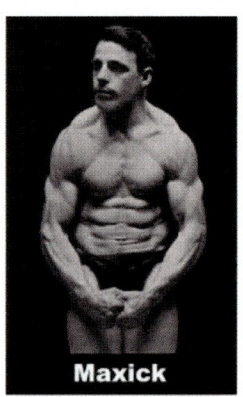

Old time strongman Maxick literally wrote the book on muscle control after discovering that the mind was the source of strength and muscle growth. Photo Affectinggravity.blogspot.com

Quality #2 How much tension you put in a muscle

The second variable in training is the amount of tension you put into a given muscle. Sometimes this is referred to how much strength a muscle has, and experts attempt to measure it with one rep maxes (1RM) or other tests of strength.

Holding more tension in a muscle is just as mental as controlling where the tension is in the first place. When you tense a muscle harder it might seem like your muscle fibers are contracting harder, but this isn't the case. Your muscle fibers are either off or on. They can't contract harder or easier when you lift a heavier weight vs a lighter weight. Instead, the total tension in a muscle is controlled by how many muscle fibers are contracting at a given time. Turning on more fibers requires a stronger neural code thus requiring more focus and concentration.

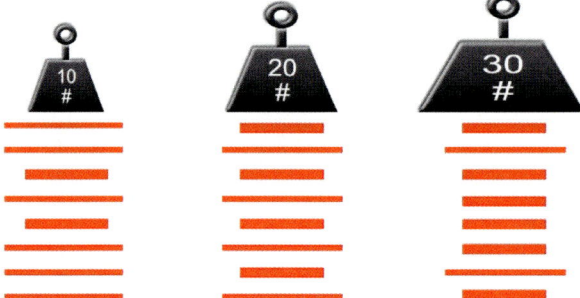

The more muscle fibers your mind recruits the more tension you create in a muscle to produce more force.

Tension is tension

Tension is tension regardless of why your mind is asking a muscle fiber to contract. To a single fiber, there's no such thing as different types of tension. If a muscle fiber in your leg is being told to turn on it doesn't matter if it's being recruited to lift a heavy weight, sprint up a flight of stairs or aid in balance. As far as that one muscle fiber is concerned, it's all the same.

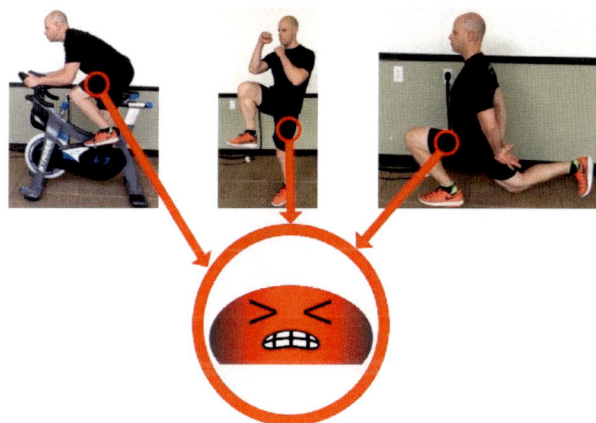

All three of these exercises are making use of the same muscle fiber in my left leg. While each exercise looks different, they are all the same to that one fiber that's contracting to make the exercise happen.

While there are different applications of muscle tension (which I discuss in the next chapter) the takeaway message is that all muscle tension is the same. There is no such thing as unproductive muscle tension. It all benefits you to at least some degree.

Don't qualify tension if you don't have to

Progressing any form of training, especially bodyweight training, requires improving your neural code which often means changing how you do an exercise. Unfortunately, there are a lot of rules out there that claim there is only one correct, or best, way to do an exercise. Typical examples include only working within a supposedly optimal rep range or adhering to one formal way to do an exercise.

When you believe an exercise is only useful if you do it a certain way, you close your mind off to the opportunity to make progressive changes. As a result, you end up spending months, even years, doing things the "right way" without ever doing things a better way.

Understanding that tension is tension regardless of why you produce it gives you the freedom to change your training in a variety of ways. You can modify your technique, rep range and a host of other variables to make progress. You won't lose ground because you're no longer strictly adhering to a narrow qualification of tension that doesn't allow you to alter your training. Instead, you'll be free to break the rules and train better because of it.

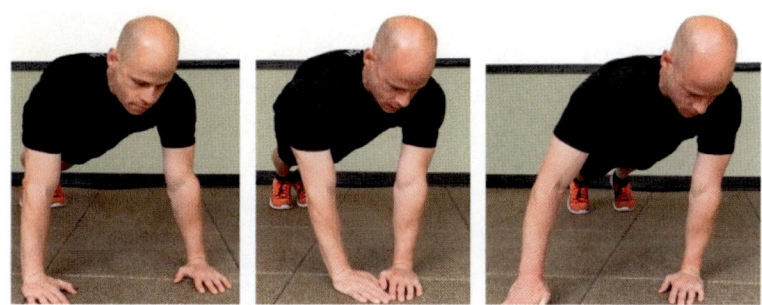

All three of these push-up variations require tension in the same muscles. It's a myth that only one of these techniques produces the "best" or "proper" tension for your goals. They are all useful for strengthening the same muscles.

Quality #3 How long you can maintain tension within a muscle

The last quality of tension is the duration a muscle can hold a given amount of tension. Unlike the quantity of tension, which depends on how many fibers are you can recruit, this variable depends more on the condition of the muscle fibers themselves.

A good way to think of this variable is to picture a muscle fiber as a sort of biomechanical battery. When that fiber contracts it starts to use up some of the energy within it. As the fiber uses up its energy, it loses the ability to contract and produce force.

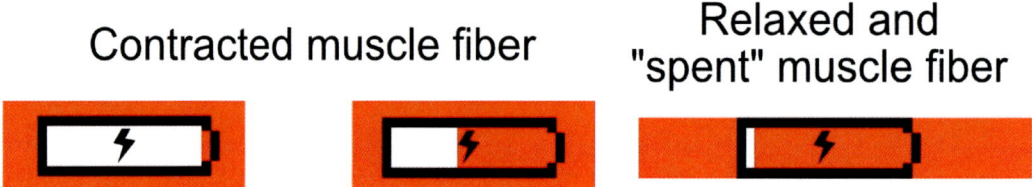

The longer you contract a muscle fiber the more you use up its "chemical energy"

Harder exercises require more muscle fibers to contract at once, so you fatigue the muscle at a faster rate of speed. Easier exercises don't use as many fibers at a time, so you don't use as much energy during each moment of training.

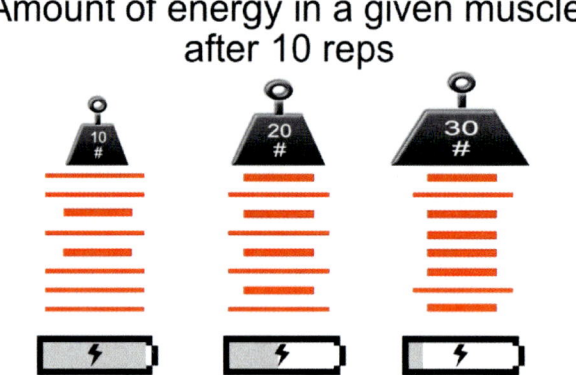

The more muscle fibers you contract the more force you produce, but you also use more total energy within the muscle in the same amount of time.

Is building muscle more about endurance than strength?

Building muscle may seem to be all about building strength, but it might also be just as much about muscle endurance.

When a muscle fiber becomes depleted, it has used a lot of the chemical energy it needs to stay contracted. When it recovers, it replenishes that chemical energy and overcompensates by putting in a little more than it had before. It's sort of like stuffing more water and acid in a battery to hold a charge for longer periods of time. Repeating this cycle of depletion and recovery is one of the primary reasons why a muscle increases in size.

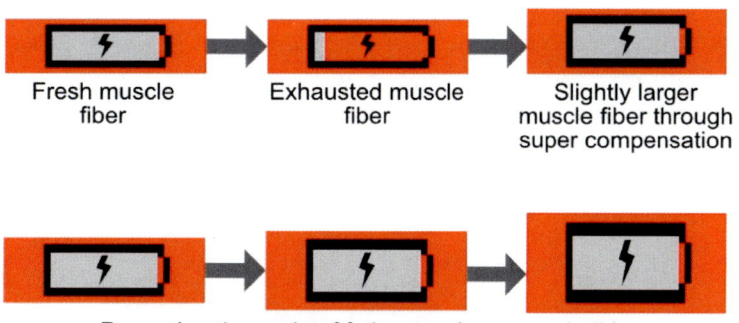

Repeating the cycle of fatigue and recovery builds bigger muscles over time

I fully admit this is a terribly over-simplified explanation for muscle growth. There's certainly more to the story including hormones and cellular damage which also play a role in stimulating muscle growth. I just wanted to share this perspective to support the idea that strength isn't the only factor contributing to muscle size and that adding some degree of volume may be helpful. This theory isn't suggesting you should only strive to add sets and reps either. Progressing both strength and endurance are important, and you shouldn't focus on improving just one or the other in your quest to build muscle.

Using the neurological feedback loop for a physical change

The neurological feedback loop between mind and muscle is what stimulates the changes you want to achieve through the natural law of homeostasis.

Homeostasis refers to the relationship between two natural elements. When the two elements are in a balanced relationship with one another they achieve a state of equilibrium. A good example is how your body reacts to external temperature. If the temperature between your body and your environment are in balance, you feel comfortable. However, if the temperature in your environment is not in harmony with your body temperature, you'll either start to sweat or shiver to regain that balance.

In the case of training, if your brain asks your muscles to do something, and they perform well enough, you have an equilibrium between the two halves of the feedback loop.

In this scenario, the mind is asking the muscles to perform an action and the muscles can satisfy that demand. This maintains a comfortable homeostatic balance between mind and body.

This scenario creates a satisfying level of comfort in both body and mind. Your mind is asking your body to do something, and your body can comply. All is fine and dandy; the only problem is this situation does not stimulate any physical change.

If you want to cause any sort of change, your mind needs to create a neurological code that asks your body to step up and do something that's little beyond what it's used to doing. When you do this, you disturb the state of homeostasis and create an imbalanced situation.

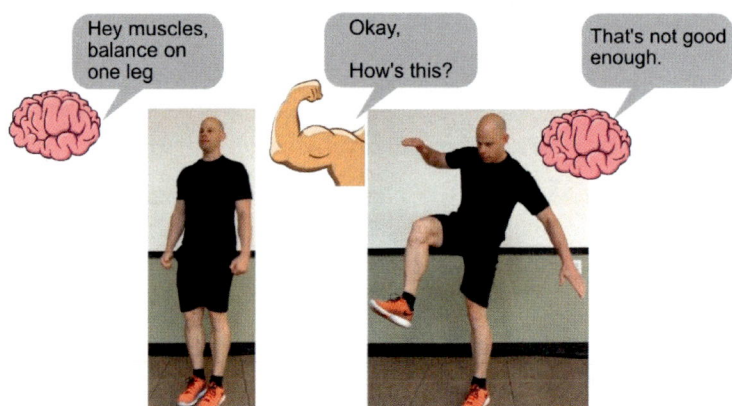

In this scenario, the muscles struggle to satisfy the functional demand the mind is creating. This creates an uncomfortable disruption between the mind-body homeostatic balance.

Homeostasis is the ultimate goal of Mother Nature. Any of the changes you want to gain from your exercise will only happen if they help you get back to a homeostatic balance between mind and body.

You can regain a homeostatic balance one of two ways. The first way is to change your thoughts which is what often happens when people feel frustrated with their inability to do something. A lot of times this involves making excuses that allow the mind to be comfortable with the body's previous level of performance. Some might blame age, genetics or just claim it's not possible. It's also easy to take comfort in the fact that they gave it a good try or worked hard and be satisfied with that. At this point, it's easy to reset the neurological code to match the current physical abilities.

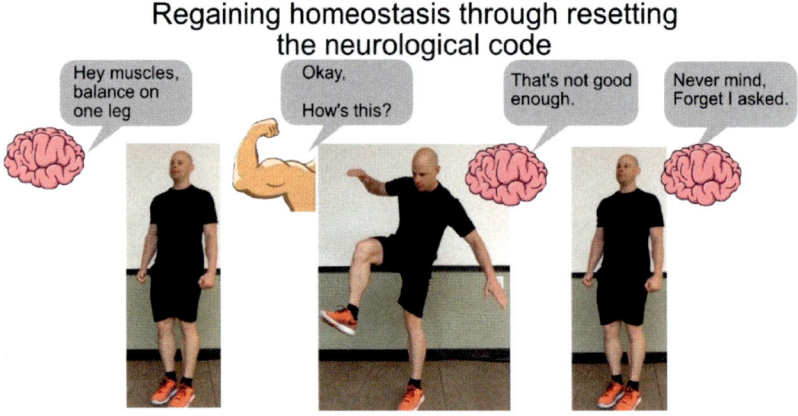

It doesn't matter what you tell yourself, the result is the same. Your mind asks your body to do something, and your body says "I can't quite do that." Then your mind says "that's okay, I'll just go back to asking you to do what you can." You're now back to a homeostatic balance by resetting your neural code to match your current level of physical ability.

The other solution is to achieve a homeostatic balance by forcing the body to change instead of the mind. While this is the preferred outcome, it's often the most difficult. It requires you to maintain an uncomfortable imbalance while your mind continues to demand a higher level of performance. Eventually, your body will adapt to regain the homeostatic harmony with your mind.

Regaining homeostasis through physical change

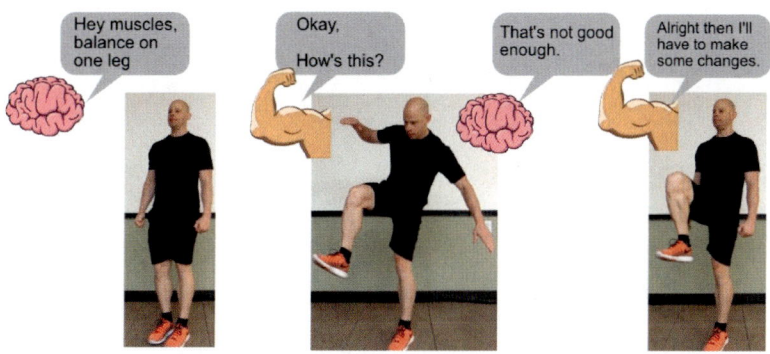

This sort of progress will take time, and it might come a bit slower than you would like, but it will happen. You're going to get back to a homeostatic state one way or another, and if your mind is strong, your body will step up to regain balance.

To sum up, all forms of training involve concentrating on using muscle tension to perform a specific task. You can change what muscles are holding tension, how much tension they are holding and how long they are holding it for. Lastly, you stimulate change when your mind instructs your muscles to perform in a way that's slightly beyond what they consider normal operation.

The final piece of the puzzle is understanding how you're supposed to use tension to accomplish your goals. I'll get right to that in the next chapter.

Chapter 4 Smart Training Part III

So far you've learned about two-thirds of the smart training principles. You know your mind creates a distinct neural code to contract your muscles and your muscles return sensory feedback that you perceive as muscle tension. The only thing left to learn is how to apply the tension feedback loop towards specific goals. For the sake of simplicity, I'm going to group all possible goals into three categories.

The Three Applications Of Muscle Tension

You can use muscle tension to burn fat, improve performance, and build muscle. Each of these goals requires you to use muscle tension in a specific way to reach your objectives. A helpful way to remember how to use tension for each goal is with the following acronyms.

S.A.I.D for improving performance

T.U.T for building muscle

I.C.E for burning fat

Let's look into each of these in more detail.

The S.A.I.D application of muscle tension for performance

S.A.I.D stands for the specific adaptation to imposed demand and it refers to how you skillfully manipulate tension throughout your body so you can improve how you do something.

A good way to think of this application is to imagine your body as a sort of musical instrument. Just like a piano, your body has numerous "keys" that can be used in a specific way to produce a result. When you play piano you hit certain keys in a specific way to get a particular melody. Even though a C flat is the same C flat in every song, how you use it is different depending on the piece you're trying to play.

Your physical keys are those motor units I mentioned earlier. While a single motor unit contracts it's muscle fibers no matter what you do, it's the specific way you use your motor units that produce the differences in performance.

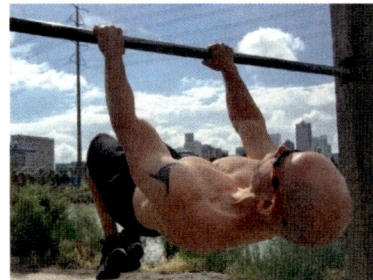
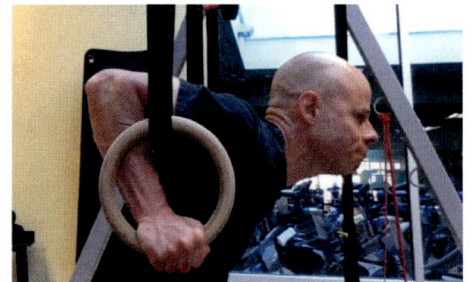

Every exercise involves concentrating on how you use the tension in your muscles. In both of these exercises, I'm concentrating on how I'm using the tension in my back muscles to do the exercise with more stability.

How to use S.A.I.D

The primary rule governing how well you perform is to challenge the performance characteristics you want to improve. If you want to be quicker, challenge your speed. If you want to be stronger, challenge your strength. If you want to improve balance, challenge your stability. By making it harder to accomplish the performance you want, your brain will be forced to upgrade your neural code to make your body work better.

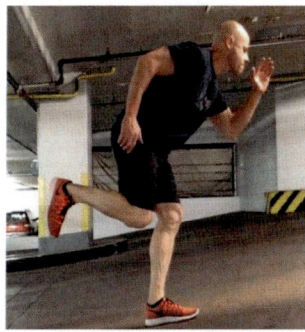
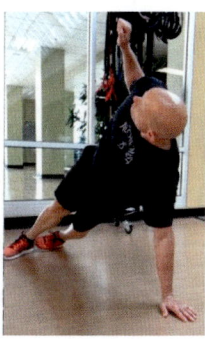

You improve the capabilities you challenge. Here, I'm challenging the power in my lower body by sprinting uphill and my shoulder stability by twisting my torso up on one arm.

You can also improve tension control by thinking about how you use your muscles during activity. So instead of just doing reps or getting the exercise done, you think about how you're using tension during those reps or exercise.

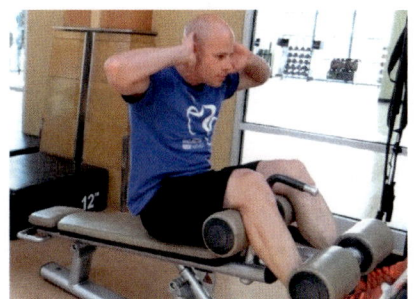

It's one thing to just sit up on a decline bench. It's another thing entirely to concentrate on putting tension in the abs, hips, quads and shin muscles while you do it.

The T.U.T application of muscle tension for building muscle

T.U.T stands for time under tension. It refers to both the amount of tension in a muscle and the amount of time that muscle holds that tension.

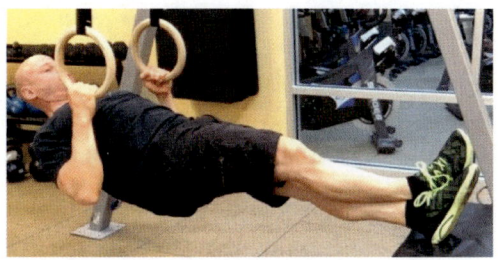

In this picture, I'm doing a row variation that requires a certain level of tension in my back and arms and I'm doing it for the amount of time it takes to do 10 reps.

How to use T.U.T

Building muscle isn't about shocking or confusing your muscles with some fancy trick or routine. It's about asking your muscles to progress their two functional capabilities which are strength and endurance.

Your muscles have a limited range of capability regarding how much tension they can hold (strength) and how long they can use that much tension (endurance). On one end of the spectrum, you can create low levels of tension for long periods of time. At the other end, you can produce large amounts of tension for short periods of time. Each end also represents the limits of your strength and endurance where you use a lot of one capability with very little of the other.

The time under tension spectrum

Low tension held for a long time
ex. 1# x 100 reps

High tension held for a short time
ex. 100# x 1 rep

All exercises are a balance between tension (red) and time (blue). The less tension there is in a muscle, the longer you can do the exercise. When the amount of tension increases the duration of time decreases.

It's important to note that you won't build any muscle with both low or high rep training if you stay within your range of capability.

In the example above, you can lift 1 pound 100 times or 100 pounds once. You will struggle to build muscle if your workout involves either of these approaches or anything in between (example lifting 50 pounds 50 times) because they are asking your muscles to do what they can already do.

Low tension held for a long time
ex. 1# x 100 reps

Med. tension held for med. time
ex. 50# x 50 reps

High tension held for a short time
ex. 100# x 1 rep

You can use any combination of time and tension in your workouts, but none of them will help you grow while you continue to work your muscles within your current range of capability.

If you want to build more muscle, you'll have to increase either the amount of tension in the muscle, the amount of time you hold tension or both.

Progression of time under tension

Low tension held for a long time
ex. 1# x 110 reps

Med. tension held for med. time
ex. 55# x 55 reps

High tension held for a short time
ex. 110# x 1 rep

In this example you increase your time under tension by increasing the amount of time on the left, the amount of tension on the right or a little bit of both in the middle.

While you can build muscle by increasing either time or tension, your best bet is to build both over time. One way you can do this is to use a strategy called double progression.

Double progression involves using a consistent level of tension while building up the time you can hold that tension over several weeks or months.

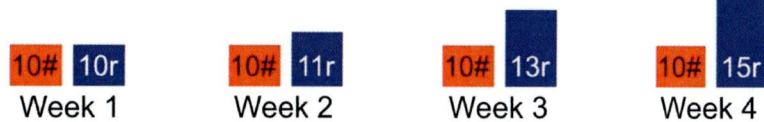

With double progression, you keep the tension in the muscle the same while increasing the time it can hold that tension for. In this example, you're creating enough tension to lift 10 pounds and increasing the time from 10 to 15 reps over a month.

After building up the time for a while, you increase the tension on the muscle. When the muscle needs to work harder, the time you hold the tension drops. You then repeat the cycle by increasing the time you can handle the higher amount of tension.

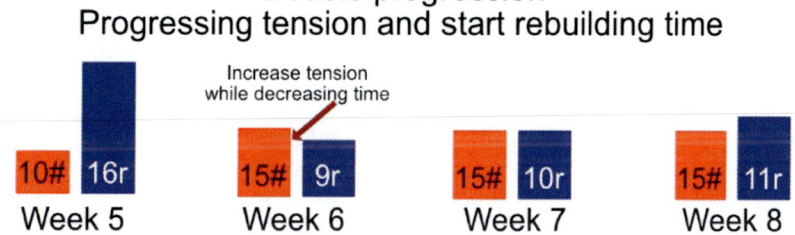

After significantly increasing the endurance of a muscle (time), you add tension (strength) and repeat the cycle by building the endurance of the new level of strength.

Eventually, you'll repeat this cycle enough to substantially increased both the strength (tension) and endurance (time) of a muscle which will make it grow.

The I.C.E application of muscle tension for burning calories

I.C.E stands for increasing caloric expenditure, which is helpful if you want to shed body fat. This application applies whenever you create muscle tension in an effort to burn more fat and calories to manage your weight.

A lot of experts discredit the importance of physical activity for weight control. Some even claim you should focus almost entirely on diet and that exercise doesn't do anything. There is some validity to this opinion because it's usually a lot easier to initially lose weight by making changes to your diet.

With that said, physical activity does have some unique weight control benefits. The first of which is increasing your physical activity is one of the best ways to increase your total calorie expenditure.

Your body burns energy for three primary reasons. The first is your base metabolic rate (B.M.R) which burns a lot of calories but it relatively slow to change.

Your total calorie expenditure

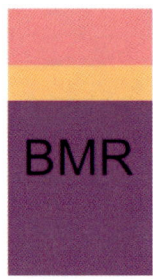

Your base metabolic rate (BMR) burns a large percentage of your daily calorie expenditure, but it's relatively slow to change and it can take months or even years to make a difference on your weight.

The second way you burn calories is your thermic effect of food (T.E.F) which is the energy you burn to consume and metabolize the food you eat. T.E.F doesn't burn a lot of calories but it can change daily due to variations in the diet.

Your total calorie expenditure

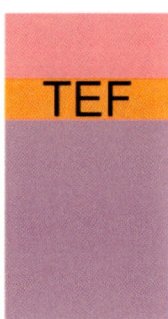

Your thermic effect of food is a relatively minor influence to your total calorie expenditure, but it can change on a daily basis due to what and how much you eat.

The third way you burn calories is your thermic effect of activity (T.E.A) which includes everything from doing a pull-up to non-exercise activity like cleaning house and walking around.

Your total calorie expenditure

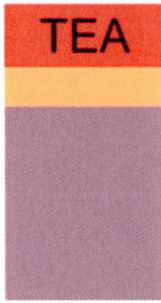

Your thermic effect of activity is a highly adjustable influence on your total calorie expenditure. It can change very quickly from one moment to the next.

Your physical activity is the best of both B.M.R and T.E.A. You can increase your calorie expenditure quickly and burn hundreds, even thousands of calories at the drop of a hat.

The highly variable nature of your thermic effect of activity allows you to potentially burn hundreds, even thousands, of extra calories in a single day.

While you may lose more weight through improving your diet at first, physical activity still plays an important role in both short term and long term weight loss.

The biggest reason is that you lose body fat by actively burning it off. Adjusting your diet mostly changes the speed at which you consume calories. It has limited influence on your ability to proactively burn the calories you're trying to lose. Physical activity gives you the power to apply the metabolic blowtorch to the very fat you're trying to lose so you can burn it by force.

In some ways, exercise can make your diet more effective. I've known plenty of folks who change their diet and lose weight, but they've already been practicing regular physical activity. In these cases, it's tempting to believe the change in diet was responsible for the weight loss, but you could also say the diet made their workout effective for weight loss.

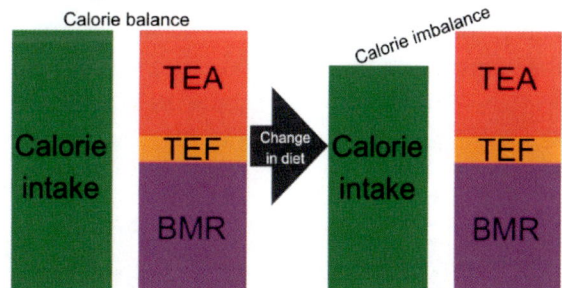

In this example, a change in diet resulted in a negative calorie balance but it was only possible through burning a lot of calories through activity. This change in the diet wouldn't have produced a negative calorie balance or weight loss if the TEA wasn't so high.

The second reason to not over-rely on diet is the fact that you can't out-diet homeostasis. Dropping weight is only a temporary situation as your body adjusts to any new diet you adopt. Sooner or later, your body adjusts to your new diet to balance your calorie intake and expenditure in order to survive. In other words, every diet ultimately trains your body how *not* to lose weight as you become conditioned to the new diet.

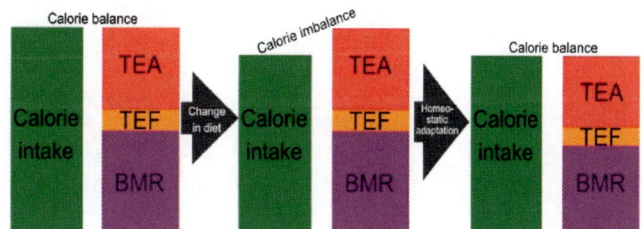

Sooner or later, all dietary changes result in weight maintenance after a temporary period of weight loss. You regain balance from your body making subtle changes in your BMR, TEF, and TEA.

Physical activity is one way you can stimulate weight loss without triggering a homeostatic adaptation. It is true that habitual physical activity, like running a mile three times a week, will trigger a homeostatic adaptation and thus weight maintenance. However, you can engage in sporadic activity, like a weekend hike, which doesn't happen often enough to cause much of a homeostatic change. You just head out, burn a bunch of calories and they're gone for good.

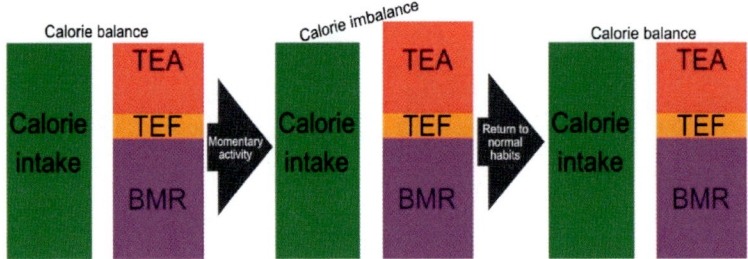

Engaging in a momentary activity like a long walk or hike proactively burns more calories than normal. This creates a temporary negative calorie balance that chips away at excess fat stores without triggering a homeostatic response.

There is more to the story of weight loss than just diet and exercise. It's not like your ability to lose, and maintain, weight depends entirely on a particular exercise routine. I just wanted to make the case that while diet may be king, physical activity plays a larger role in weight loss than many diet experts realize.

How to use I.C.E

I.C.E may be the simplest application to use out of the three. All you need to do is move your body any way you can. Tension is tension, and all of it burns calories regardless of how you're creating it. So just do something, anything at all, and you'll be burning calories at a faster rate.

But let's say you want to maximize how fast you can burn fat and calories. How would you do that? Like with muscle building, don't worry about needing some fancy or complicated plan. Burning fat faster is as simple as creating more tension. You can do this by progressing the three quality of muscle tension I mentioned in the last chapter. You'll burn more calories when you either use more muscle, work at a higher intensity or move for longer periods of time.

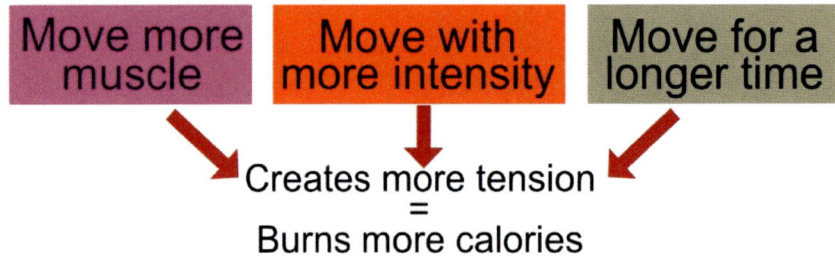

Don't worry about what sort of activities burn fat and which ones supposedly don't. As long as you're creating some form of muscle tension, you're increasing your rate of calorie expenditure.

The S.A.I.D, T.U.T, I.C.E hierarchy

It's impossible to do anything that only uses tension for S.A.I.D, T.U.T, or I.C.E. All physical activity uses tension in a specific way to create time under tension which burns calories. The key is to use a strategy that focuses on whichever application is most important for your goals. I'll be covering just how to do that a little later on.

Meanwhile, the interconnection between all three applications is important to understand because they form a bit of a hierarchy. Even if you're only interested in building muscle, shedding fat or improving performance, all three applications play a role in helping you achieve your goal. Understanding this hierarchy can help you identify weaknesses that may be holding you back.

The muscle tension hierarchy

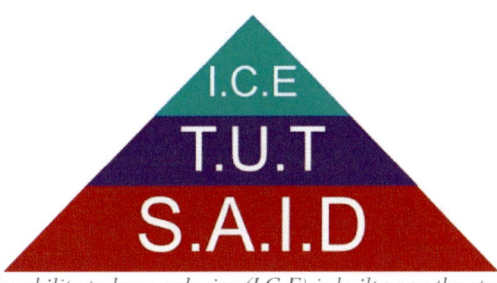

The muscle tension hierarchy shows how the ability to burn calories (I.C.E) is built upon the strength and endurance of your muscles (T.U.T) and that's built on your foundation of using tension in a specific functional way (S.A.I.D).

The muscle tension hierarchy shows how your ability to reach your goals depends on all three qualities.

Starting at the top, your ability to I.C.E is built upon the foundation of your T.U.T or the strength and endurance of your muscles. It's easy to understand why this is the case. It's very hard to burn even a modest amount of fat when your muscles are weak and quickly fatigue. It's a lot easier to burn more calories when you can work your muscles harder and for longer periods of time.

The foundation of your strength and endurance is based on your ability to use tension in a specific and functional way. This is especially the case with calisthenics training. There's just no way you can build strong and capable muscles when you lack the functional skills to use those muscles in an advanced way.

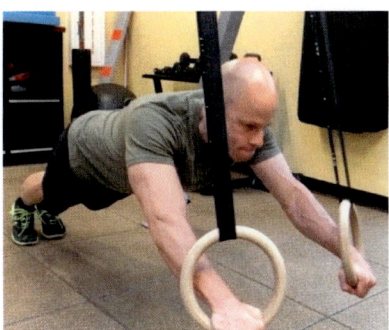

Ring planks are one of the best exercises for building super strong abs as long as you have the functional skill to keep your abs tight and shoulders stable.

So even if you only want to build muscle or burn fat, it's important to recognize how the three applications of tension relate to each other. The more you improve your functional capabilities the more you can increase your time under tension. The more you increase your time under tension, the easier it will be to burn a lot of calories.

Smart training wrap up

At this point, you have a much better understanding of how to train smarter than even most experienced athletes and gym rats. Getting an effective workout is all about mentally focusing on manipulating the three qualities of tension to satisfy S.A.I.D, T.U.T or I.C.E.

How to train smarter
Use focus and concentration....
To manipulate the three qualities of tension....
To progress S.A.I.D, T.U.T and I.C.E
Where's the tension
How much
How long
I.C.E
T.U.T
S.A.I.D

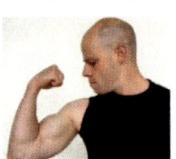

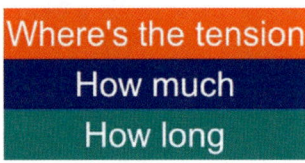

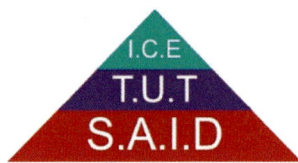

This lesson applies to all forms of exercise, not just bodyweight training. Not only can you use this approach to make the exercises in this book work for you, but any other training methods you learn for the rest of your life.

So with that said, let's get into the meat of how to use this three-step system to progress your bodyweight training.

Chapter 5 The Elements Of Progression

Progression is the essence of what makes your workout effective. When you use tension to improve performance, time under tension or energy expenditure, your training will be more productive regardless of how you arrange the details in your routine or program.

The biggest challenge with bodyweight training is understanding how to progress it. A lot of methods use a step-by-step approach for advancing calisthenics. While this can work very well, I've come to use a bit more of an exploratory approach. I take this view because progressing exercise isn't just about working harder or learning a few tricks. It's ultimately about learning how to use your body better. Sure, you'll be able to make some initial progress by just pushing yourself while you're a beginner, but no one ever achieved mastery in anything through hard work alone. To reach even moderate levels of success you need to improve how well you use your own body, not just how hard you use it.

Doing this is not something you can always plan within a set system that works perfectly well for everybody. You have your unique abilities, strengths, and weaknesses making your path to success as unique to you as your fingerprints. I can't lay out the perfect plan for you which is why the progressions in the following pages are only a rough template and are by no means a complete progressive system. There are well over 100 different ways you can progress just your push-ups alone.

I encourage you to play around and explore how well you can use your body so you can discover your own path to success. To better understand how to do this I've created a table of progressive elements that you can mix and match with your training.

The Table of Progressive Elements

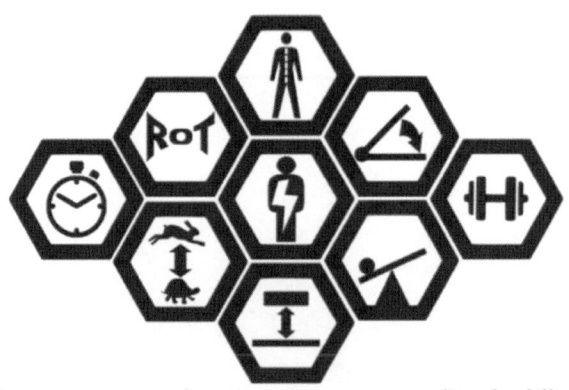

The table of progressive elements represents the primary ways you can adjust the difficulty of nearly any exercise.

Just like the periodic table of elements in chemistry, each exercise uses a combination of these various elements to adjust the difficulty of any exercise. Let's look at each item in detail.

Element #1 Tension control

The first element is at the heart of the table because controlling muscle tension is the focus of smart bodyweight training. While creating tension is the objective of your training, it's also an element you can progress through improving how you control tension throughout your muscles. It's represented by the figure with the bolt because tension control is about controlling electrical signals running through your nervous system.

Element #2 Centerline

Just as all rivers lead to the sea, all tension must be directed in toward the centerline of your body. Martial artists are familiar with working with the centerline that splits the body between the left and right side. Understanding it is the key to achieving balance, power, strength, and leverage which gives the martial artist their incredible capabilities.

This centerline principle doesn't just apply to kicking and throwing but to all human movement. It helps you build strength, flexibility, balance, and muscle control. If you look at the majority of muscles, you'll notice that almost all of the muscle fibers are arranged to direct tension in towards your centerline. Even muscles that don't drive tension inwards, direct it towards muscles that eventually turn toward the centerline.

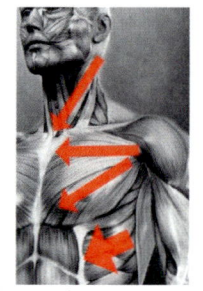

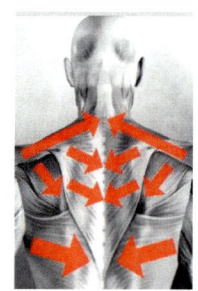

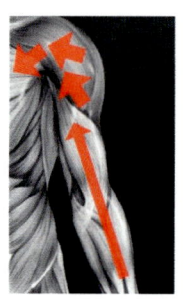

These images show how the muscle fibers of many muscles direct tension in toward the centerline. Even the muscles in the arm direct tension toward the shoulder where tension can flow further inward.

From a mechanical perspective, this makes sense. If you want to move your body, you have to apply force towards your center of gravity. Even a seemingly outward projection of energy like throwing a punch is made possible by driving tension inwards.

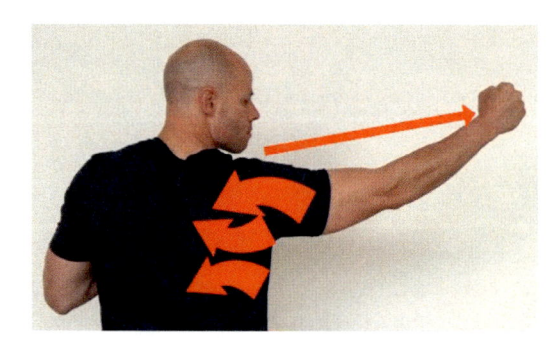

In this image, the muscles in my back and shoulder pull in toward my centerline to help me strike out with the back of my fist.

This inward flow of energy is why many of the calisthenics progressions involve driving force inwards rather than just forward or backward.

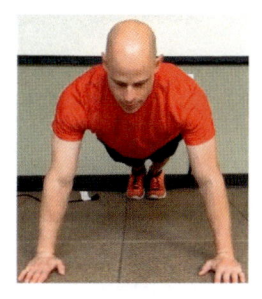

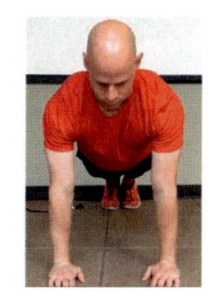

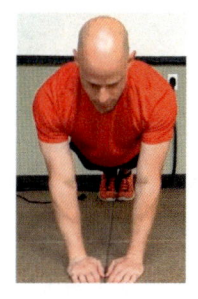

Moving the working limbs closer to the centerline is one of the most common ways to progress basic exercises.

The centerline element is also effective for adjusting your base of support which can either add or remove stability during the exercise. The less stable you are, the more tension you will need to generate in your muscles to maintain control.

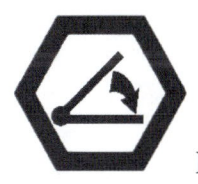

Element #3 Angle to gravity

You can create more resistance against your muscles through adjusting the angle you're working against gravity. The more you move directly against gravity, the more resistance you receive.

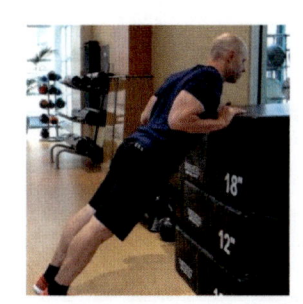

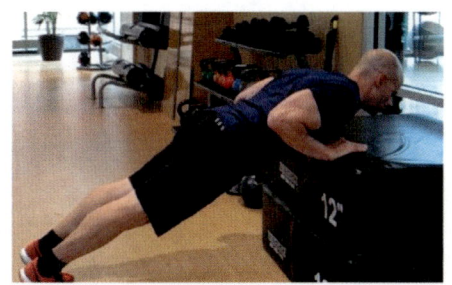

Pushing against a higher or lower surface is a common way to adjust your body's angle to gravity.

Adjusting the angle to gravity is just like adjusting the weight on a barbell. Both methods are just a different way to adjust the resistance on your muscles which requires more muscle tension.

Element #4 Extension

Leverage is a fascinating thing. You can use it to make light objects impossibly heavy, and heavy objects light as a feather. It's also an excellent way to make your muscles very strong through adjusting the length of your body as it moves against gravity.

A classic example of this element in action is when you extend your legs, during a leg raise. The more you straighten your legs, the more difficult the exercise becomes for both lying and hanging versions of this exercise.

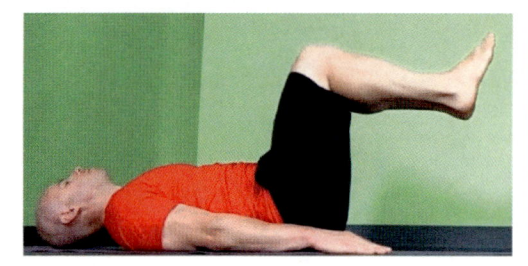

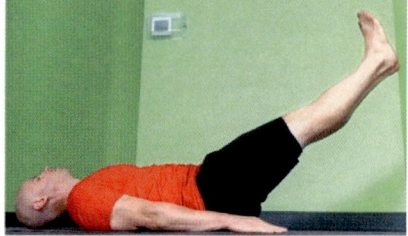

Extending the legs during abdominal exercises is one of the most common uses of the extension element. In this example, extending the knee is adding resistance to the hip and abdominal muscles.

Just as the angle to gravity element adjusts the resistance you create against gravity, the extension element also creates more resistance against gravity thus requiring more tension in the muscle.

Element #5 Range of tension

The resistance of a muscle often changes as you move through a range of motion. For example, there is often less resistance on your triceps at the top of a push-up, but it increases as you lower yourself to the floor.

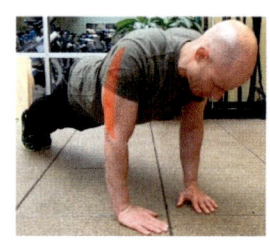

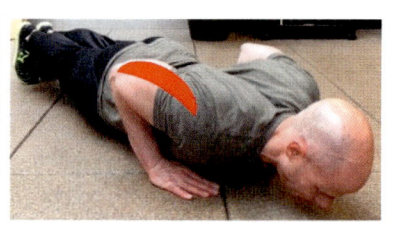

The resistance on my triceps muscle at the top of the push-up is significantly less than when the elbow is bent at the muscle is elongated at the bottom of the push-up. This is why moving through a deeper range of motion can increase the resistance on a muscle.

Because the intensity of an exercise can change through the range of movement, you can adjust the difficulty of any move by changing how much you move within each rep.

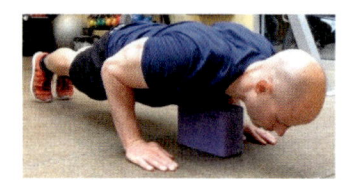

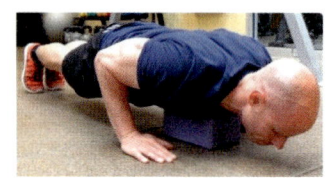

I like to use yoga blocks to quantify and adjust the range of tension in pushing exercise because they offer 3 different heights in one handy block. The lower the block surface is the more range of tension you use.

Powerlifters are known to do this with boxes while doing squats and boards on their chest while benching. These devices change the range they can move in and thus the influence on their muscle tension.

There's also a tendency to relax a muscle as it stretches out. Typical examples include relaxing the biceps and shoulders at the bottom of a pull-up or relaxing the abs in the lower part of a leg raise. By working to keep a muscle tense at the elongated position, you'll improve your tension control and place more tension in the muscle.

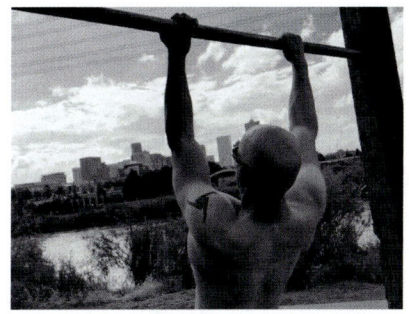

Maintaining tension at the bottom of a pull-up can be more challenging than relaxing in a dead-hang position.

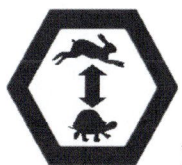

Element #6 Speed

Adjusting the speed you move at can influence your muscle tension in a couple of ways. In some cases, you'll benefit from moving slower. Other times moving faster may be more challenging. Sometimes, not moving at all can be best as in the case of isometric exercises.

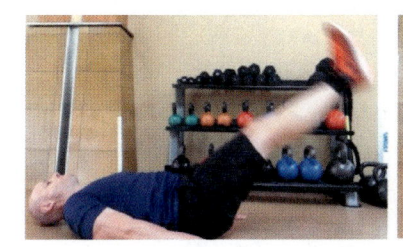

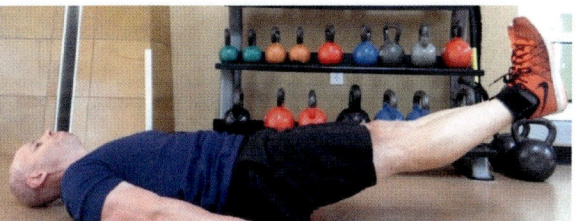

It's fun to mix various lifting speeds within a single workout or even a single set. Here, I do 20 fast leg raises followed by a 20 seconds isometric hold.

Adjusting the speed and tempo of your training can challenge your tension control as well. Moving slower can substantially increase the time you spend during each repetition. It can also help improve muscle control by forcing you to not rush through weak points in each rep. On the other hand, moving fast can increase the amount of tension in a muscle as you need to recruit more muscle fibers to move faster. Moving faster can also potentially increase your calorie expenditure and stamina.

You can improve your tension skills to satisfy the functional demands of S.A.I.D depending on the way speed influences your performance. In Taekwon-Do, we would practice kicking very slowly to improve control and coordination. We would also kick sheets of paper in an attempt to tear the paper by kicking it as fast as we could.

You can also move faster or slower to progress your I.C.E. A slow-paced exercise, like walking, can help you burn a lot of calories because you can do it for a long time. Moving fast, like running up a hill can increase your tension which burns calories by the truckload.

Element #7 Time

This one is simple. You can progress anything you do by spending more time doing it. Typical examples include adding reps or sets in your strength workout, or the amount of time you do an exercise like running.

Sometimes you can make progress by using less time to do an activity. If you can run around a track in less time that means you're getting faster. The same is the case for completing 100 pushups in less time.

Element #8 Weight shifting

Even though your total bodyweight may not change, you can add weight to some muscles through shifting your weight onto one limb.

One of the most common examples is shifting your weight more onto one arm when doing an exercise. Placing more weight on one arm will make the muscles in that limb work harder even though your total bodyweight doesn't change.

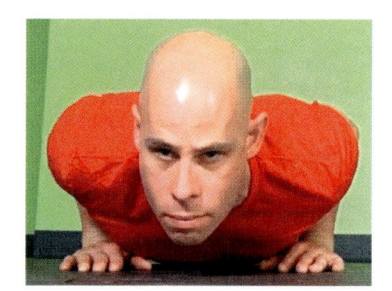

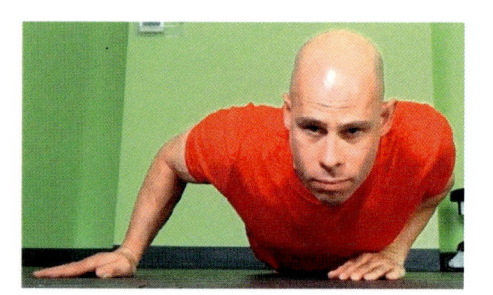

In this example, I'm reaching out with my right arm to place more weight on my left arm.

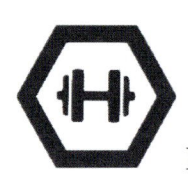

Element #9 Weight adjustment

Just like any form of weight training, you can adjust the weight you lift in calisthenics. Adding or subtracting weight from the body is a common practice for athletes who want to change the resistance of the exercise without modifying technique.

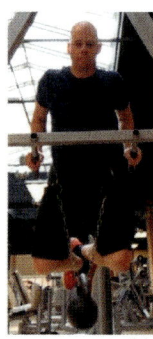

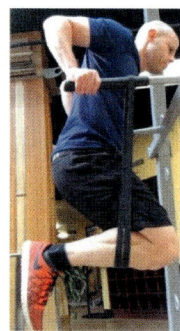

You can add or subtract weight from the body just as you would weight on a barbell. In this example, I've added 30# to a dip belt and I've removed about the same amount of weight while using exercise bands to lift me up on the same exercise.

Just like the table of chemical elements, these are grouped together to show a relationship between one another. At the center is the element of tension since that's the focal point of all of your training. All of the elements influence both time and tension, the elements on the left are more of an influence on the amount of time you do an exercise. The elements on the right are a bit more of an influence on the resistance and tension in your muscles. The centerline and extension elements influence both time and tension pretty equally.

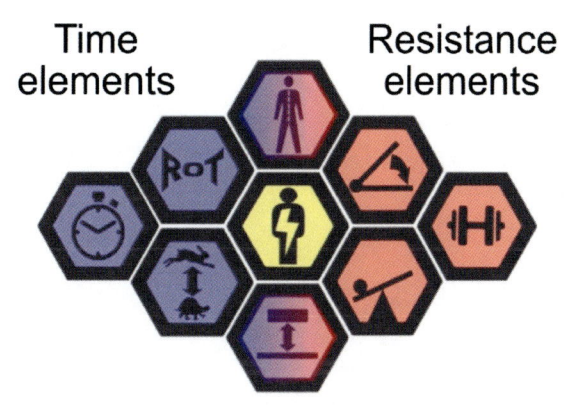

All elements influence time and tension, but the ones on the left have a greater influence on time and the ones on the right have more influence on the resistance on the muscle.

Each of the elements also influences the elements next to them. For example, the extension element influences both the speed with which you do an exercise and the weight you shift around your body. The time element is influenced by both your range of tension and the speed elements and so on.

Mix and match

I like to think of these elements like ingredients in a kitchen pantry. You can mix and combine them in various ways with each exercise to create the perfect level of difficulty for you.

Take the classic push-up as an example. On the one hand, you can progress it through the angle element by doing a push-up on a different incline. You can also adjust the difficulty through the centerline and weight shift elements.

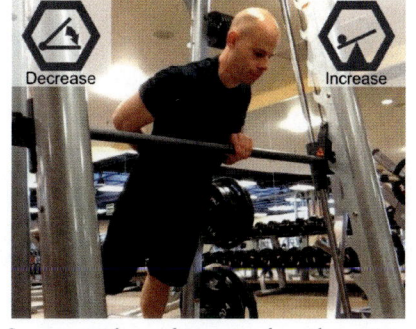

Almost anyone can do one arm push-ups. Here, I use a smith machine to reduce the resistance on my muscles through regressing the angle to gravity. This allows me to progress the weight shift element so all of the resistance is on my left arm.

In this case, you're not progressing your angle to gravity, but you are using the weight shift element.

Let's explore a little more how you can manipulate a few of the progressive elements with push-ups. In the example below, you've been doing knee push-ups (A) and are looking for a new challenge. You can use the extension element to do them on your toes (B), or you can stay on your knees and use the centerline element to bring your hands closer together (C). But let's say you like the idea of doing "real push-ups" on your toes and you find them to be a bit too difficult. Not a problem, you can slightly regress the exercise with a yoga block to decrease the range of tension (D). Now you're feeling like you're working at the appropriate level but after a few weeks, you feel like you're almost bouncing out of the bottom position. It's kind of hard on your joints so you use the time element and hold the bottom position for a full 2-second count (E).

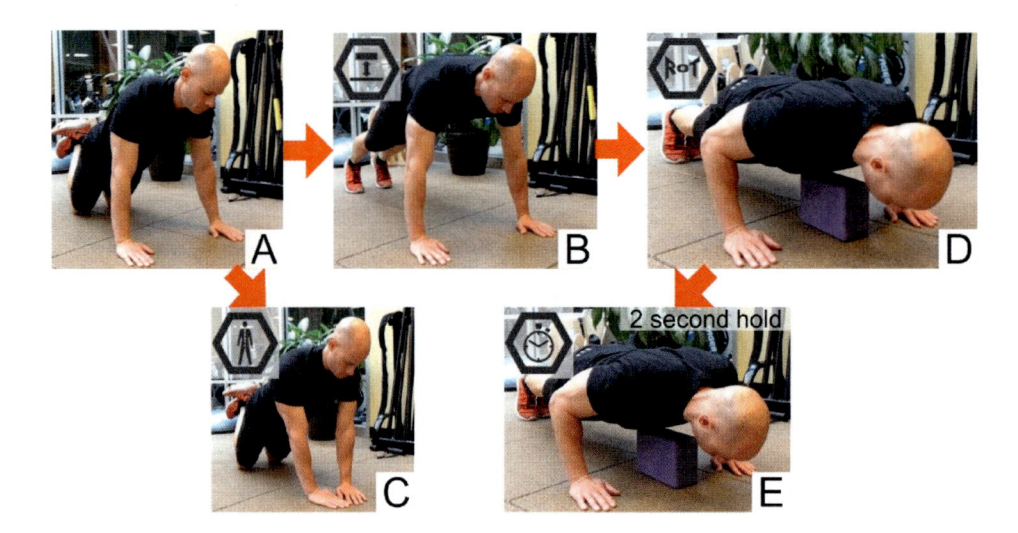

Being able to mix and swap progressive elements is one of the biggest advantages of calisthenics. You're not limited to changing just weight and reps so you can customize any technique to perfectly fit your needs and capabilities.

Measuring Progression

Understanding the elements of progression allows you to quantify your calisthenics training just as well as you can quantify weightlifting. All you need to do is quantify how much you use each of the elements. Let's take a look at how you would do this with each element.

#1 Quantifying Time

Time is easy to quantify with a stopwatch or smartphone app. Reps are another way to quantify time. If you increase the number of reps, you're increasing the time under tension provided you don't change the amount of time it takes to do each rep.

#2 Quantifying ROT

This one is also simple. You can use objects like books, bricks, or anything you wish to quantify the range of motion you're using in an exercise.

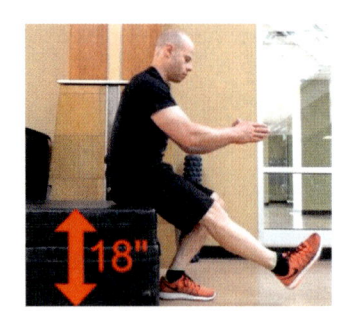

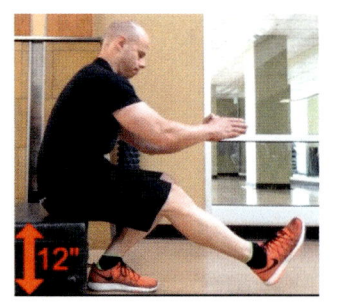

Using box heights is a good way to quantify your squat depth. You can also use seats or chairs at different heights as well.

I've used wooden blocks cut from 2x4s to measure the distance I'm using for push-ups and handstands. Yoga blocks are also handy for this purpose since you can stand them up at 3 different heights.

#3 Quantifying speed

You can time your speed by measuring how fast you can run around a track. You can measure your explosive power by how high you can jump.

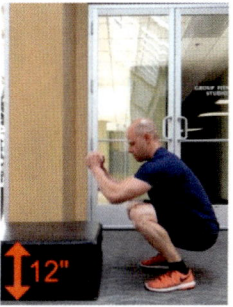

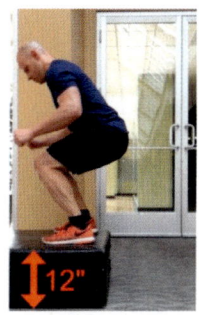

Quantifying how high you can jump is one way to measure explosive power in the legs. You can also pay attention to how far you are from the box so you jump further instead of just higher.

#4 Quantifying centerline

This element is quantified by measuring the distance between your hands or feet. You can get the job done with a tape measure or even floor tiles.

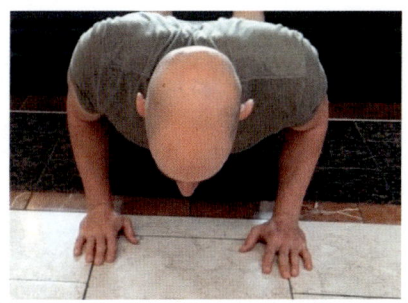

I like to use lines on the floor to measure the width of my hands during push-ups. You can change the width by changing which fingers are on the line or how many tiles your hands are apart.

#5 Quantifying lever length

Sometimes, this one is easy because your body can only change its length in steps like when you do push-ups on your knees or toes.

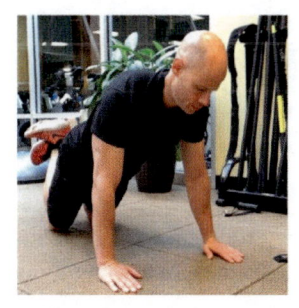

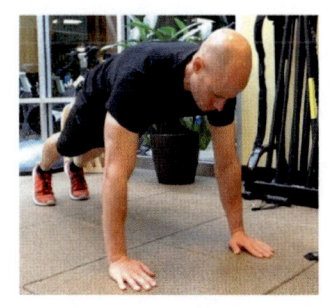

Some exercises are more challenging like how far you extend your legs out while doing leg raises. You may be able to place a wall or object at a measurable distance away from you to gauge how far you extend your lever.

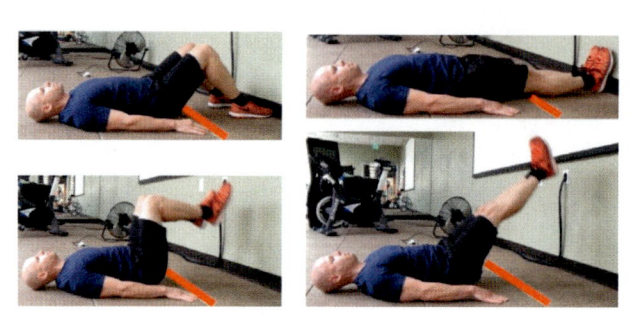

In this image, I'm using a line on the floor (highlighted in red) to quantify the length of my legs during leg raises. When my fingers are on the line my legs are bent when my toes touch the wall. Moving away from the line allows my legs to extend and increase the resistance.

#6 Quantifying angle to gravity

This element is easy to quantify when you measure the height of the surface you place your hands on. For example, you might do push-ups on the kitchen counter. Then, you might do them on the lower kitchen table. Then the chairs, then the lowest step on the stairs and finally the floor. The changes don't have to be equal and uniform in their progression. As long as you're making general progress over a series of elevations you're good.

I've also used a Smith Machine or adjustable barbell rack at the gym for quantifying the height at which someone does push-ups and rows.

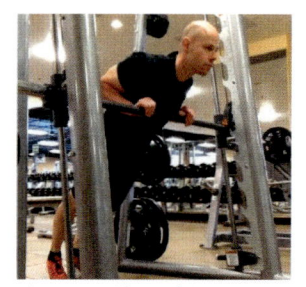

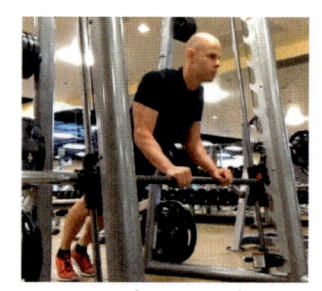

The classic smith machine is a great way to quantify your angle to gravity.

Suspension straps make angle adjustment particularly easy since you can quantify the height of the handles based on a measuring tape. You can also measure height based on physical points like knee height, thigh height, waist height and so on.

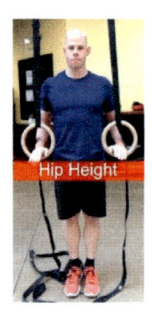

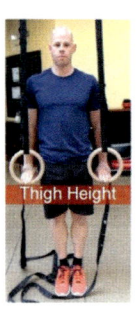

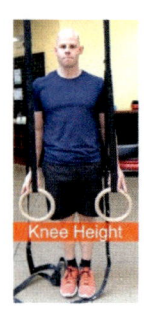

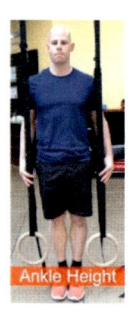

Some rings and suspension straps come with numbers on the straps to quantify their height. If you don't have numbers, you can quantify the height in relation to your body.

#7 Quantifying weight distribution

There are many ways you can quantify this element. One of which is to measure the distance between the primary working limb and the assistance limb. The further apart the two become, the less assistance there is to the main arm or leg. You can use the same method of using floor tiles like with centerline push-ups.

Another way to measure the assistance is by how many fingers you use on the assistance arm. The less of your hand you're using to assist, the more resistance there is on the working arm.

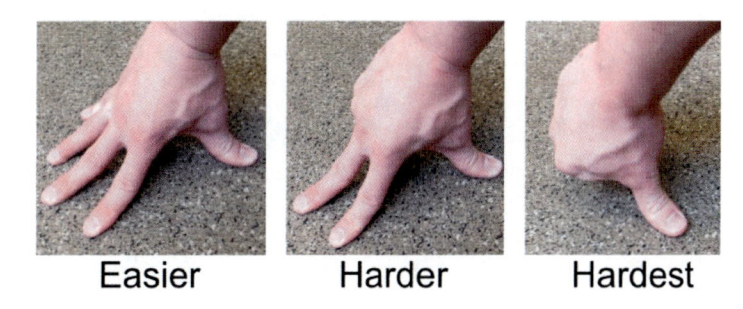

Easier   Harder   Hardest

#8 Quantifying weight

Weight is easy to quantify because you can measure it in pounds or kilograms which is why it's an ideal choice for many athletes.

#9 Quantifying tension

Even though there are many ways you can quantify your training, none of these methods directly measure the one thing that matters most: the actual tension in your muscles.

Unfortunately, there isn't much you can do to quantify muscle tension directly. All of these elements, including weight and time, are merely influences to your muscle tension but they are not a perfect indication of how your mind is sending tension throughout your body. This inaccuracy is why you don't want to focus too much on any single quantifiable measurement. Getting hung up on how many reps you can do or how much weight you can lift distract you from focusing on how you're using your muscle tension.

Albert Einstein once said "not everything that counts can be counted and not everything that can be counted counts." This point is particularly the case in fitness and exercise. While you can attach a number to many influences in your exercise, some of your success will not come from variables you can plot on a spreadsheet. Your neural code and muscle tension is a good example. It's almost impossible to quantify your thoughts and mental focus during a workout.

While you may not be able to put a number on muscle tension, you probably don't need to. Just consider many of the disciplines that people have excelled in despite a lack of numerical quantification. Think of the chef who can expertly improve a recipe through using a refined pallet. Or the sculptor who can improve the visual balance of a statue through visual perception. Even writing this book has been a progressive process, yet I didn't use numbers to improve the grammatical structure of this sentence.

Numbers are great, but it's what's behind them is what's most important. When you're struggling to progress the things you can quantify it may be time to focus on the things you can't quantify.

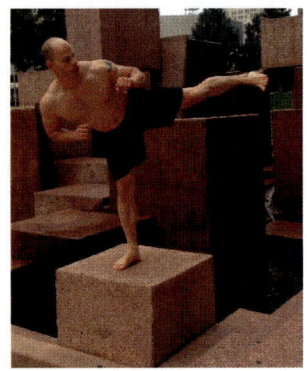

It's hard to attach a number to how well someone can throw a sidekick but you may not always need to. I know a kick is stronger or weaker by how it feels against a heavy bag or how it looks in a mirror.

How To Master Your Training By Becoming A Technician

My Taekwon-do instructor always told us "You want to become a technician! Anyone can throw a punch or kick and I expect you to bring your skills up to a higher level than that."

As a hormone-saturated teenager, I didn't quite understand just how deep this lesson was. I thought gut-busting effort was the path to success. Eventually, I started to understand what being a technician was about and it has changed everything from how I move to even how I talk.

Let me be very blunt about this. Technical proficiency is the foundation of your success. Everything from the exercises you practice to the equipment you use is pretty much worthless if you do not strive to improve your technical proficiency. I even made a graphic representation of technical proficiency in the logo for the Red Delta Project to serve as a constant reminder of its essential nature.

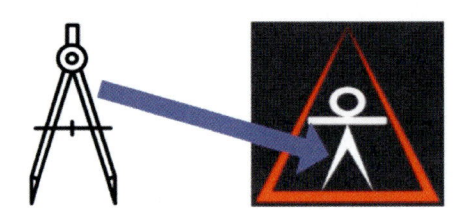

Just as your legs are your foundation when standing, technical proficiency is the foundation of your training success.

The legs of the figure were inspired by a compass tool which is used in drafting and navigation applications that require a high level of technical accuracy. Just as the legs are the foundation of a strong body, so too is technical accuracy the foundation of your training.

Becoming a technician is the essence of smart training. The more technically proficient you become, the better your results will be even if you put in a fraction of the effort. It's not difficult to become a technician, but here are a few key points you should understand.

#1 A technician is focused on the process

The goal of the technician isn't to just win the trophy or championship. Instead, they strive to improve how they practice their respective discipline.

One of the best examples of this is the legendary basketball coach John Wooden. Despite winning ten national championships within 12 years, his focus was always on the process of practicing the game. Even years after his retirement, he said he missed planning and implementing his practices more than anything else about his coaching career.

#2 A technician is immersed in the sensation of training

A technician is a connoisseur of their body and the sensations flowing through it. Distractions like TV and small talk are unwelcome annoyances. They savor the burn in their muscles and how their hands feel when they grab onto a pull-up bar. They understand the more they embrace these feelings, the more feedback they can receive to progress their neurological code.

#3 A technician is always looking to do things better

The technician understands it can be limiting to label a particular technique as either right or wrong. Saying a technique is wrong can be frustrating and self-defeating. Claiming something is being done the right way can quench the thirst for improvement.

By keeping their mind on the continuous progressive process, a technician can find progressive value in even the most amateur movements. This mindset helps to ensure they always move forward without self-defeating criticism or blinding arrogance. This point is also why the figure in the R.D.P logo is white as it symbolizes a "beginner mind" that's always eager to learn and grow.

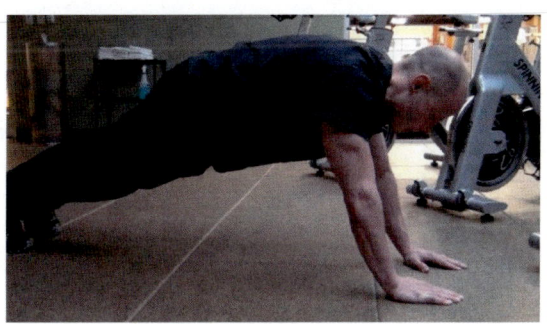

A technician never grows tired of the basics. Even simple isometrics, like the plank, offer endless opportunity to learn and grow.

#4 A technician is detail oriented

The technician understands that no detail is too trivial to consider. They pay attention to their hamstrings while doing pull-ups. They take note of small shifts in weight during push-ups. They even pay attention to how the tension in a single muscle might change throughout a range of motion. While such details may not make a big difference, they contribute to the process of progression.

#5 A technician is self-compassionate

It's impossible to create a positive outcome when you're coming from a negative place, both mentally and emotionally. Hardly anyone has reached their goals by beating themselves up with negative self-talk and abuse. The technician understands this and strives to be understanding of their situation. They don't admonish themselves for eating too much chocolate or skipping a workout. Instead, they recognize the habits that prevent them from reaching their goals and they learn from them. While others may pout and give in to self-pity from a mistake, the technician will step back and analyze the situation while creating a plan for the future.

#6 A technician values hard work, but doesn't rely on it for success

Most importantly, the technician understands that while hard work is very important, it's not the secret to success. A good example of this is in the art of breaking in Taekwon-do. Smashing a stack of boards may seem like a demonstration of might and strength, but it's actually a test of mental and physical technique. I've seen people try to work their way through boards and bricks to no avail. They literally shed their blood, sweat, and tears only to continue smashing against an unyielding object.

I've also seen people smash through a seemingly impenetrable layer of wood or concrete with hardly any effort at all. The difference has always been in the technical proficiency they brought to the punch or kick they used. The lesson is, spend your time and effort to refine your technical skills. Doing so will bring you far greater results than doing ten times the grunt work without working to improve your technical proficiency.

How Plateaus Fuel Your Progress

One of the biggest myths about progression is that it's supposed to happen in a continuous linear pattern. You may have run across ideas like you should be losing about 1.5 pounds a week or adding 5 pounds to your primary lifts every ten days. This type of thinking presents growth as a constant process that doesn't end.

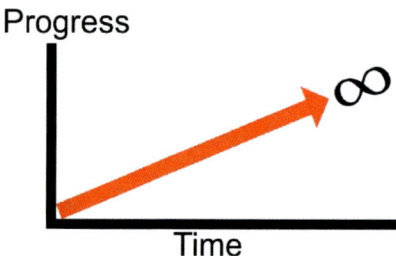

While making endless progress at a steady pace sounds pretty good, it's not something you can do.

As promising as steady improvement may seem, it's pure science fiction. Plateaus and even temporary regressions are all part of growth and progress. Few things just grow and develop endlessly over time. While plateaus may seem frustrating, they help fuel your long-term progress. Both body and mind undergo a lot of stress when you change during a homeostatic imbalance. A plateau is Mother Nature's way of allowing you to rest and get used to the new level you've acquired.

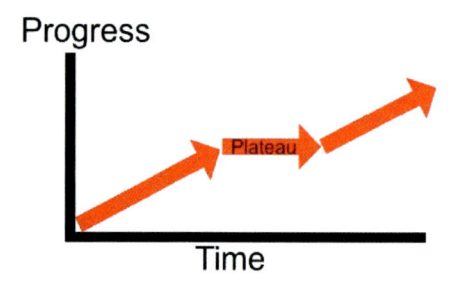

Plateaus give both your body and mind a chance to acclimate to your new level of fitness. Once you're comfortable with your new level of progress you'll find it's easier to continue making progress.

Don't make the mistake of believing that something is wrong just because you've hit a plateau. If anything, your plateau means you're on the right track. So sit for a spell and allow yourself to acclimatize to your new level of fitness. Once you've spent some time getting used to it, you'll be ready to continue to make progress.

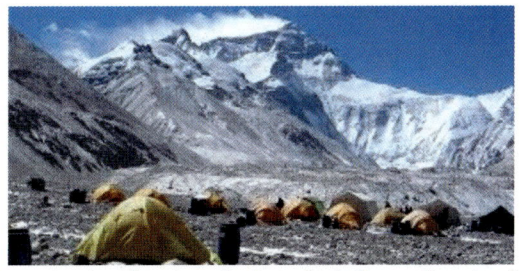

A plateau is like stopping at the Everest base camp to allow your body and mind to acclimatize. It may seem like you're not making progress, but it's a necessary break to reach your goals. Photo: thenepaltrekingcompany.com

Progression is a creative process

Getting in shape is more of a creative process than people realize. The popular notion is that success comes through obediently following the perfect plan that leads you by the hand to the results you want.

The path of progress is different for everyone. We all have our own history, preferences, resources, genetics, and abilities. Because of this, getting in shape requires you to accomplish your goals in a unique way that no one has ever used before. Improving your fitness is not unlike creating the next Oscar-winning screenplay or the next big trend in technology. No one knows for sure how to go about doing it and we're all kind of making it up as we go along.

No one knows for sure what's the best way for you to make progress. If you want to be successful, you're going to have to get creative and figure out the best way to do this for yourself. That's what the Table of Progressive Elements can do for you. It gives you the freedom to progress your training in a way that works for you rather than take a gamble on a plan that may or may not be a good fit.

It's fine to use other people's plans for ideas or as a starting point, but don't be afraid to break the mold and change things as you like. The best plan for you is the one you're going to create through trial and error. So roll up your sleeves and get busy experimenting. You don't have to know for sure what's best for you. All progression requires is to improve just a little bit each day, week or month.

Chapter 6 Chain Training

Training success is just as much mental as it physical. In some cases, most of your progress will come from how you think about your training rather than how to physically practice it. Over the years, I've adopted a form of mental imagery that can make your training simpler and more efficient. I call it Chain Training, and it's a practical way of thinking about how to use the body.

Chain Training isn't anything new. Instead, it combines two ways most people look at their training. Let's explore these two methods and the pros and cons of each.

Method #1 Muscle Training

Muscle training is when your mind focuses on placing tension within a particular muscle, or muscle group. It's very common in bodybuilding circles with exercises designed for the arms, legs, chest, back and so on.

It's also commonly practiced in healing disciplines like physical therapists and chiropractors who train muscles to correct imbalances.

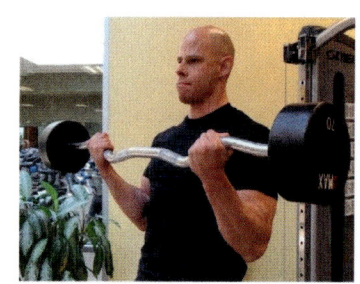

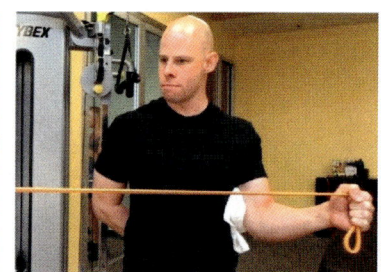

Targeted muscle training is practical for improving aesthetic balance, like curls in bodybuilding, and shoring up injury causing weaknesses like with rotator cuff work in physical therapy.

Advantages of muscle training

Muscle training is an excellent way to improve tension control within a given muscle. It can strengthen physical imbalances and weaknesses that can impede health and performance. It's also a good way to work on proportion and aesthetic balance.

Disadvantages of muscle training

Muscle training is a fragmented approach to tension control. It focuses on placing tension in specific parts of the body while neglecting tension in other areas. This fragmented approach to can condition the mind to only create tension in select muscles while neglecting others which can leave you vulnerable to weaknesses and imbalances.

Fragmented training can also be a costly way to train since it requires more exercises and workouts. Breaking up your leg workout, to focus on 5 different muscles means you need to do 5 different exercises. Each exercise may also require a separate piece of equipment and series of sets and reps which increases the cost of the workout.

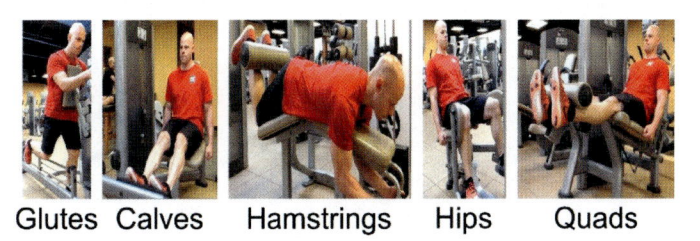

Fragmented training can cost a lot of time and energy. Each of these 5 lower body exercises focuses on a specific muscle group while neglecting the others. This requires you to do many exercises which take a lot of time and energy to cover everything.

Another disadvantage is while training muscles can improve tension control in individual muscles, that control may not carry over to large movements that require the coordination of several muscle groups.

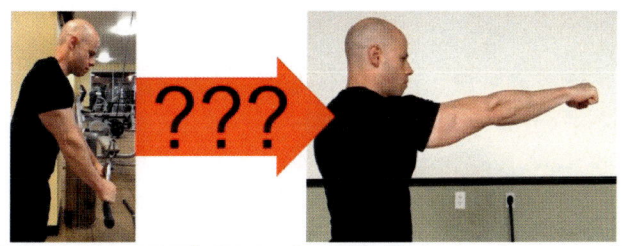

Isolated triceps exercises can make the triceps bigger and stronger, but how effective are they are teaching you how to use your triceps with your shoulders and chest when you throw a punch?

Method #2 Movement Training

Movement training is when you focus on performing a basic movement instead of working a set of muscles. For example, instead of focusing on working the quads or hamstrings you might work on squats, lunges or jumping.

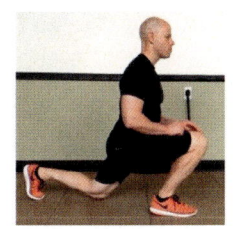

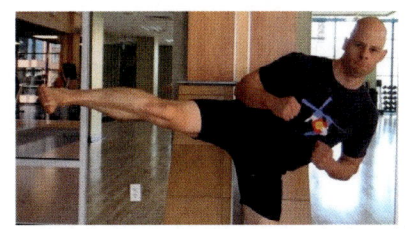

In these images, I'm thinking more about performing the movement of a lunge and throwing a kick and less about what muscles I'm using to make those actions happen.

Advantages of movement training

Movement training is very efficient. Basic movements use a lot of muscles at once so you can train your whole body with a handful of exercises.

Training in basic movements also teaches your mind how to coordinate multiple muscle groups to work together which can improve functional carryover.

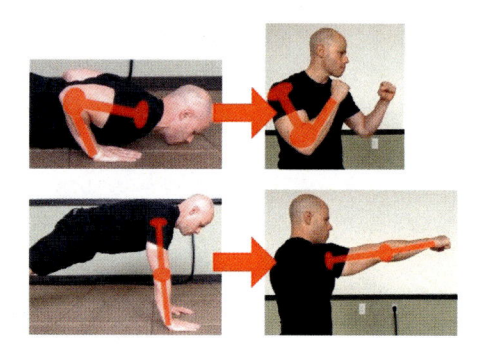

It's easy to see how a compound pushing movement, like the push-up, can have a lot of functional carry over to punching.

Disadvantages of movement training

Movement training makes the mistake of assuming your mind always knows how to optimally use tension while doing basic activities. It would be nice if just doing push-ups and lunges was enough to create optimal muscle tension, but this is rarely the case. The mind has an incredible ability to compensate for weaknesses especially when your focus is on just accomplishing the activity at hand. It doesn't matter if lunges are supposed to work your hips. Your mind will find a way to get the exercise done without much hip strength one way or another. Over time, these compensatory patterns lead to muscle imbalances, injury, and impede performance.

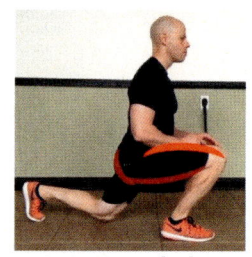

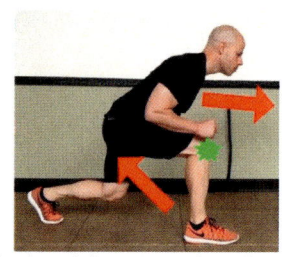

A lack of tension in the glutes and hamstrings causes the hips to move back and the torso to lean forward during lunges. This prevents the front leg from producing much force while placing stress on the front knee but you might accept it if your goal is just to perform the lunge movement in order to complete a workout routine.

Chain Training is the combination of muscle and movement training. It uses large full body movements while concentrating on placing tension within specific muscles. In this way, you gain the benefit of both types of training without the disadvantages of either.

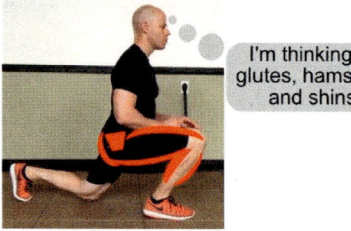

Chain Training is a way to mentally focus on how you produce tension in individual muscles during functional compound movements.

The whole idea behind Chain Training is that your muscles can potentially carry more tension when your mind asks them to work together as one cohesive unit. When you try to isolate the tension in one muscle you create a relatively weak neural code that inhibits the total amount of tension your brain sends to that muscle. While that muscle might feel like it's working super hard, the total amount of tension within it is relatively low.

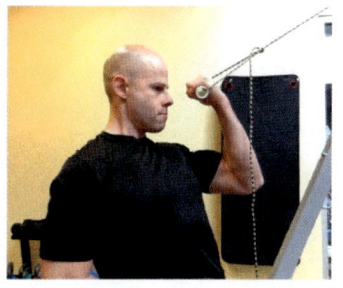

Bicep curls on suspension straps are a great supplemental exercise to pull-ups and rows. They are very effective at concentrating tension into your biceps.

Working your muscles as a collective unit helps you create a stronger neurological code that allows you to place more total tension in a given muscle. So even if it doesn't feel like a single muscle is working as hard, it's probably holding a lot more total tension.

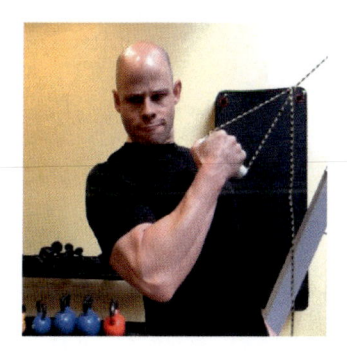

Single arm rows may not feel like they concentrate tension as well as curls, but allowing the biceps to work with your back and shoulders allows more total tension to flow into the biceps.

Holding more total tension in a chain helps each individual muscle grow bigger and stronger which is why you may get better aesthetic results than if you tried to train your muscles solely in an isolated fashion. At the same time, producing more total tension along a muscle chain can help you move stronger and generate more power. This is why Chain Training may help you build both a better look and better performing body than with just training muscles or movements alone.

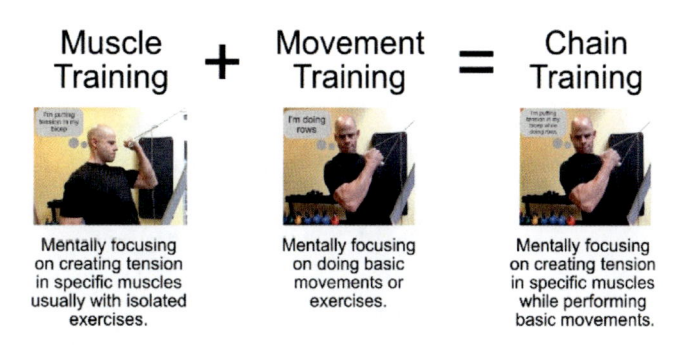

Muscle Training + **Movement Training** = **Chain Training**

Mentally focusing on creating tension in specific muscles usually with isolated exercises.

Mentally focusing on doing basic movements or exercises.

Mentally focusing on creating tension in specific muscles while performing basic movements.

You can quickly experience this phenomenon for yourself by trying to squeeze your wrist between your pointer finger and thumb. Try to isolate the tension to just that one finger by keeping the other fingers as relaxed as possible. Now squeeze your wrist with all of your fingers. You'll notice you not only produce more total force while using your whole hand but there will be more tension in your pointer finger as well.

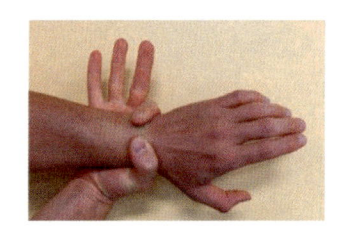

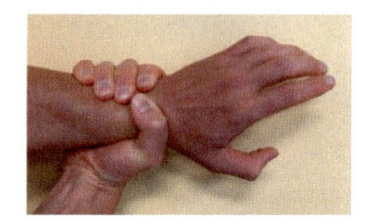

Grabbing your wrist with one finger vs the whole hand is a good way to experience how much stronger you are when you use your muscles together rather than one at a time.

The Six Muscle Chains

Okay, enough with what makes Chain Training work. Let's get into the nitty-gritty of what Chain Training is so you can start using it. First, let's explore the six-movement chains. Here they are in no particular order.

The Six Muscle Chains

Push Chain	Flexion Chain
Pull Chain	Extension Chain
Squat Chain	Lateral Chain

Each chain is made up of a group of muscles responsible for that respective movement. The three chains listed on the left are the "limb chains" as they primarily move the body through the motion of the arms and legs. The three on the right are the "body chains" since they run the full length of the body from head to toe. Let's take a look at them in more detail.

Push chain

The push chain includes the muscles in the upper body responsible for pushing your hands away from your torso. It includes the muscles in the chest, triceps, shoulders and the extensors in the forearm and hands.

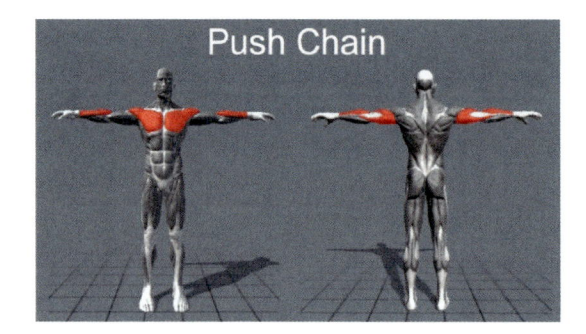

Pull chain

The pull chain is composed of the muscles responsible for pulling your hands closer to your torso. These include the muscles in your back including your latissimus dorsi, traps, rhomboids, and infraspinatus. Other muscles include the shoulders, biceps and the majority of your grip muscles in your forearm and hand.

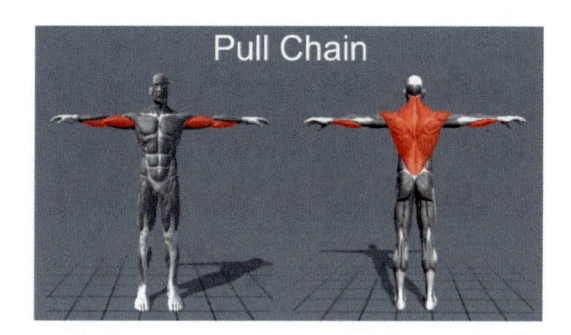

Flexion chain

Sometimes referred to as the anterior chain, the flexion chain involves the muscles on the front of the body that bends your body forward. These include the abdominals and core muscles, hip flexors, quads and even the muscles in your shins and the top of your foot. The muscles in the front of your neck are also part of this chain.

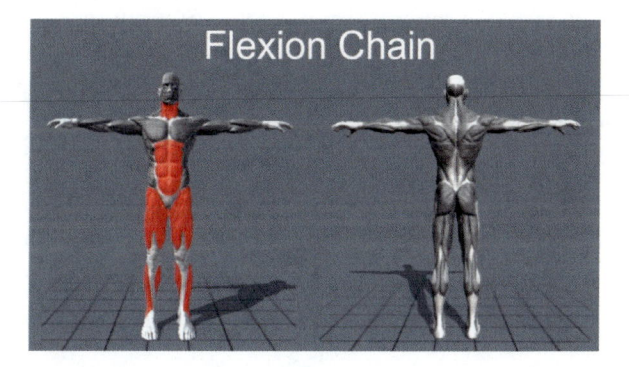

Extension chain

Often called your posterior chain, the extension chain is used to extend the body from a flexed position. Muscles include the calves, hamstrings, glutes, the lower back, and the muscles on along the spine and neck. The lats are also sometimes considered an extension muscle for the torso.

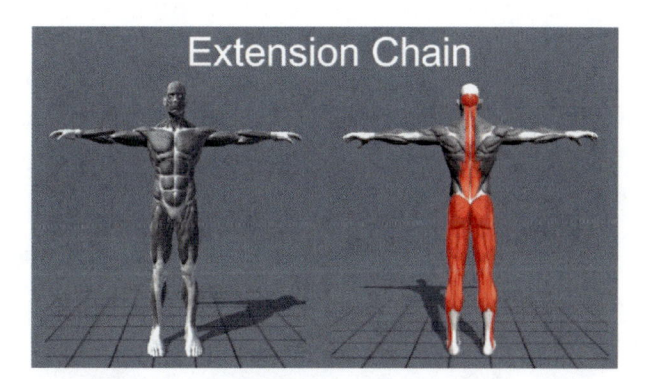

Squat chain

The squat chain includes every muscle from the waist down and is responsible for all of your lower body movements especially squatting, lunging, jumping, walking and running. Major muscles include your hips, quads, hamstrings, calves and the muscles along your shin.

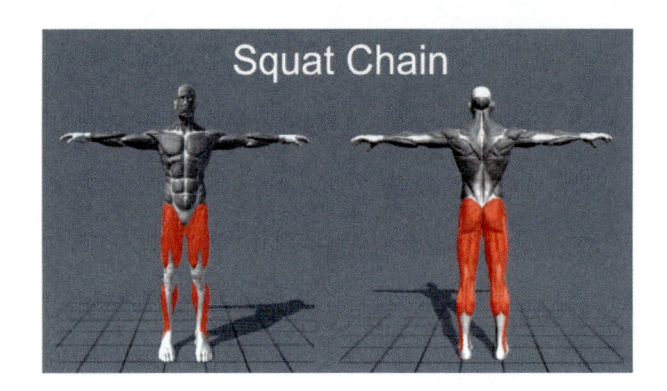

Lateral chain

Your lateral chain is essentially a lateral combination of all five chains. There aren't many specialty muscles for this group, but lateral chain work does hit the inner and outer hip muscles as well as your obliques and lats. It's usually trained for support and stability which carries over to improvement in training the other chains. It's also heavily involved in twisting and rotation motions like a golf swing.

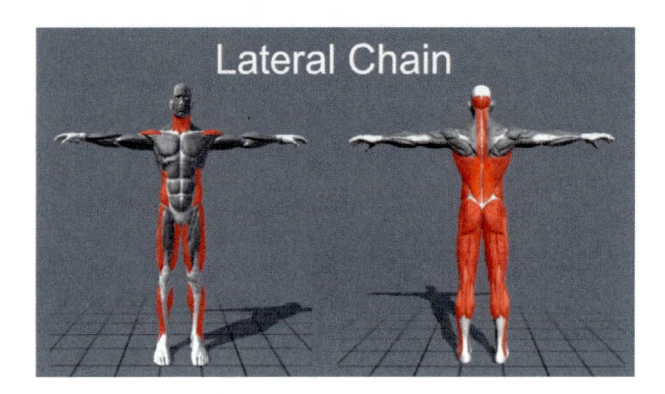

Many muscles play a role in multiple chains sort of like how the muscles in your core are used in almost every basic movement you do. The important thing isn't to isolate a muscle chain but to use it as a target for most of your muscle tension while training. Even though your squat chain may be the primary muscle group you use while sprinting up a hill that doesn't mean your abs and arms are not involved.

Technically, you have 12 muscle chains because each movement chain is also split between a right and left side. For example, you have a right squat chain (your right leg) and a left squat chain (your left leg.) Understanding this is important because you'll be using both right and left chains in different ways with some progressions later on.

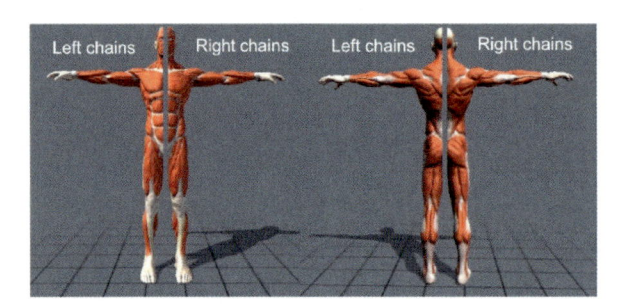

How Do You Use Chain Training?

Chain Training is not a particular way to train or exercise. It's a way to think about your training and exercise. It a mental filter, or template, you can apply to any exercise in order to optimize your neural code.

You don't have to always distribute tension evenly through each muscle in a chain, but your goal is to make it more uniform over time. Eventually, it should feel like the entire chain is one big muscle rather than a collection of smaller muscles. The more you even out the tension in your muscle chain, the safer, more comfortable and beneficial your training will be.

You don't have to tense all of your muscles as hard as possible.

One of the biggest misconceptions of Chain Training is that you need to tense all of your muscles as hard as possible. While adding more tension to a muscle chain is the goal, you don't have to keep everything super tight, especially when you're starting out. Sometimes, it's not ideal to tense every muscle as much as you can. Athletic activities like running or kicking require a lot of relaxation. Too much tension makes you slow and wears you out. Even though you don't want to tense your leg as hard as possible during a kick, you do want to concentrate on using the muscles in that leg as one collective unit.

P.T.R For Perfect Sets in Every Workout

A helpful technique I've used to establish tension along a chain is something I call the P.T.R, or "Peter," method which stands for Position, Tension, and Resistance.

I created it because tension can be difficult to manipulate once you apply resistance to a muscle. P.T.R only takes a second or two, but it can significantly improve the tension quality along any muscle chain.

Step #1 Get into position

The first step is to get yourself into the physical position you want to do your exercise. Pay attention to where you place your hands and feet as well as the position of your hips and shoulders.

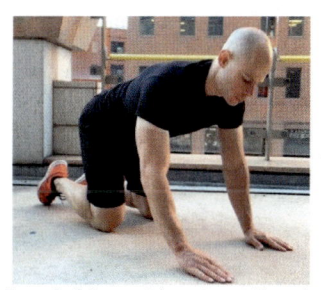

Getting into push-up position requires thoughtful consideration of hand and foot placement and body alignment.

Step #2 Apply tension throughout the movement chain

Once you're in position, contract your muscles to apply tension throughout the muscle chain as well as any other muscles that play a role in the exercise. It doesn't need to be as much tension as possible. It just needs to establish the flow of tension along the chain without leaving any gaps.

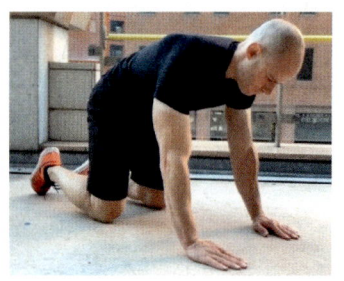

Tense up the muscles in the push chain especially the arms, chest, and shoulders. Also, tense the abs and back since those muscles play a supportive role.

Step #3 Apply resistance

Last, apply resistance to the exercise by lifting off the floor, or shifting your weight, so gravity is pulling on your body.

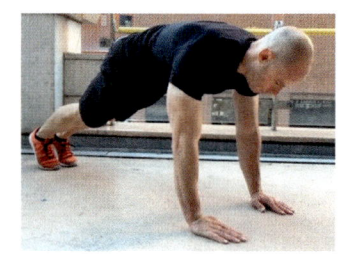

Picking the knees up off the floor transfers more weight onto the arms to create resistance on the push chain muscles.

P.T.R works because it can be tempting to jump into an exercise without optimally setting up your position or muscle tension. If you drop down into a push-up without much thought, you're rolling the dice on the quality and effectiveness of the exercise. You might get halfway through the set before your mind starts to contemplate how to put more tension on certain muscles or feel like your hand position was a little too narrow or wide. You might also wonder why your wrist is starting to hurt or why you don't feel your pecs working. At that point, you're just hoping to finish the set to get it over with, and you struggle to get the last remaining reps. Taking a moment to apply P.T.R before each exercise will help you avoid this scenario and increase the quality of your workout.

Chapter 7 Extension Chain

This first muscle chain may be the single most important muscle group in your entire body. This chain runs the full length of the back of your body starting at the bottom of your feet, wrapping behind your ankles, running up your calves, hamstrings, glutes, low back, running the length of your spine, and the back of your neck. Some folks even claim the muscles that raise your eyebrows are part of this chain.

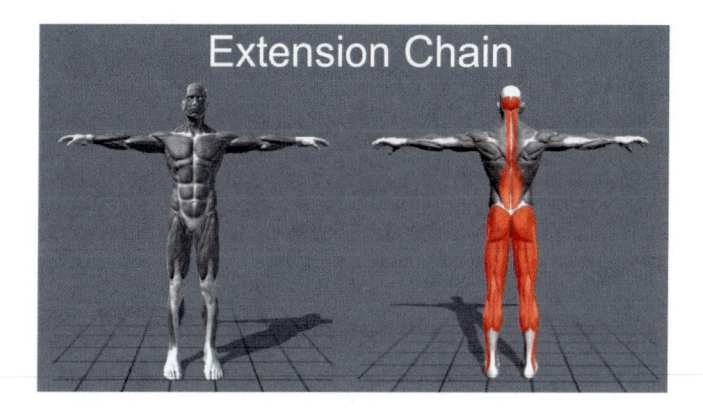

Your extension chain plays a vital role in your health and fitness, but it's sadly one of the most neglected and deconditioned muscle chains for many people. You use it for virtually everything you do yet it doesn't receive much attention, especially when it comes to bodyweight training. Maybe it's because exercises like bridges and hip extensions don't get to sit at the cool kid's table along with push-ups and pull-ups. It could also be because understanding how to train it isn't common knowledge. It's time to turn the tide starting with the following reasons why building a strong extension chain could be the best thing you ever do in fitness.

#1 It enhances your physical appearance

Keeping your backside healthy is essential in maintaining your appearance and physical attractiveness. It's ironic how the mirror muscles or trouble spots of the body get a lot of attention while a strong extension chain is much more important when it comes to looking your best. It doesn't matter how toned your abs are or how big your biceps grow. Walking around all stooped over sends a subliminal message that you're weak, shy and lack confidence. When you have a "commanding posture," your muscular development can be modest, but everyone will know you're a strong and capable person, both inside and out.

#2 It improves your ability to do everything

Every motion you do requires at least some tension in your extension chain. Even building strong biceps and abs require a well-conditioned extension chain.

The reason is simple; all muscle tension has to flow around and through your back and hips. Many people look to the core as the foundation for health and fitness, but this is a bit of a myth. A fully capable extension chain (which includes parts of your "core") is the real foundation of your physical movement.

I learned this lesson the hard way one cold day when I jumped into a Taekwon-do class without warming up. When I threw my first punch, I instantly felt a shot of pain and a sensation like a rubber band was tightening up the left side of my spine. I had strained one of my spinal erectors, and it made me feel like an old man for the next couple of days. Every movement I did was weak and stiff. Even opening a jar or standing up from a chair was difficult. I had no power or strength in even the smallest of movements. It was a powerful lesson in how the extension chain plays a significant role in everything I do.

#3 It plays a vital role in your health and wellbeing

There're many reasons for back pain, and if you're suffering any such pain, you should certainly consult a medical professional. Never accept pain as a part of training or life because it will always hold you back.

The common mistake is to assume that low back pain is due to weakness in the lower back. This assumption leads to practicing ineffective exercises in an attempt to isolate and work or stretch that area.

Low back pain is a classic case of stress pooling into that area because tension is not flowing through the rest of the muscular chain. You usually don't have overstressed back muscles because they are weak. It's often because the other muscles in the chain aren't engaged enough to pull the pressure off that area.

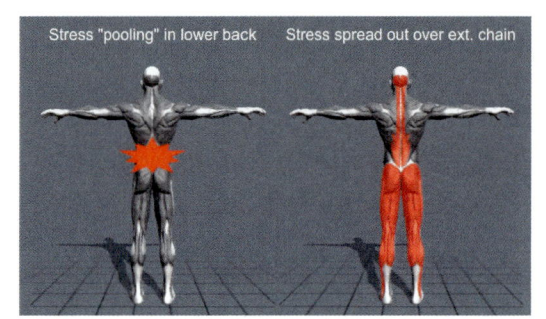

When the muscles in the back of the legs and spine are weak, the low back becomes a pinch point where stress pools and overloads the small muscles. Engaging the other muscles helps spread the stress so it doesn't cause pain or discomfort.

Your extension chain also plays a significant role in keeping your other joints healthy. The strength of your hamstrings and glutes can reduce stress on your knees and ankles. Strong calf muscles can help lessen the risk of plantar fasciitis while controlling your upper back helps protect your shoulders and elbows. I've even had clients reduce the occurrence of tension headaches through improving their posture and lessen the strain on their neck muscles.

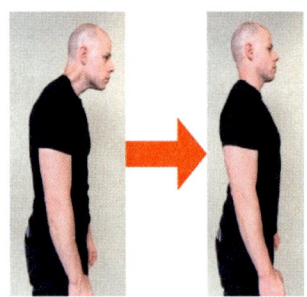

Poor posture can wreak havoc on your physique, performance, and health. Extension exercises, like bridges, can be a valuable part of the solution.

Joint stress isn't the only health risk that can be reduced by a well-conditioned extension chain. Your breathing, which can influence many aspects of your health, is also influenced. Modern living has turned even serious athletes into "chest breathers" where they breathe as if only using the top third of their lungs. Most of the extension exercises in this chapter are designed to "open your lungs" and stretch your abdominal cavity making it easier to breath deeper.

#4 Your extension chain is under daily attack

Your extension chain suffers daily abuse from tension fragmentation and neuromuscular amnesia. Much of this is from sitting for extended periods of time. With your extensors asleep, tension flows in fragmented segments which hurt your health, posture, and performance. It's also why many people suffer from back pain.

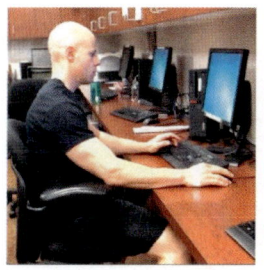

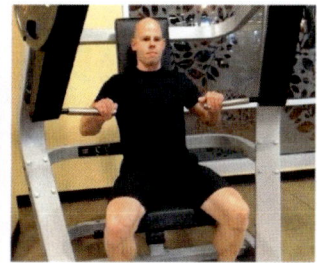

Sitting is one of the biggest threats to your extension chain. Is there any wonder why we struggle with poor back health when we sit so much?

#5 It will improve every other exercise you do

Your extension chain influences the strength of every muscle in your body. If you want abs, you need strong spinal erectors. If you want bigger arms and wide shoulders you need a stable extension chain. Even your calf and grip training can be affected by how well you use your backside. So even though you may not see the muscles in your extension chain, you will notice their influence over every inch of your body.

I'm placing this chapter first in the Chain Training section to put an emphasis on this muscle chain. Please don't merely play around with these exercises or consider them a fancy party trick. They can bring a lot of benefits but only if you take them as seriously as you would any other exercise.

Okay, lecture over. Let's get down to the business of training your extension chain.

Turning On Your Extension Chain

These isometric exercises are meant to wake up sleepy muscles so you can get tension flowing through your extension chain. You may not feel much when you first try them but give it time. Tension control is a skill, and it can take a lot of practice to get the hang of it.

Standing extension with arm torque

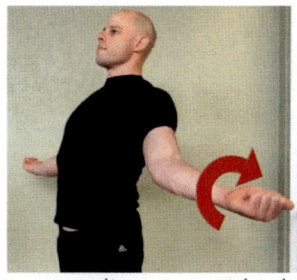

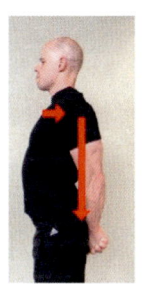

Standing and extending your back is a great way to relieve stress and wake up the muscles along your spine. Torqueing your arms back, like in the image on the left, can help you keep tension through your upper back. Clasping your hands behind your hips and pushing your shoulders down is another popular variation.

This exercise is ideal for anyone who works at a desk. It opens the chest and engages the extension chain all the way down to the floor.

Stand up and extend your spine up and back as far as you comfortably can without straining. At the same time, rotate your arms as if your trying to point your thumbs down behind you. Tuck your shoulder blades down and in toward each other while tensing up every muscle from your upper back to your ankles.

Hold for a few moments and release the tension while taking note of how your body eases into your old posture. This move is not meant to be a hard exercise nor is it supposed to create a lot of fatigue. It's gentle enough to do multiple times every day which I highly recommend.

Staggered stance hold

The other exercise is a staggered stance hold where you're trying to pull the floor apart with your back foot.

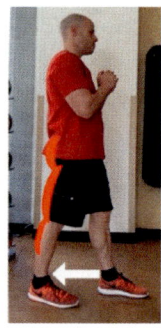

The simple staggered stance exercise is a great way to wake up the glutes, hamstrings, and calves. Just isometric tense the back of your rear leg like you're trying to pull the floor apart between your feet. Hold for 5-10 seconds.

This drill teaches you how to turn on the muscles in the back of your legs and hips. Place your legs apart as you would when taking a small step forward and push into the heel of the back foot. It should feel like you're trying to scrape your foot against the floor by using the muscles in the back of your leg. Be sure to create tension in your glutes, hamstrings, and calves. Like the standing spinal extension, you can do this anytime you're standing.

Extension Chain Exercises

Bridges are one of the most popular extension chain exercises in calisthenics. They work the entire chain while targeting weak areas. They also stretch the front of your body and are the natural antidote to the effects of sitting.

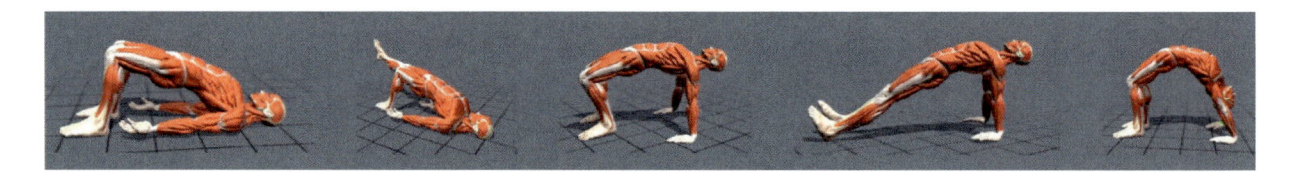

You can practice bridges in both a dynamic and isometric fashion. Doing an isometric bridge can help program your neural code to engage your whole extension chain. A dynamic variation is ideal for learning how to control your tension through a range of motion. It also does a lot to fatigue your muscles and stimulates muscle growth.

Hip bridges

The first three bridge variations are what I call hip bridges. While all bridges work your hips and hamstrings, these focus on using your glutes and hamstrings to lift your pelvis off the floor. Your spinal erectors and shoulders are also working to extend your spine.

Lying Bridges

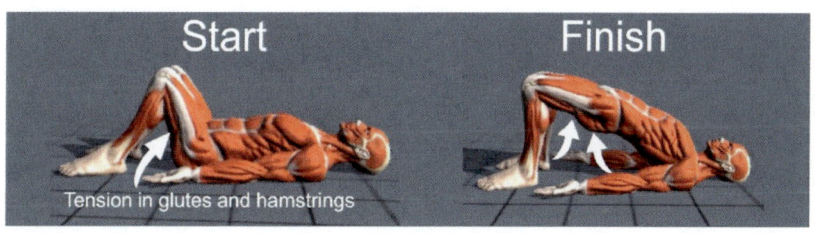

Place feet flat on the floor near hips with arms flat on the floor palms up. Drive your hips up by squeezing your glutes and hamstrings and pulling your heels into the floor.

Lying bridges are a great introductory exercise. They help stretch out the front of your hips and allow you to work on turning on your extension chain.

It's common for people to push into their feet like they are trying to press the floor apart. While not a bad technique, you'll get a lot more tension in your hamstrings when you pull your feet into the floor. This motion should feel like you're trying to pull the floor together between your feet and shoulders. It also helps to drive your knees forward as you lift up.

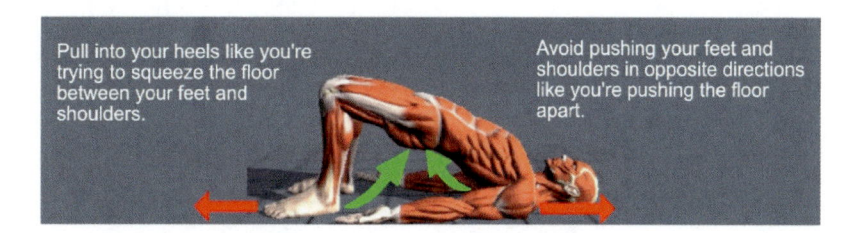

Lying bridges are also a good way to learn how to use your spinal erectors to arch your back. Imagine lifting your chest up to your chin as you lift your hips. Be sure not to make your lower back muscles do all of the work. Try to spread the tension evenly throughout the erector muscles along your spine.

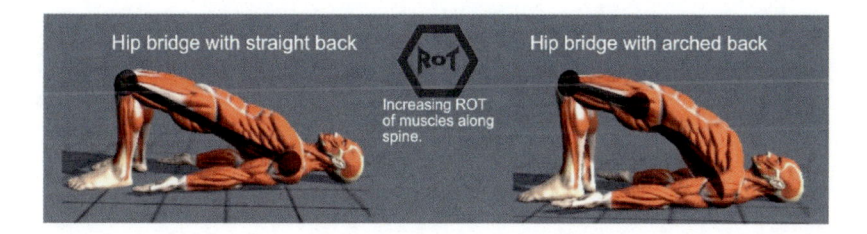

Some people find their hamstrings cramp up when they first learn how to pull into a bridge. If this happens, don't lift your hips as high for the first few workouts. You can increase the range as your muscles become more used to the increase in tension.

Table bridges

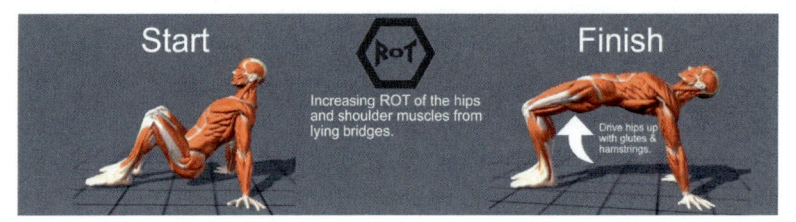

Start sitting with your hands and feet flat on the floor. Place tension along your entire extension chain and drive your hips up with your glutes and hamstrings. Pause at the top and then lower your hips back to the floor while maintaining tension in your extension chain.

Table bridges are one of my favorite exercises, and I do them almost daily. They place more tension in the upper back than lying bridges while also working on the mobility of the shoulders. You'll also find they use more range of tension in the hips than lying bridges.

Doing bridges on your hands gives your shoulder blades more freedom of movement compared to lying on the floor. This upper back work makes the table bridge a good way to learn how to pull your shoulder blades down and back.

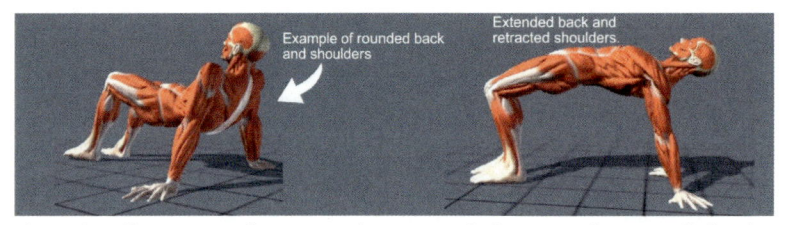

Once again, try squeezing the floor together or at least applying tension straight down into the floor instead of pushing outward. I also recommend trying to squeeze the floor together between both hands and feet. I like to picture pulling the floor together to a central point under my tailbone.

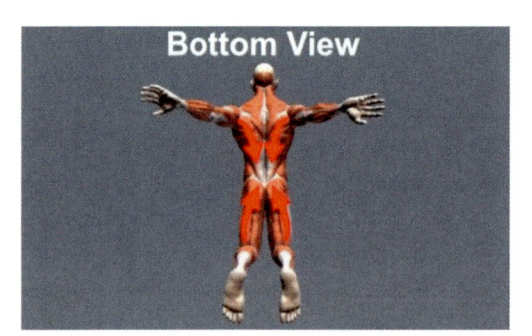

Driving tension in toward the lower back can improve tension control and stability in many bridge exercises.

Table bridges have a couple of fun variations depending on where you drop your hips at the bottom of each rep. These changes can slightly change where your mind places tension in your extension chain.

The most common variation is to drop your hips straight down between your hands and feet. This technique creates an even distribution of tension through your back, hips, and hamstrings.

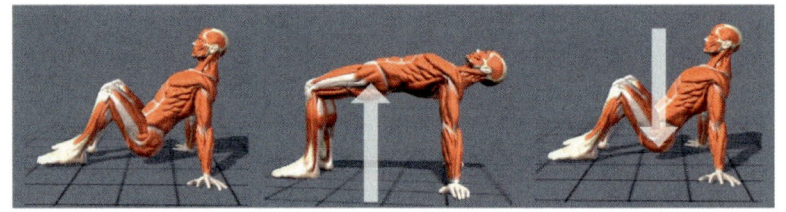

Start with equal weight between your hands and feet with your hips near the floor. Drive your hips straight up while squeezing the floor between hands and feet. Pause at the top and then lower your hips straight down while maintaining tension in your extension chain.

The next variation involves dropping your hips down closer to your hands. This motion requires slightly straightening your legs as you move into a seated position. You'll be pulling a little more with your hamstrings as you bend your knees when you lift your hips.

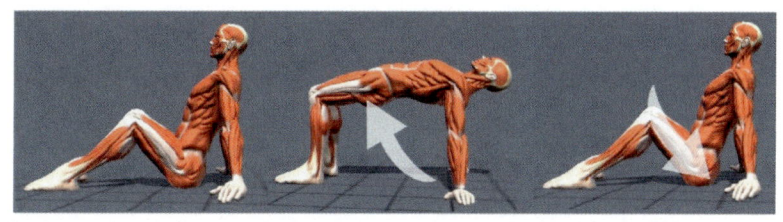

Start with most of your weight on your hands and your knees bent at a 45-degree angle. Pull your hips up with your hamstrings and glutes while keeping a straight back. Pause at the top and lower your hips down and back toward your hands.

Lastly, you can drop your hips down toward your heels while shifting your weight more to your feet. This position requires more mobility in your hips, shoulders, and wrists. You'll use a little more tension in your glutes as you extend your hips up and back.

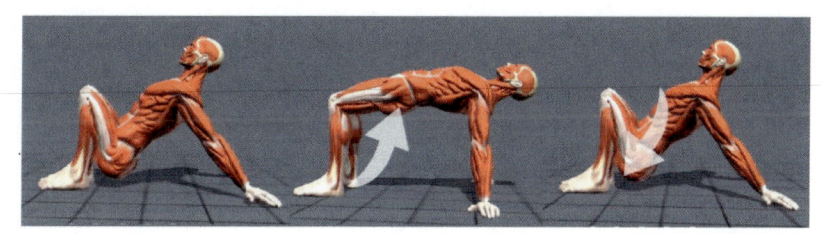

Start with your hips behind your heels and most of your weight on your legs. Drive your heels into the floor while shifting some weight onto your hands so your weight is equally spread out. Pause at the top and flex your hips to pull your hips back to your heels while maintaining tension in the back of your legs.

Straight bridges/ reverse plank

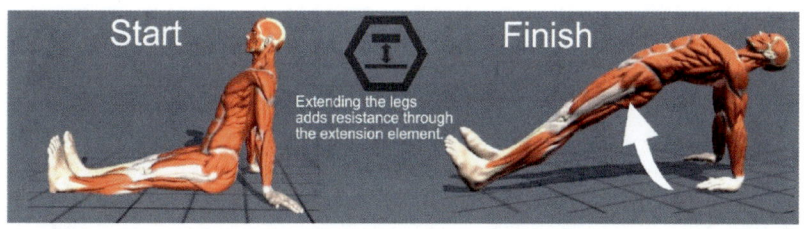

Start sitting on the floor and slightly leaning back onto your hands. Drive your hands and heels into the floor while using your glutes and hamstrings to drive your ups up. Pause at the top and lower your hips back to the floor while keeping your extension chain tense.

This move uses the extension element and the more you extend your legs, the more difficult the exercise becomes.

You can also experiment with foot angles. Some people prefer to point their toes forward, and others like to point them up. My experience is pointing the toes up is a little harder while pointing them forward is a little easier. Experiment for yourself and see how it feels to you.

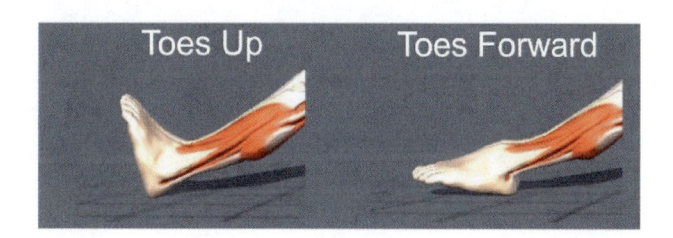

You might find this exercise to be a little easier on your shoulders and upper back due to the lower position of your hips on the slant. Elevating your feet, even slightly, will make your muscles work more against the pull of gravity.

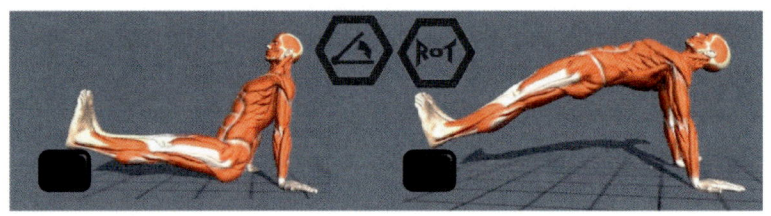

Elevating your feet during hip bridges increases the range of tension in the shoulders while also placing more weight on your hands by changing your angle to gravity.

You don't have to jump right from the table bridge to the straight leg bridge. You can gradually progress by straightening your legs over time and add resistance gradually.

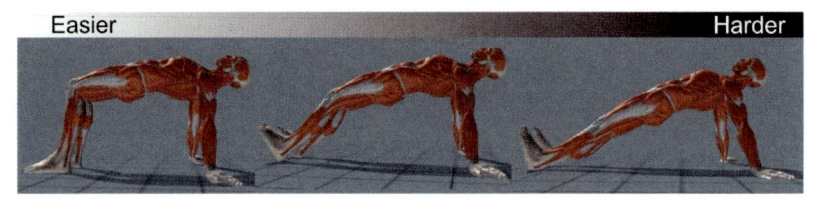

You don't need to jump right from the table bridge to the slant bridge in one leap. Inching your feet forward can help you fine-tune the resistance to your fitness level.

Common hip bridge progressions

You can progress all three of these bridges with the centerline and weight shifting elements. The easier variation of all three is to lift up with your legs about shoulder width to provide stability. From there, you can progress by moving your feet closer together toward your centerline.

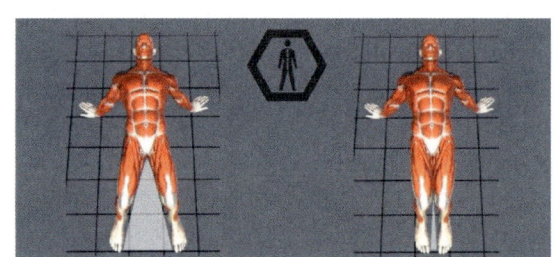

Placing your knees and feet close together will make your hip bridges more difficult through the centerline principle.

Once you're comfortable with bridges on the centerline, you can start to shift your weight to one leg by crossing at the ankle or knee. From there you can place all of your weight on one leg while you hold the other above the floor.

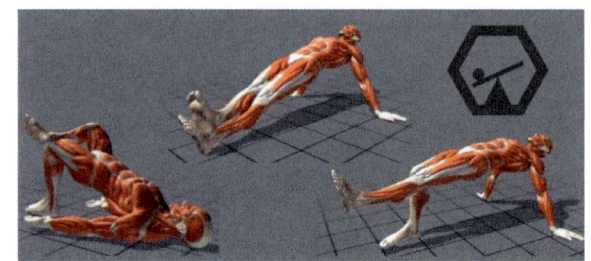

Some examples of unilateral hip bridges that use the weight shift element to place more resistance on one leg. Crossing at the ankle or knee allows one leg to assist in the movement while keeping a leg off the ground or from touching you places all the weight on one leg.

Shoulder bridges

These bridge variations involve more spinal extension than hip bridges. This motion increases the range of tension along your spine, increases shoulder mobility and strength while strengthening your arms and shoulders. Even though these bridges use your upper body more, try to maintain the same tension in your hips and hamstrings that you would use with hip bridges.

Strap bridges

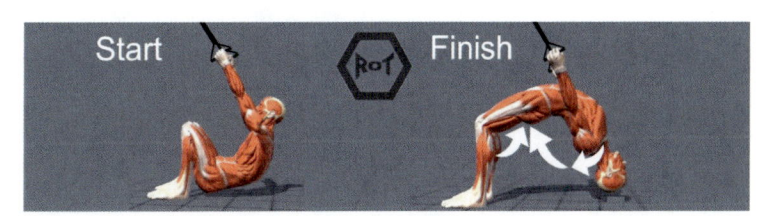

Start with your hips by your heels and your back flexed. Try to maintain tension in your back and hips. Pull your hips up with your glutes and hamstrings while extending your spine with your spinal erectors. Be sure to tuck your shoulders down and back and let the tension flow up the back of your neck. Pause at the top and return to the start position while maintaining tension in your muscles. Try to spread tension throughout yours whole extension chain rather than have it pool into your lower back.

This exercise helps introduce you to a greater range of tension in your hips and torso without requiring much range or strength in your upper body. They are an excellent way to learn how to retract and depress your shoulder blades as you pull your upper back closer to your feet.

The range of tension is the primary progressive element you'll use with this exercise as you work to increase the height of your hips and the arch in your back. You can also progress through the center line element by placing your hands or feet closer together.

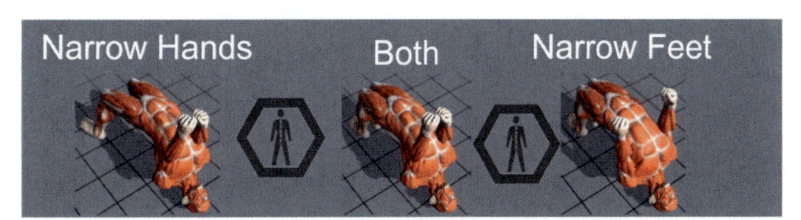

If you're using a suspension trainer, you can adjust your resistance through the angle you work against gravity. Starting with the straps angled towards your feet allows gravity to assist your movement. Moving your feet forward removes this assistance until the angle of the straps provides some resistance against your bridge.

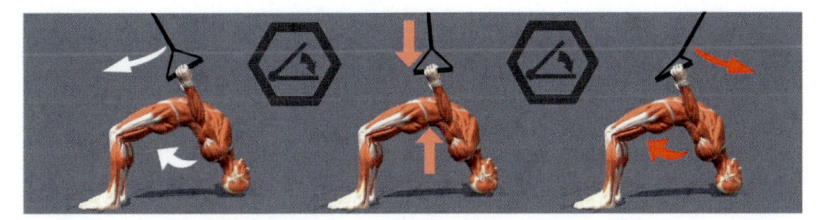

Angling the straps uses the angle to gravity element to change the resistance on your extension chain. In the image on the left the straps assist with pulling into the bridge. In the middle, they play a neutral role when the straps are vertical. Angling the straps away from your feet adds resistance against your extension chain as you can see in the example on the right.

As with all bridges, you may feel a pinch in your lower back if you're trying to place too much tension in your lumbar muscles. Be sure to tense your entire extension chain including your hamstrings, hips and spinal erectors to distribute tension over the whole back side of your body.

Bench bridges

Practicing bridges on an elevated surface, like a weight bench, makes it easier to develop the shoulder strength and mobility you'll need to reach behind your head.

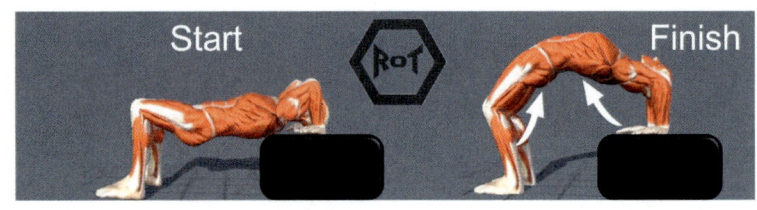

Start with your shoulders and head resting on a surface that's about knee height. Reach your hands back while pointing your elbows up and slightly back while pressing your palms straight down into the bench. Press your hands into the bench with your upper back and shoulder muscles while also contracting your hamstring and glutes to elevate your hips. Pause at the top and lower your upper back to the bench while maintaining tension in your arms and extension chain.

Be sure to keep your hands on either side of your head and drive your elbows back as you press. Failing to do so will place more strain on the wrists which is a common issue with back bridges. Also, don't let your elbows flare out to the side as this will also create stress on the wrists.

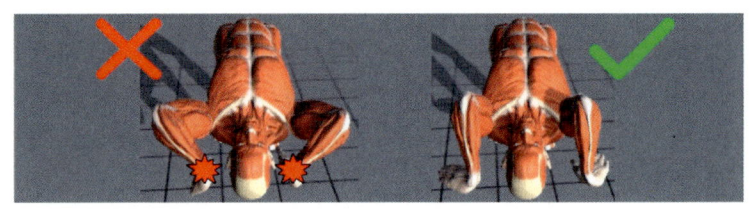

Placing your wrists too high or letting your elbows flare out to the side can place a significant strain on your wrists. Keep your shoulders tucked down and back while driving your elbows in and back can ease such stress while making your muscles work harder.

Floor press bridges

This is the common back bridge exercise. You'll start off laying on the floor with your knees bent and your feet flat near your hips. Your hands reach back next to your head and your press up into an arch while engaging your extension chain.

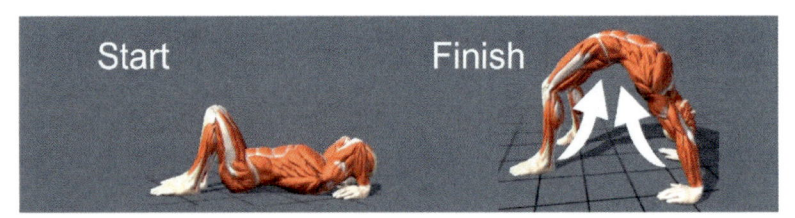

Lay on the floor with your feet flat near your hips and your hands on either side of your head. Drive your feet into the floor to place tension into your hamstrings and glutes while pressing into the palm heel of your hands to turn on your back and shoulders. Continue to press into the floor while pressing open your hips and shoulders as you lift your body off the floor. Lift as high as you comfortably can. Pause at the top and lower yourself back onto the floor in a controlled motion.

The range of tension element will probably be your primary element of progression for this exercise as you strengthen your extension chain and mobilize your flexion chain. Strive to lift yourself higher off the floor while opening your shoulders and hips over time.

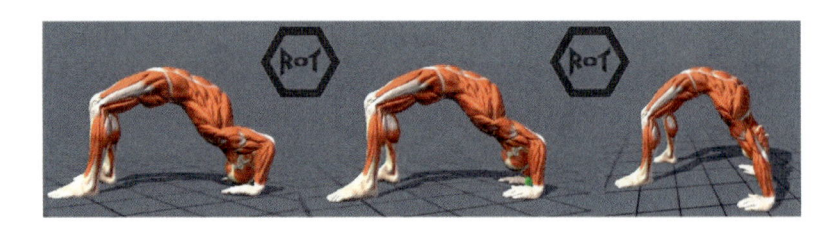

Initial press bridges may give you just enough range to tilt your head back. Progression is accomplished by further extending your hips, flexing your shoulders and extending your elbows while also extending your spine. Be sure to not force your range of motion.

Press, or back bridges, involve a wide range of motion at a number of joints including your hips, spine, shoulder, elbow, and wrist. It's not uncommon for at least one of these joints to be tight and the surrounding muscles to be relatively weak. If you find a weak, or stiff link in your chain, be sure not to force it to catch up to your other joints. It's tempting to overextend the spine when your shoulders are stiff or to extend the wrists too much when you're not extending your hips high enough. This can cause strain and stress to pool into the weak and stiff joints. Be patient and gently work on strengthening and opening up all of the joints involved in the exercise to build complete strength and mobility.

While you can do this exercise for reps, you'll probably progress your range of tension faster if you hold at the top as an isometric. This way, you're using the time element to place more emphasis on the strength and flexibility you need to increase your range of tension.

Bridge stepping or crawling on the floor

This variation uses the weight shifting element as you move your weight so you can pick up a hand or foot off the floor. Start off with stationary stepping where you pick one limb off the floor for a second before placing it back down. Progress to crawling bridges where you can move forward, backward and sideways.

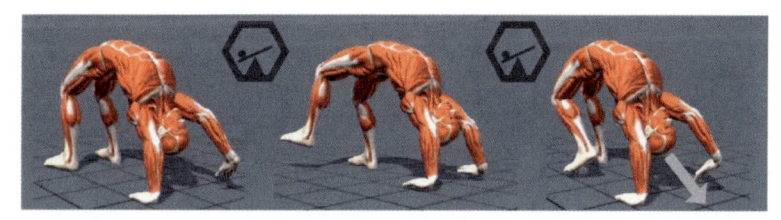

Picking up a hand (left) or a foot (middle) is a great way to use the weight shifting element to place more resistance on one arm or leg in a bridge position. Doing both in a smooth controlled motion is more difficult but it can produce more strength and tension control along your extension chain especially when crawling along the floor (right.)

You can also apply this crawling method to the table bridges with a "crab walk." This exercise is a great workout for your hamstrings as you pull yourself forward by flexing at your knee.

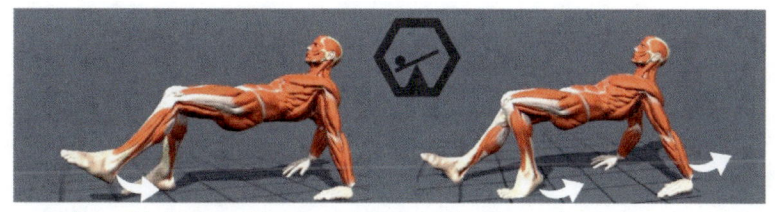

Classic "crab walks" are just crawling table bridges. Start by reaching one leg forward and use your hamstrings to pull your body toward your foot while pushing your arms back. It's basically traveling hamstring curls!

You can also adjust the difficulty through lifting your hips higher (harder) or keeping them close to the floor (easier).

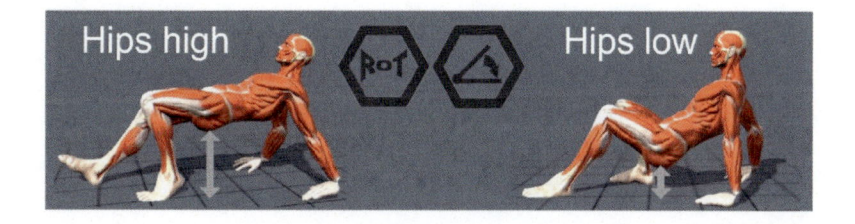

Adjusting the height of your hips changes both the range of tension and your angle to gravity in several joints including your hips, knees, shoulders, and spine.

Bridge crawling on a wall

Another fun progression is to walk yourself into a bridge position by crawling up or down a wall. Naturally, this uses the angle to gravity to adjust the difficulty of the move.

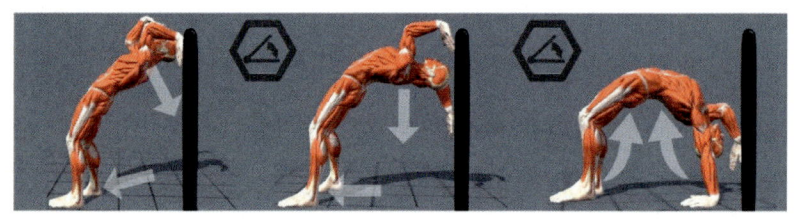

Arch your back and bend your knees while pressing your hands into the wall behind you. Slowly walk your hands down the wall as you step your feet forward. Once you reach the bottom of the wall place both hands on the floor in the classic bridge position while using your extension chain to press yourself up. Reverse the process to crawl back up or lower your hips to the floor and stand back up for another set of downward crawling.

It's easier to crawl down the wall than up it, so it's customary to spend time on just walking down the wall and then standing back up before crawling down again. Once you can comfortably do this more than ten times you may want to start on the floor and walk your hands up the wall out of the bridge position.

Once you can walk up the wall, then you may want to play with walking up and down the wall in one shot.

Back-bend Bridges

One of the hardest bridge variations involves bending back into a full bridge without any support on the upper body until you reach the floor. Once you're in the bridge, you come back up to a standing position.

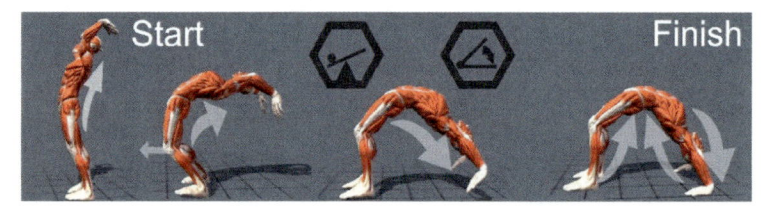

Start standing upright and reach overhead while pressing your hips forward. Bend at the knees while shifting your weight forward to counterbalance your weight as you continue to bend backward. Continue to flex your shoulders and straighten your arms to reach toward the floor. Allow your weight to shift to your arms once your hands reach the floor and pause in the bridge position.

This move requires a lot of strength and control in your extension chain plus a pretty good amount of strength and flexibility in your flexion chain as well. The key is to do this in a graceful movement where you shift your weight forward as you bend back to maintain balance on your feet. You don't want to fall into the bridge position which can cause stress and strain on your joints.

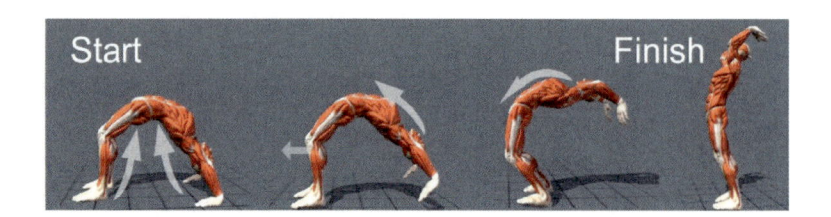

Standing back up is the reverse motion of bending back. Start in the bridge position and shift your weight to your feet. Slightly press off your hands and use your flexion chain to pull yourself upright while using your extension chain for support.

Hip extensions

This exercise requires a special piece of equipment that holds your lower body in place. You might also be able to find someone to hold your legs down as you drape yourself over an exercise ball or weight bench.

Hip extensions focus a lot of tension on the glutes and hamstrings since they primarily move at the hip joint while keeping your spine stable.

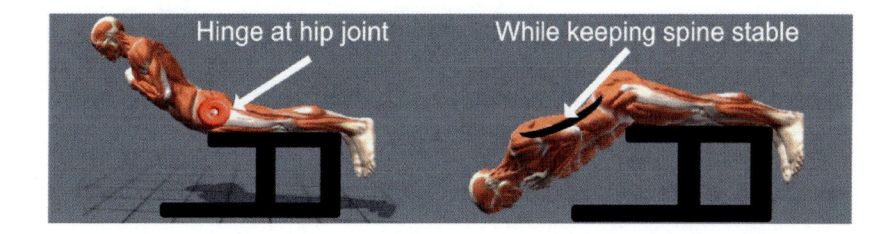

You can progress your hip extensions different ways including the lever, angle and weight element. Using the angle element requires finding a different piece of equipment, so your body is parallel to the floor when you fully extend your hips.

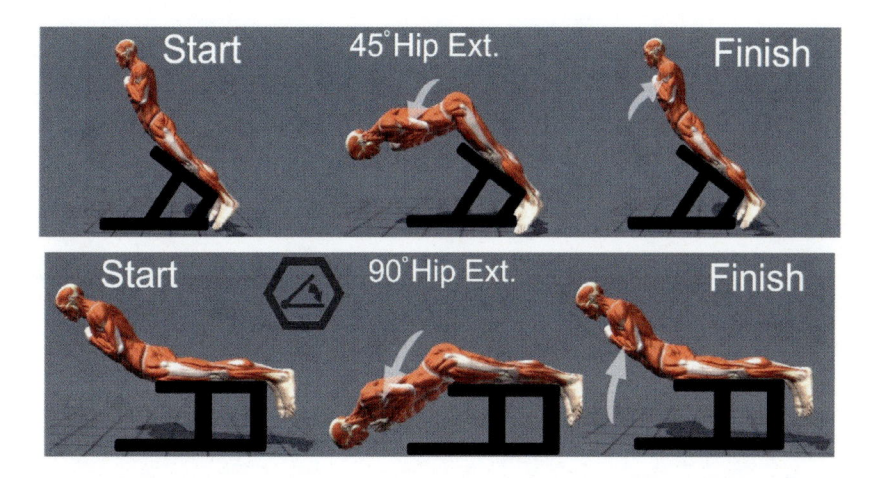

The extension element is the easiest to use since it involves extending your arms further overhead. The easiest variation is to hold your hands behind your back with the hardest progressing your arms overhead.

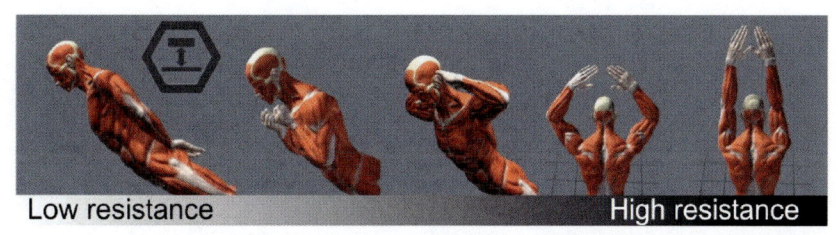

Lowest resistance is hands behind the hips. Resistance increases as your hands reach higher to extend your lever from hands across chest, hands on ears, reaching overhead and finally fully extending arms overhead. Pulling the elbows back also increases resistance on your shoulders and upper back to strengthen your traps and rear deltoids.

Hip extensions are a popular exercise to do with extra weight since it's easy to hold a weight in your hands. The most popular version is to hold heavier weight on the chest or near the torso. I've always preferred to use a lighter weight with my arms fully extended since it doesn't require as much direct load on the back. Overall, both variations can work since they only change the resistance of the exercise, but it's the tension in the muscles that actually makes you stronger.

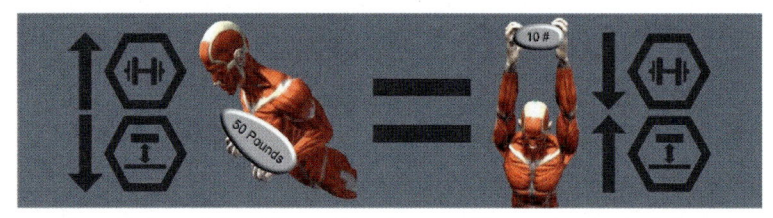

Both variations control resistance through the weight and extension elements. The version on the left uses more weight but less extension when holding weight to the chest. The variation on the right increases resistance through extension but decreases weight. Both variations can produce the same resistance on the extension chain despite using a different technique and weight.

Spine extensions

Spine extensions may look similar to hip extensions, but they use a different neurological code. Instead of stabilizing your spine and moving at your hip joint, you're now stabilizing your hips and moving your spine.

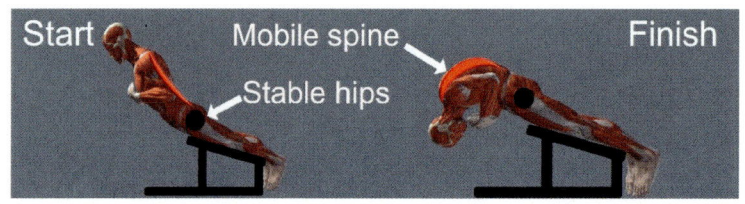

Start in the same position as hip extensions with your spine and hips extended. Curl your torso downward while flexing your spine while limiting the motion in your hips. Pause at the bottom and extend your spine back up to extension in a smooth and controlled motion.

Be careful with this movement. You don't need a lot of resistance, and it is easier to strain your erectors and lower back compared to bridges. I recommend always doing this exercise in a slow and controlled motion.

You can progress this move with the same progressive elements you would use with hip extensions with the angle, lever and weight elements. Just be aware that you won't need nearly as much resistance to sufficiently work your erectors.

Elevated lying hip extensions

Elevated lying hip extensions are bridges with your feet on a ledge or suspension straps. It's a great way to teach your hamstrings to pull into a bridge.

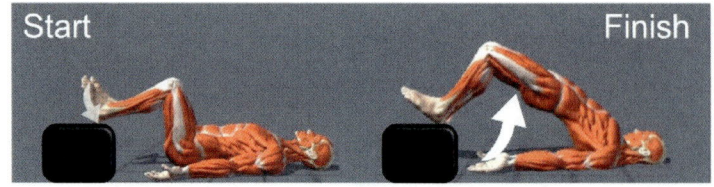

Lay on your back with the back of your heels on a sturdy elevated surface like a weight bench. Drive your heels down and slightly back to put tension into your calves, hamstrings, and glutes. Continue to press until your hips are fully extended. Pause at the top and lower your tailbone back to the floor while controlling the tension in the back of your legs.

Doing hip extensions with your feet on suspension straps is a great test to see if you push too much into your feet. You'll instantly know this if your knee straightens a bit as you lift your hips.

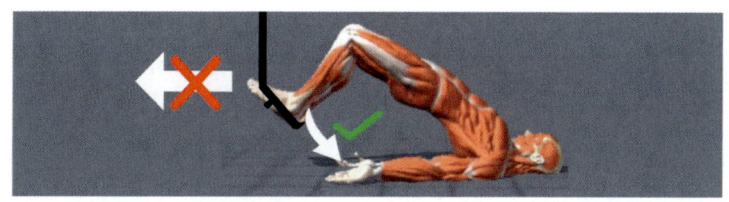

Be sure to pull into your heels when extending your hips. This will bring more resistance to your hamstrings and glutes while easing stress on your lower back.

One of my favorite hip hinge variations is to do them while a partner holds your feet up while placing their hands on the back of your heels. This position allows your partner to feel how you're using tension through each rep. They'll know if you're pushing, pulling or even rotating your feet by how your heels press into their hands.

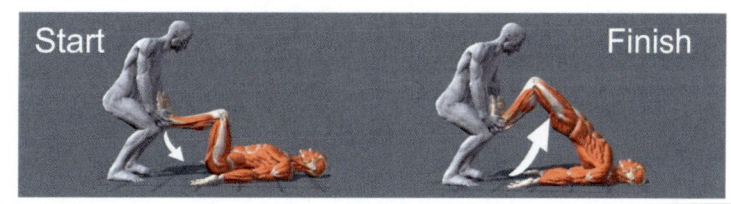

Start by laying on the floor while your partner assumes a half squat while holding the back of your heels. Make sure your partner is ready and places tension along their own extension chain so they can support your weight. Press your heels into their hands while lifting your hips up off the ground. Pause at the top and return your hips back to the floor in a controlled motion. Afterward, discuss how you were applying tension and force into their hands and explore changes you can make.

Accessory Moves For Extension Chain

Hamstring curls

You can do this exercise on a set of suspension straps or an exercise ball. They just may be one of the best hamstring exercises because they use your hamstrings for both hip extension and knee flexion.

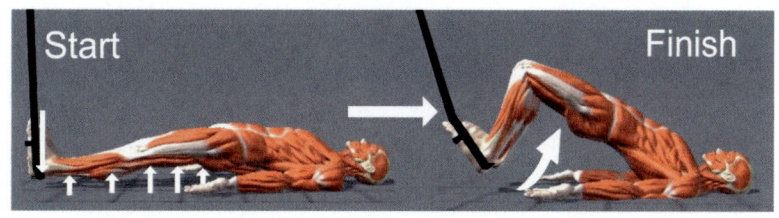

Lay on your back with your heels in a suspension trainer about 3-4 inches off the floor. Drive into your heels to elevate your body above the floor except for your shoulders, arms, and head. Begin the rep by flexing your knees to pull your heels toward your butt while elevating your hips. Pause at the top and extend your knees while lowering your hips within a couple of inches off the floor.

You can progress these hamstring curls the same ways you can progress any other bridge work. The first is to work on how high you lift your hips as you flex your knees. The higher you lift your hips at the top of each rep the harder your hamstrings will work.

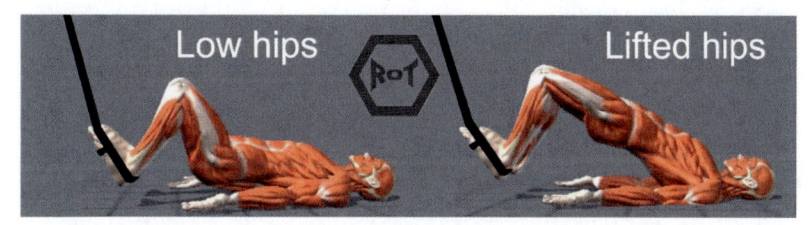

Your hips are the weight you lift when doing bridges and hamstring curls. Pulling your feet closer to your butt without lifting your hips creates less resistance while lifting your hips as you pull in creates more.

You can use the centerline element by pressing your feet together. Holding a pillow or yoga block between your knees help force more tension into your inner thigh hamstrings.

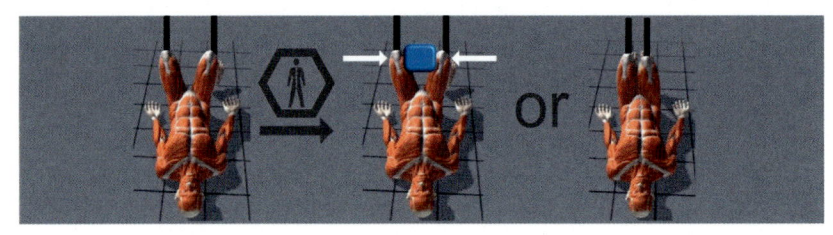

You can also progress your hamstring curls through the centerline element by placing an object, like a yoga block, between your knees or moving both your knees and feet closer together.

You can shift weight onto one leg by crossing your legs with the bottom foot in the strap. It's easier to pull with your feet crossed at the ankle, and more difficult crossed at the shin and knee.

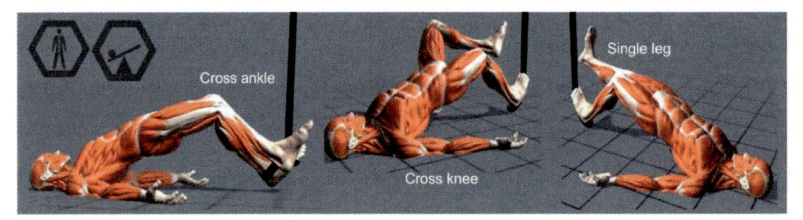

You can progress hamstring curls just like with all hip extension bridges with crossing the ankles, crossing at the knee and finally progressing to single leg curls. Be sure to keep the working foot and knee close to your centerline so they don't wing out to the side.

Lastly, you can use the weight shifting element by holding your hands on your hips instead of on the floor. This technique adds weight to your hips as you lift them up while removing the assistance your arms provided by pushing into the floor. You can also hold a weight on your hips to increase the weight you lift.

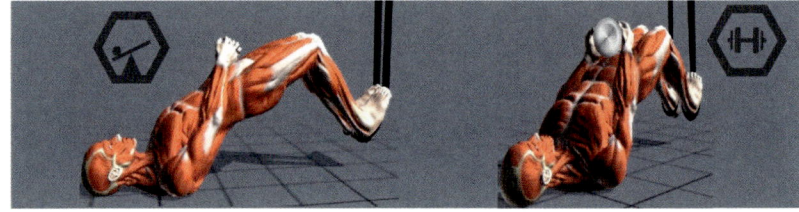

Placing your hands on your hips uses the weight shifting element to remove the support of your arms and places their weight on the part of your body which you lift against gravity. You can also add weight to all hip extension bridges by holding a weight on your hips.

Points To Ponder

There's almost an infinite number of things to consider while doing even the most basic exercises. That's why I'm including this section at the end of each chain chapter as a resource for things you may want to think about while doing your exercises to improve your workout. I certainly don't expect you to try and apply all of these points in a single session. Just pick one or two and work on them for a few weeks until you do them automatically. Then, you can move onto a couple of other points.

Use this list as a source of ideas on what you can work on if you feel stuck with a given technique. You can also refer back to this list to remind yourself of any points you may have forgotten about.

1. Pay attention to weight distribution between your toes and heel while doing bridges with flat feet. Notice how pressing into the floor with your toes or heel can influence the tension in the back of your legs.

2. Look for knee movement while moving up or down with each rep. If your knees are tracking inward work to press them outward and vice versa.
3. Be sure to breathe smoothly at the top of each rep and not hold your breath.
4. Notice if the tension in your hamstrings or glutes fades toward the bottom of each rep and try to maintain tension throughout the full range of motion.
5. Watch your shoulder movement during each rep. Experiment with allowing your shoulders to hunch forward at the bottom of each rep while pulling them back at the top. You can also try to keep your shoulders back and locked in place during each rep as well.
6. Work on hand position especially during hip dominant bridges. Notice how the exercise feels different depending on where you point your fingers either forward, back or to the side.
7. Cramping hamstrings is often a sign that your glutes are not engaged enough to help with hip extension.
8. Low back stress is a sign that your glutes and abs are holding enough tension to maintain a neural pelvis without any anterior or posterior tilt.
9. Imagine pulling your shoulder blades together as you lift up to provide support for the upper back. This includes keeping the upper traps tense as if you're shrugging up your shoulders.
10. Be mindful of the tension in your calves as that can be a common link in the extension chain that doesn't get engaged enough.
11. If you're struggling to do many reps of a particular exercise try, for a few weeks, holding the top position as an isometric exercise. You can also reduce the range of motion and do half reps until your muscles get used to the motion.
12. Don't force yourself into position. Doing so might cause a strain on the back or pull a muscle that's not quite ready to move that much. Instead, work on gradually increasing the range you can control in small increments.

Chapter 8 Squat Chain

Your squat chain contains every muscle in your lower body, and it may be one of the most important muscle chains to train for the following reasons.

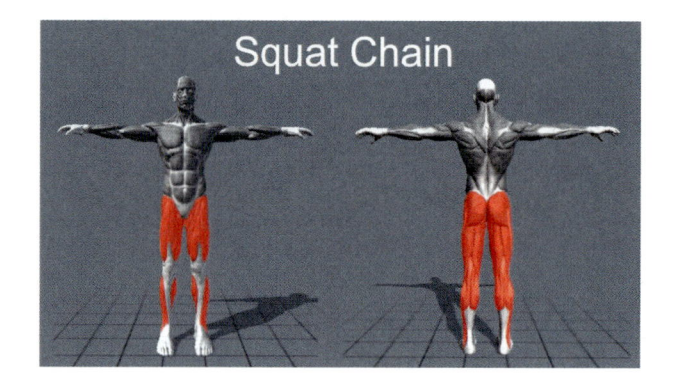

#1 Strong legs improve performance in just about everything

I can't think of many activities that don't require strong legs. Even seemingly upper body dominant exercises like punching or throwing require powerful legs to drive force into the ground. Just try hitting a punching bag on your knees or throwing a football while sitting in a chair. It won't matter how strong your upper body is, you won't have much power when your legs are out of the picture.

It's not just the shear strength that your legs provide. It's also the variety of ways they can perform. Your legs are designed to work for both endurance and strength. You can use them for graceful balancing movements one minute and explosive power the next. Progressive calisthenics exercises develop not only every muscle in your legs but also a wide spectrum of physical ability. Yes, you will build strength, but you also develop stability, power, balance, and flexibility as well.

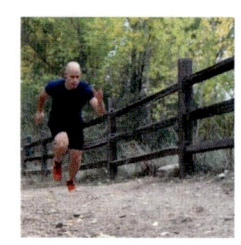

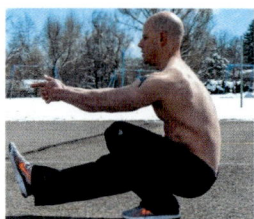

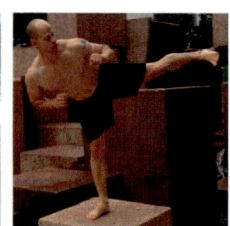

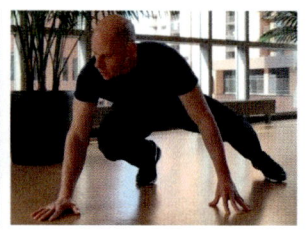

Your legs are capable of a wide range of performance. It only makes sense to train them accordingly.

#2 Muscular legs look great

Strong legs improve your appearance in the same subliminal way a strong extension chain does. It's not an area of the body that people usually show off, but the shape and use of your legs tell everyone you're strong and can handle yourself. Big legs also keep you from falling victim to the idea that you're working out just for vanity reasons. There's a reason why people make fun of guys who skip leg day.

On the other side, strong legs command respect. Before I was into strength training, I had built my legs up through cycling and skiing. My lower body development even impressed a former Mr. America winner who would ask for my advice on calf training.

#3 Strong legs help you burn fat

Strong legs are your secret weapon in the war on fat. When your legs are strong, you can torch calories faster while exercising for longer periods of time at higher levels of intensity. Not only will you be working longer and harder, but you'll also burn fat with less effort compared to someone doing the same activity with weaker legs.

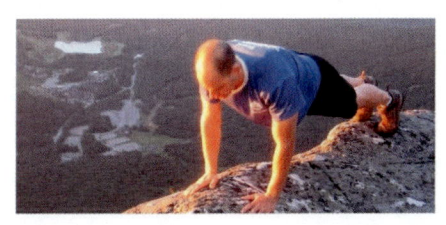

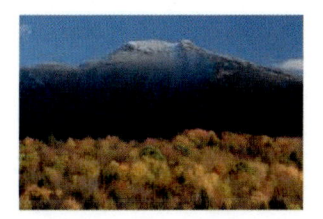

The old photo on the left was taken of me at dawn on the peak of the tallest mountain in Vermont, Mt. Mansfield. Its peak is 4,393 feet above sea level so it's not exactly Everest but it will help you burn loads of calories provided your legs are strong and resilient.

Strong legs are also crucial in helping you maintain a high energy level. If you're on your feet at work, you'll be tired and unmotivated to train at the end of the workday. If you have strong legs, you'll have no problem working overtime and still have plenty of energy left over for a workout.

#4 Many aches and pains come from deconditioned legs

Weak legs are the plague of modern life. Many issues ranging from back pain to poor balance, originate from weakness in the lower body. Chances are, no matter what your goals are, or what issues you're facing, strengthening your lower body will make a substantial improvement.

Why Do Bodyweight Leg Exercises Usually Suck?

A lot of people are skeptical about building strong legs with bodyweight training. Even a lot of calisthenics enthusiasts head for the leg press and squat rack on leg day.

When I got into bodyweight training, I figured I might maintain my current level of leg strength at best. You can imagine my surprise when after a few months of just calisthenics training, my legs improved more than any other area of my body. It confused me at first, but I learned my newfound leg strength had less to do with my workout and more to do with my office chair.

The cast of sitting

It's no secret that people are sitting an awful lot these days. We sit at home, at work, and in the car when we go between the two. We sit when we have fun, and when we socialize. Some people even sit more than they sleep.

All of this sitting locks your lower body into right angle compliance. It causes your ankles, knees, and hips to hold a right angle position and maintains that position for extended periods of time.

The chair you're sitting in also supports you in that seated posture. When a structure is supporting your body, you don't have to create muscle tension to hold yourself in place. Over time, your neural code becomes deconditioned which causes all sorts of problems from stiffness to fragmented tension patterns.

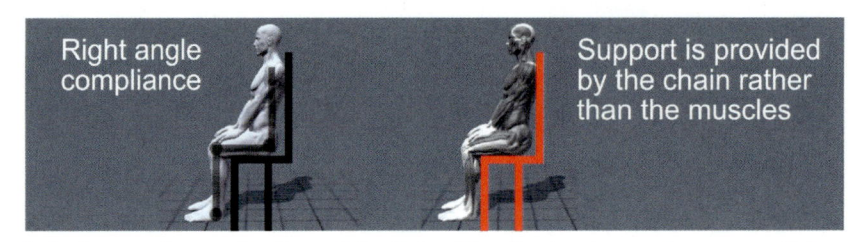

Sitting in a chair causes the body to conform to the shape of the chair while allowing the muscles to turn off due to the external support.

This same type of deconditioning happens when you suffer an injury and have to immobilize a part of your body. If you've ever had to suffer through wearing a cast you know what happens when the cast comes off. You find the limb is stiff and the associated muscles are weak. It may even be difficult to use those muscles due to neuromuscular amnesia. Such stiffness and weakness is the natural result of keeping a part of your body immobile for extended periods of time.

Sitting does the same thing to your lower body as a cast on your leg. It doesn't completely restrict your movement and muscle activation, but it does significantly reduce it. The result is the muscles in your lower body become stiff, weak and hard to turn on.

Training to sit stronger

Sitting has not only influenced how people work, travel and play, it's also heavily influenced how they exercise as well. Many modern leg training techniques have succumbed to the influences of sitting which further endorse the adverse effects.

The most prominent examples are the leg machines in a modern gym. Leg presses, hack squats, leg extensions and even calf machines are designed to maintain that right angle compliance.

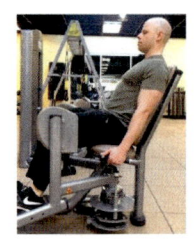

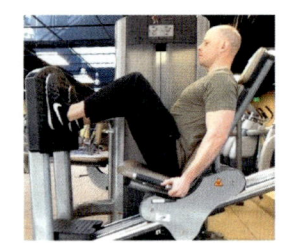

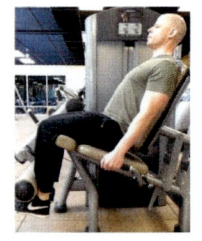

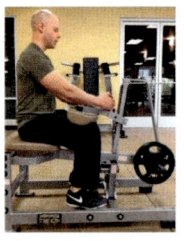

Some lower body weight machines are designed to maintain a seated posture.

It's not just weight machines that have fallen victim to the influence of sitting. Many experts teach athletes to maintain right angle compliance while using free weights. Coaches and trainers tell them to "sit back with the hips" and "don't let the knees go in front of your toes." Even seemingly obvious rules like "keeping your weight on your heels" are all about conforming to the habit of sitting in a chair.

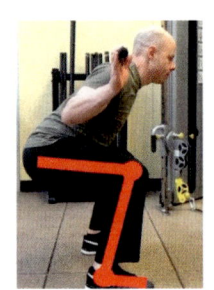

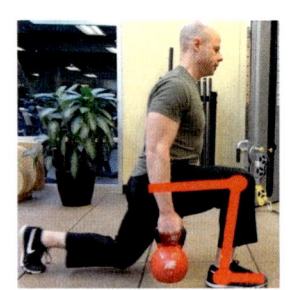

Even natural movements like squatting and lunging have fallen under the influence of right angle compliance.

The rules of right angle compliance are recommended for the sake of safety and performance and for a good reason. It's not safe to tell a patient to take a boxing class right after they have had a cast removed from their arm. Likewise, it's much easier and safer to conform to the influences of sitting than to risk discomfort and injury by doing extreme leg exercises. The result is people are using exercises designed to strengthen the limited capabilities they've adopted through sitting.

One of the biggest advantages of working within right angle compliance is that it creates an easier technique. Sure, folks can move a lot of weight or do a lot of reps, but that's not always a good thing. It doesn't require a lot of strength or effort to do shallow leg work which is why you need a lot of weight to sufficiently challenging your muscles.

That's the biggest reason why most people never get very much from calisthenics leg training. When they start practicing bodyweight leg exercises, they bring the rules and techniques that governed how they use machines and free weights with them. Without the heavy iron, there isn't enough resistance to promote the necessary tension in the muscle, and their results suffer. Even worse, their joints and muscles haven't been conditioned to operate safely outside of those rules so the risk of injury increases. It's no wonder athletes who try bodyweight leg training end up weaker and sometimes injured, so they run back to the leg press while telling everyone it's not possible to build strong legs with calisthenics.

The cure for sitting and right angle compliance

Sitting is a big part of modern life, and it's probably going to remain so far a long time. That's okay because the solution to the adverse effects of sitting isn't to sit less, but to squat more!

Sitting and squatting may look similar, but they quite different in several respects. The biggest difference between sitting and squatting is the range of motion at the ankle, knee, and hip. While sitting is about keeping the joints at a right angle, squatting is about maximizing your range of tension at all three joints.

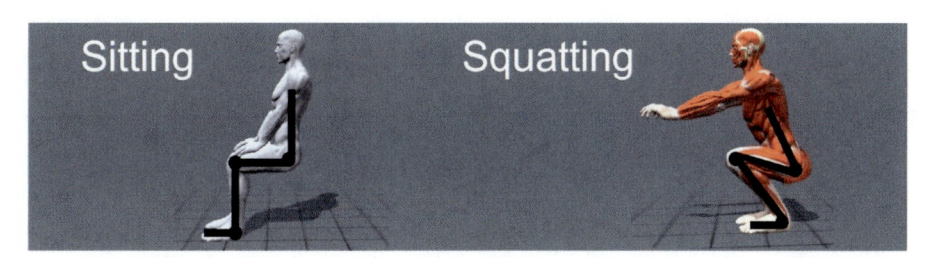

Squatting uses a greater range of motion at the hip, knee, and ankle joint compared to sitting.

Using a greater range in a squat frees you from the restriction of right angle compliance. It helps "lube" your joints improves range of tension in the muscles and requires more muscle strength.

The other notable difference in squatting over sitting is the synergistic use of muscle tension. Sitting exercises use a weight or an external support to prevent you from falling over backward.
When you squat, you use the tension in your muscles to hold you up just as nature intended. The muscles in your shin and the top of your feet pull your knee forward. Your lower hamstrings flex your knee, so your hamstrings press into your calf. Third, your hips pull your torso forward into the top of your thigh. This muscle activation is why a good squat involves not only triple extension but also triple flexion as well.

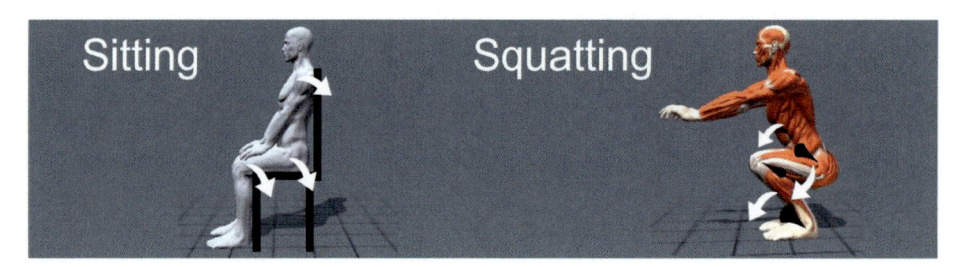

Sitting causes the front of your body to turn off as your weight "falls" into the chair. A deep squat involves triple flexion where you flex your hips to pull your torso closer to your thigh, your knees to pull your hamstrings closer to your calves, and you flex your ankles to pull your knees over your toes.

The use of both triple flexion and extension is what makes squatting safe and effective. The only challenge is learning how to make this happen when you've been sitting and exercising with right angle compliance for many years. Trying to jump into aggressive squat training can be very difficult, and even unsafe for some people. It would be no different than telling someone to start punching a heavy bag right after they had a cast removed from their arm. That's why I recommend the following exercises.

Turning On Your Squat Chain

First off, it's important to be able to place tension on your squat chain proactively. You can do this in both standing and squatting positions.

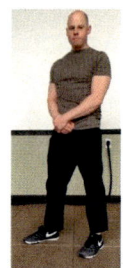

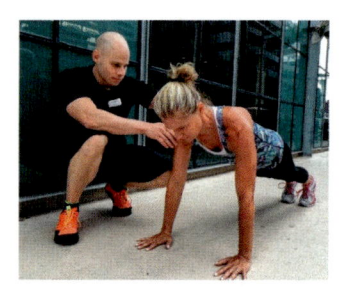

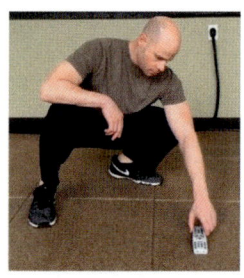

It's easy to practice tension control in the squat chain since we use our legs every day. I practice the squatting motion when I need to get low to train clients or pick things up from the floor. I even practice tensing my squat chain and it's individual muscle while just standing in place.

The key is to try and apply tension throughout every muscle in your lower body. Don't just tense up your quads or your glutes. Include smaller muscles like the front and side of your hips, your hamstrings, calves, and even your feet. Imagine slipping on a pair of nylon stockings. Everywhere those stockings cover is an area you should feel some tension. It's also good to practice applying tension on one leg at a time. Shifting your weight on one leg at a time cuts the neural workload in half, so your mind doesn't have to engage as much muscle. It also makes it easier to detect discrepancies from one leg to the other.

Shifting from sitting to a squat position

Another handy exercise is to practice shifting from a sitting position into a squat position. This can help your mind understand how to pull into the squatting position. It's also a simple form of practice you can apply many times as a matter of habit throughout the day.

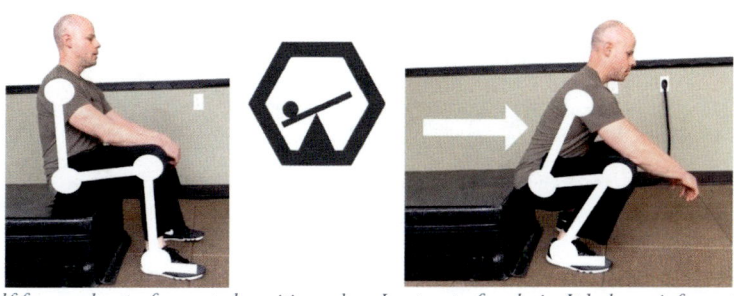

I make a habit of pulling myself forward out of a seated position when I get out of a chair. It helps reinforce the pulling motion used in a squat even if I only pass through a half squatted position for a split second.

You can also do this with lunges since the back leg can support your hips. Lower yourself down with your weight equally between the front and back leg. Then pull your weight forward with your front leg. Hold for 5-10 seconds and then shift your weight back so you're balanced between both legs. From there, you can repeat for another rep on that side or switch legs.

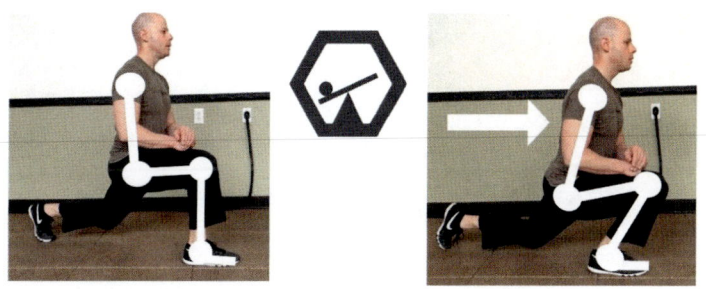

Lunges are essentially single leg squats with back leg assistance. Shifting your weight from your back leg to the front builds the strength, stability, and mobility you want for strong, capable legs.

Shifting from a sitting position into a squat is a helpful warm-up for your squat workout. Be sure to pay attention to how you're creating tension in your muscles and look for areas when you lack tension. You don't need a lot of tension in the whole lower body, and it doesn't need to be evenly spread out over all of the muscles. You're just trying to keep some tension throughout the lower body without any gaps.

Squat Chain Exercises

Working your squat chain is simple; you just squat and then stand back up again. The key is understanding how to do this progressively so you can start at your own level and grow from there.

Upper body assistance squats

I always recommend folks start with an assisted style of squats to develop the mobility and stability they will need later on. You can use your upper body to assist with squatting exercises by grabbing onto a sturdy supportive object. Upper body support squats are a great warm-up exercise, or they can be used to work on tension control in a supportive setting.

You can practice these by grabbing onto a pole or countertop with your arms bent. As you squat down, your arms will straighten while pulling slightly to keep yourself upright. You can also use a set of suspension straps or a partner for assistance.

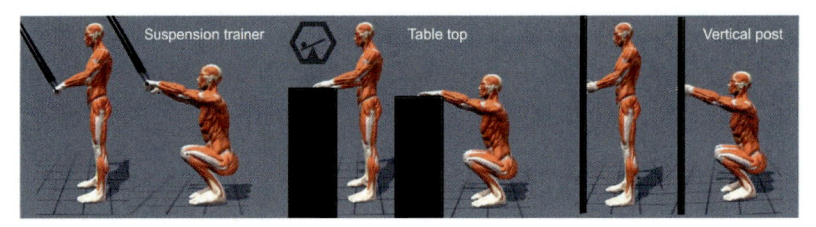

Holding onto something while squatting uses the weight shifting element to transfer some of your bodyweight into your arms. This allows you to work on improving the tension control and range of motion in your squat chain. It also gives you additional stability so you can confidently work on driving your knees forward as you bring your hips closer to the back of your heels.

Upper body assist squats help you to break out of the habit of sitting by allowing you to progressively squat deeper with ease and confidence. You may need to rely on your upper body a lot to hold you up at first, but you won't need to pull as much as you improve the pulling strength and range of tension in your lower body. Suspension straps are a good tool to use because they can sag slightly as you improve your ability to pull into your squat.

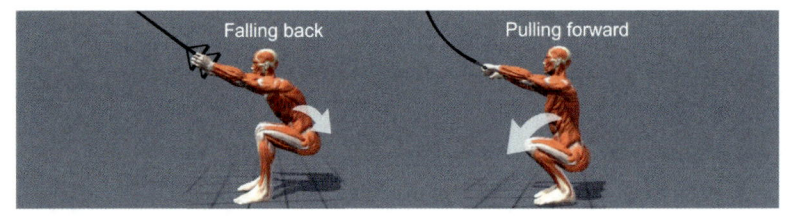

Suspension straps can sag as you improve your ability to pull yourself into a squat with your hip flexors, hamstrings and shin muscles.

Lower body assistance squats

You can also adjust the difficulty by providing support to your lower body. The most common of these are box squats where you lower your hips onto a ledge. This technique modifies your range of tension while providing stability at the bottom of each rep. The lower the box is, the more difficult the exercise becomes. You can also make each rep easier by "sitting" on the box and allowing your weight to transfer into your hips just like when you sit in a chair. You can make it a little more difficult by only allowing your hips to "kiss" the surface of the box before standing back up.

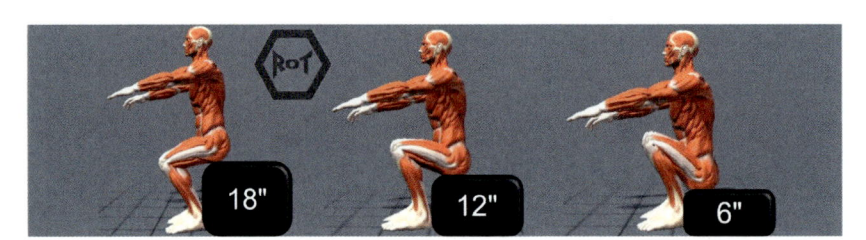

Box squats give you a dedicated range of motion to ensure you're squatting at the same depth every rep. They also "catch" you if your muscle tension can't hold you up.

The other version of lower body assistance is to stand on a weight plate or an incline. Doing this requires a little less flexion at your ankle since gravity is slightly pulling you forward. This makes it easier to gain more range of tension at your knee and hip joint. The more you elevate your heel the easier the exercise is while lowering your heel will make it more difficult.

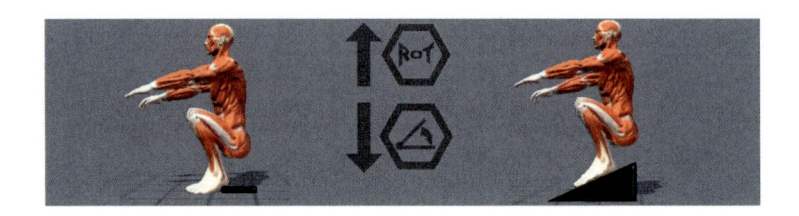

Elevating your heel changes your lower leg's relationship to gravity. The higher your heel raises the more gravity pulls you forward.

Stance width

It's easy to use the centerline element to adjust the difficulty of your squats. A wider stance provides a broader base of support while a narrow stance tends to be more difficult.

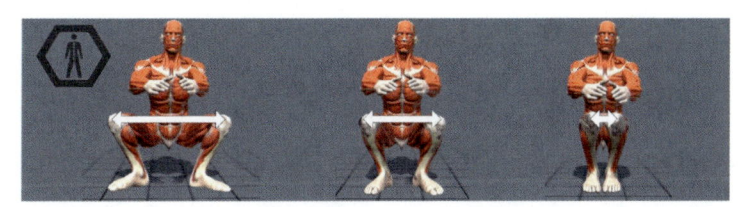

In general, the centerline element will make your squats more difficult when you place your knees and feet closer together. The narrower you squat the more mobility and pulling strength you will need. Wide squats are also a great mobility exercise for the muscles in the inside of the leg.

Close or narrow squats are a great exercise to build the stability and control you need for more advanced squat exercises. I highly recommend working up to being able to do them by gradually narrowing your stance until your feet are touching or about 1 inch apart.

Be sure to pay attention to the direction your knee position with various stance widths. Your thighs should point more outward the wider your stance gets so allow your feet to do the same. This adjustment can help alleviate stress on the knees and allow you to sink deeper into the squat.

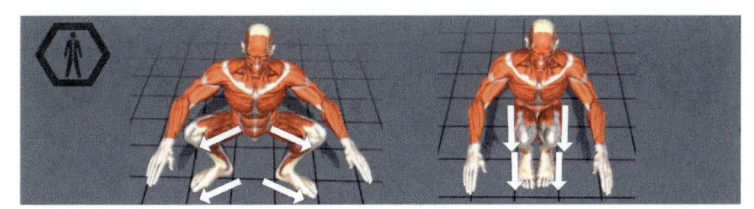

Your thighs naturally point outward the wider you squat so allow your feet to do likewise. Bring both feet and thighs inward when your squat becomes more narrow.

Shifting squats

Shifting squats employ the weight shifting element by moving your weight around while in a squat position. You can do this many ways but the most common is to shift your weight side to side as you load one leg and then the other.

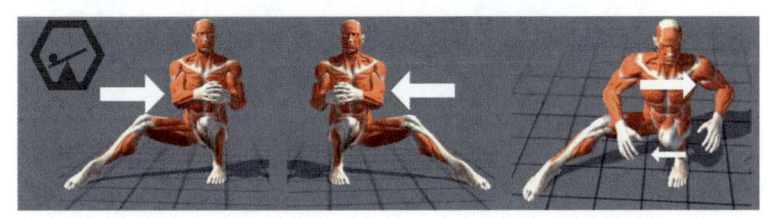

Shifting squats load more weight onto one leg at a time. The wider your stance, the further you shift your weight. Making your stance narrower won't use as much shift and the exercise will be easier. Be sure to pull your knee onto your centerline as you shift. This will keep your balanced and reduce strain on your knee.

Shifting squats will help you build a strong "foundation of strength" so you're stable in a variety of positions. Shifting also loosens tight muscles and improves tension control. Be sure not to allow yourself to relax into the bottom of a squat. Keep your muscles at least a little tense to prevent stress from flowing into your joints.

You can do shifting squats with upper or lower body assistance as well like when you hold onto a suspension trainer. Play around with these for a warm up to your squat routine or when loosening up after sitting for a while. Just be sure to move in smooth and controlled motions. Avoid quick bouncing movements that can potentially strain a muscle.

Split squats and lunges

Split squats and lunges can be a functional and challenging exercise. They help weed out imbalances between your two legs as well as improve balance and hip control.

Start by standing with one leg in front of the other about a shoulder width and a half in length. Be sure your weight is 50/50 between your two feet. From there, bend your back knee and squat down onto your front leg. Pause at the bottom and stand back up without moving your feet.

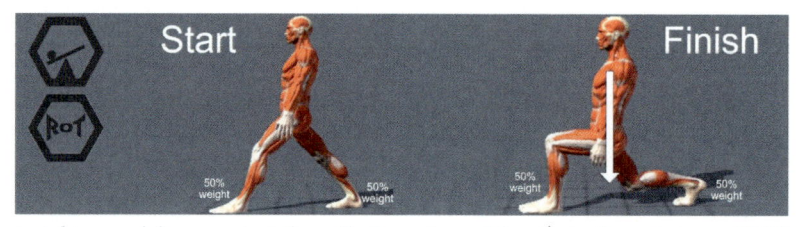

Split squats move the body straight up and down against the pull of gravity and they typically maintain a 50/50 distribution of weight between both legs. They are a good way to start learning how to control your weight distribution and range of tension with one leg in front of the other. As with squats, the resistance on the muscles increases the lower you squat. Just be sure to gently "kiss" your knee to the floor if you go that low.

Pay attention to the length and width of your stance. A longer stance may challenge your mobility and strength a bit more while a narrower stance will progress your balance and stability. Start off with a stance length and width that feels comfortable for you.

Progression can be made through the weight shift and range of tension elements by shifting more of your weight onto your front foot. Doing this makes the exercise a bit more like a single leg squat with the back leg being used as assistance. Be sure to "pull" into your heel by keeping your glutes and hamstrings engaged to prevent stress on your front knee.

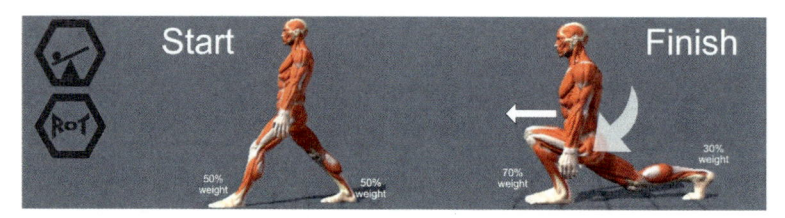

Shifting split squats place more weight on the front leg as you squat down. You can do this by either shifting your weight forward as you squat down, or you can keep a 50/50 weight distribution until you're at the bottom and then shift forward in the bottom position.

You can also shift more weight to your front foot by elevating your back leg. Be sure not to place your front leg too far forward, so you don't push too much weight on your back leg.

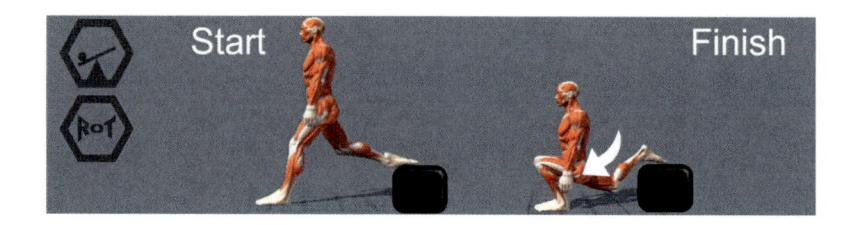

Elevating your back leg makes your front leg work harder by increasing the range of tension and shifting more weight onto it. The higher your supporting foot is the more range and weight will shift to your front leg.

Lunges

Lunges are a little more difficult from split squats because you need to control the momentum of your bodyweight while stepping. They are still very much a form of squat because one leg is doing a squat while the other is providing support and balance.

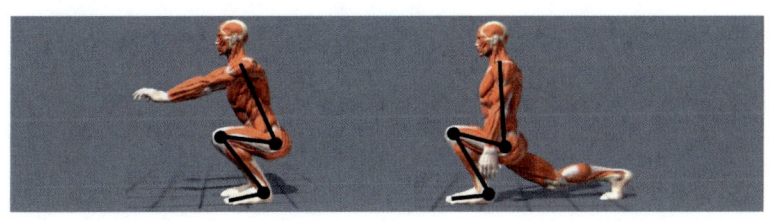

Lunges are essentially single leg squats with back leg assistance. They both use your squat chain in almost identical ways so the difference between the two should be minimal over time.

I recommend starting out with spot lunges. These involve stepping out from a standing position into a lunge, pausing for a second and then returning to the same standing position you started in. You can do these forwards, backward or to the side.

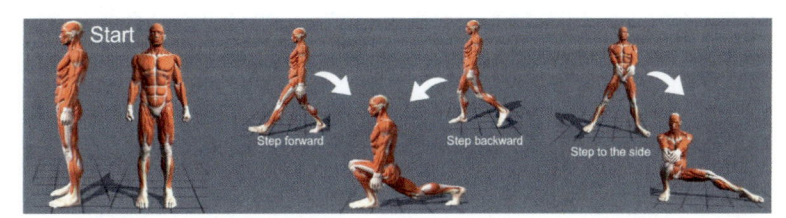

There are as many lunges as there are points on a compass. Forward, back and side tend to be the most popular but feel free to play with moving at diagonal directions as well. Just remember to treat each step like a squat on the dominant working leg.

Backward lunges are a good technique to start with because most of your movement is straight down into a squat while your support leg reaches back. You won't have to deal with a lot of forward or lateral momentum with each step.

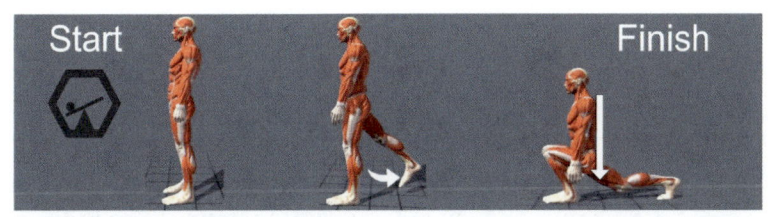

Back spot lunges involve stepping back with one leg while maintaining most of your weight on the front leg. This helps minimize backward momentum and makes the front leg "squat" more into the lunge position.

I also like back spot lunges because they don't take up a lot of room and they teach you how to pull yourself up and forward with the glutes and hamstrings of the front foot.

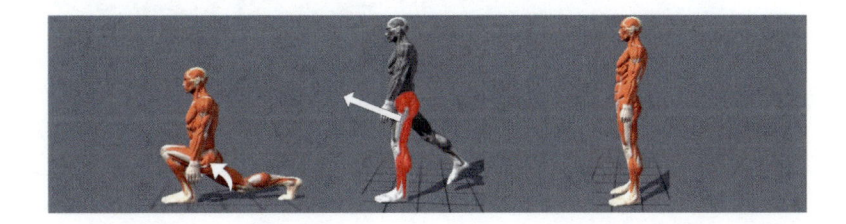

87

Back lunges are a great way to teach you how to pull yourself forward with the glutes and hamstrings of your front leg rather than pushing off of the back foot or leaning forward too much. Not only will learning how to pull save stress on your knees but it improves performance for activities like running.

Front lunges are the next order of business as you step forward onto your front leg while the back leg offers support. Some people have trouble with this technique as they tend to "fall" into each step with forward momentum. This excess forward energy can cause stress on the front of the knees.

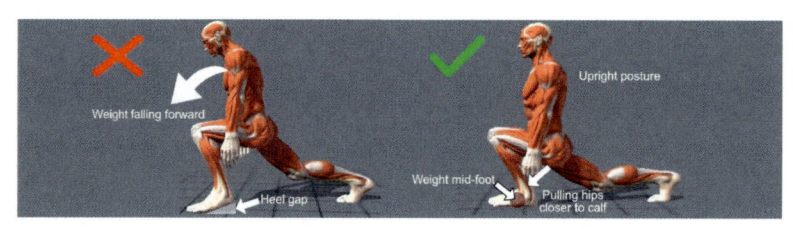

Even though you're lunging forward, you don't want your weight to fall forward and onto the ball of your foot. Instead, take a step forward and then pull your weight onto your front foot.

Instead of falling into each step, start by placing your foot forward and then pull your weight forward and down through triple flexion. Lunging this way will maintain the tension in your hips and other flexing muscles which improve balance and control.

Side lunges are a great tool to test the flexibility in your ankle and hip. Since the support leg is out to the side, the muscles in your squatting leg need to work very hard to pull your hips forward so you don't fall over backward.

You can do side lunges either as a squatting motion where you step out with your assistance leg and "squat" down or as a stepping lunge where you step to the side and squat down onto that leg.

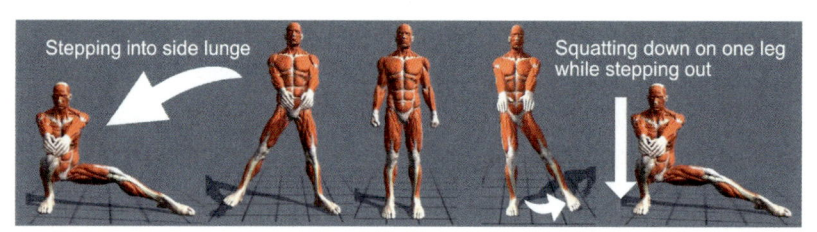

Side lunges require a lot of mobility and strength. The further you step the harder the exercise will be since there is more weight on one leg.

Walking lunges

Performing lunges in a walking motion is an excellent way to condition your legs for strength, flexibility, balance, and endurance. They are also a nice break from the traditional rep counting style workouts since you usually do them for distance. You can do walking lunges backward and to the side but forward walking lunges are the most common. I also prefer forward walking lunges because they have a lot of functional carryover to stepping activities like walking and running.

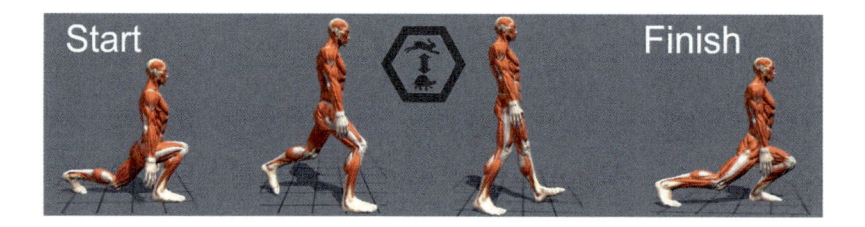

Walking lunges use the speed element to string multiple reps together while creating more momentum which you need more strength and stability to control. Remember to pull yourself forward with your front leg rather than push off of your back leg to optimize the tension in the hamstrings and glutes.

The two most popular walking lunges are stop lunges and step through lunges. Stop lunges use a pause at the top of each step with your weight equally distributed between your two feet. This stop makes it easier to balance and give the muscles a bit of rest. Step through lunges do not involve this stop at the top, and your back foot passes right by your stationary foot as you step forward into your next rep.

Both types of walking lunges are a great opportunity to learn how to use the tension in your glutes and hamstrings to both pull yourself forward as well as using the same muscles to absorb force when you step forward. Learning how to do this will do wonders for easing stress off of your knees and lower back while hiking and running.

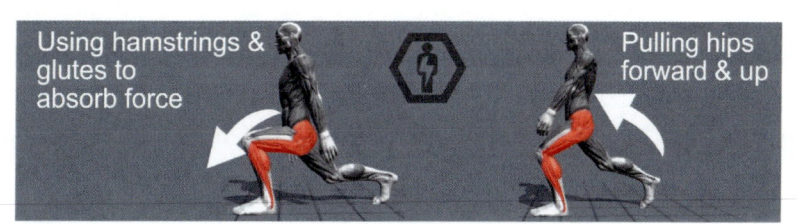

The muscles on the back of the leg play an important role in both propelling your body forward as well as absorbing force with each step. Lunges are a great way to learn how to use tension in this way since they are basically an exaggerated step.

A word on stance width

You can vary the width of your lunge stance to adjust the difficulty with the centerline element. A wide stance is easier while a narrow stance is more difficult. Note that narrow lunges involve placing your foot and knee closer to your centerline, so this will require angling the thigh of your front leg slightly inward.

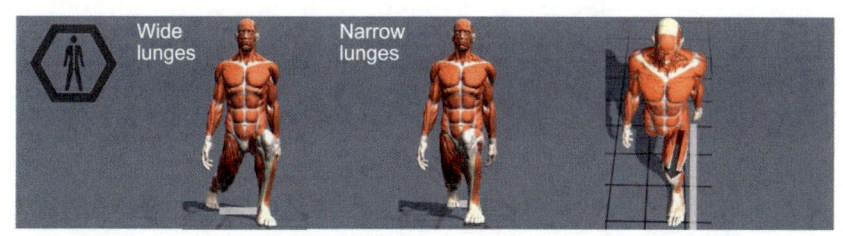

Your stance width uses the centerline element to challenge your range of motion, stability, and strength. As always, the more narrow you work the more challenging the exercise will be. The image on the right demonstrates the slight inward angle your thigh makes while using a narrow stance.

If you use a wider stance, I recommend using an outcurve step. This move involves sweeping your stepping leg in closer to your support leg as you stand up and then back out as you step forward.

This curving step is a slight motion, but it helps maintain balance during the transition from one lunge to the next. It also keeps you in control, so you don't fall forward into the next step.

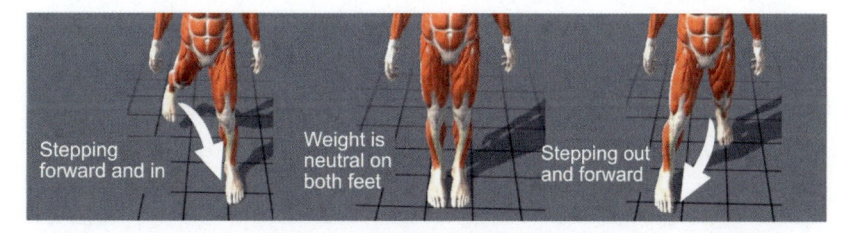

Outcurve stepping can help you maintain stability when doing wide lunges.

As I mentioned before, you'll gain more from your lunges if you pull yourself forward with your front leg instead of pushing off of the back leg. Doing this requires a lot more work from the front leg, especially the upper hamstrings and glutes. Instep lunges are a great way to learn how to pull yourself forward since you can't push off your back foot.

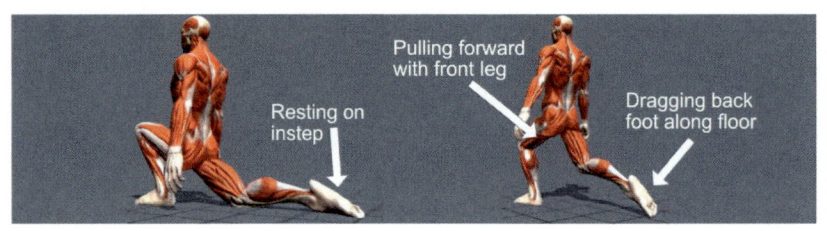

Instep lunges remove the mechanical advantage of pushing off your back foot. This forces you to pull more with your front leg to better train your glutes, hamstrings, and calves.

Single leg squats

The single leg squat is one of the most admired exercises in calisthenics, and for good reason. It requires a high level of leg strength and coordination to even attempt squatting down and standing back up on one leg. You can get away with a lack of mobility or coordination on a leg press or even some types of lunges, but single leg squats will expose every lower body weakness you have. It's for this very reason many people don't practice them very much and claim they are somehow unnatural or unsafe. So be sure to check your ego at the door when practicing them.

I do recommend becoming proficient with closed stance squats and narrow lunges before venturing into single leg squats. Those exercises require you to use your legs close to your center line which develops the strength and mobility you need to do pistol squats.

The first thing to know about squatting down on one leg is to be mindful of where you place your foot, knee and hip when squatting on one leg. You'll need to keep both your foot and knee close to your centerline which requires your thigh to point inward slightly. You'll also find it's important to shift your hips to the side so your squatting foot is on your centerline. Failing to adhere to these tips will result is the risky, yet funny looking "splat effect" where your limbs flail outward.

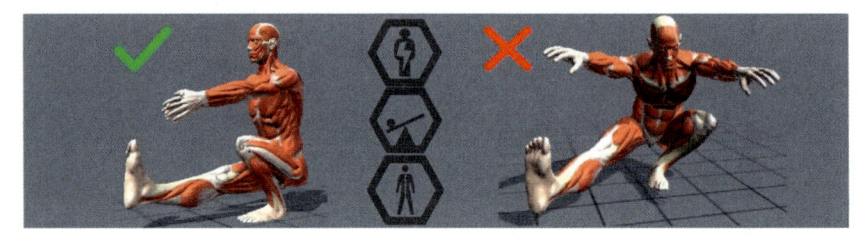

A strong single leg squat is all about control. Most of the points involve pulling your limbs in close to your centerline. This includes pulling your legs together and keeping your hands touching or at least close together. Beware the tendency to let the knee of your squatting leg point out to the side which creates a lot of torque on the knee especially as your other leg and arms flail about in an effort to gain control. This flailing can also be hard on your lower back as your torso reaches forward while twisting around.

Single leg squats are one of those classic calisthenics exercises that a lot of people can do, but few put in the time and effort to become truly proficient in. It's also common for ego-driven guys (like myself) to rush into single leg squats and fall into the habit of doing a single leg squat increasing the risk of injury and poor results. That's why I highly recommend using the following exercises to gradually build the stability and mobility you'll need to really master the single leg squat.

Upper body assisted single leg squats

You can use your upper body to handle some of the resistance and control of a single leg squat. By doing this, you can employ a number of progressive elements like weight shifting, centerline and lever length to vary the workload of the working leg. There are many ways you can use your upper body for assistance, but here are some of the most common.

Horizontal bar assist

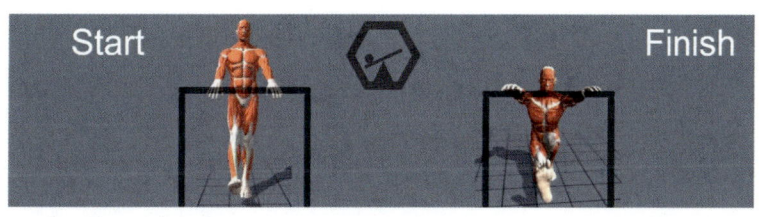

Practicing single leg squats on a fixed bar or handle uses your upper body to assist your squatting leg.

The smith machine at your local gym is perfect for this but you can also use playground bars and countertops. Just be sure whatever you're grabbing onto is very sturdy and is not going to move around on you.

Horizontal bar assists allow you to use your arms to pull you into the squat as well as pull you back up to a standing position. They can be progressed with the centerline elements by placing your hands closer together for more difficulty. You can also make the movement harder by changing the height of the bar. The lower the bar goes the less your upper body can assist so your legs work harder.

A third option is to hold onto the bar with just one hand. This makes the move less stable and, you need to compensate by stabilizing with more tension in the working leg.

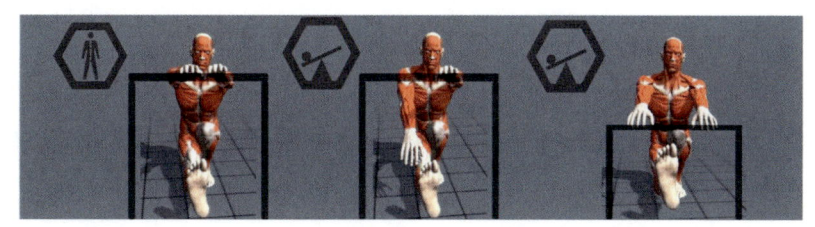

These are just a few ways you can progress horizontal bar assisted squats. You can bring your hands closer together (left), use one hand (center) or lower the bar so you can't put as much weight into your hands (right.)

Pole assist

Using a vertical pole or door frame is a similar option to a horizontal bar but, it's a little less stable. You can start off with two hands on the pole while keeping the pole aligned with your centerline. This should allow the nonworking leg to move just to the side of the post. You can then progress to holding on with one arm.

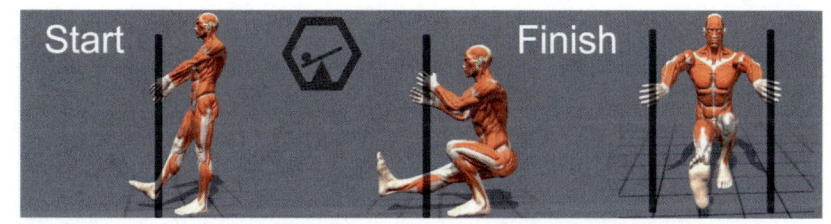

A vertical post is ideal for learning how to do single leg squats. It's easy to progress by adjusting how high you grab the pole or how hard you grab it. Door frame squats (right) are also ideal as the frame provides a sturdy set up upright supports you can grab onto.

This option will test your ability to stabilize and control your body on one leg. It will also expose weaknesses that make your body twist and torque through each rep. Be super vigilant about where you're creating tension in your lower body and look for areas where you're relaxing as you get lower.

One of the best things about post squats is they are easy to adjust. The lower you grab on the post, the more difficult the exercise becomes. Some athletes will allow their hand to slide up and down the post to adjust the difficulty through each rep.

Suspension assist

Suspension assist squats use a suspension trainer or gymnastics rings for support, but they are not as stable as a fixed bar or post. They expose more weak links and imbalances as you move and shift through each rep.

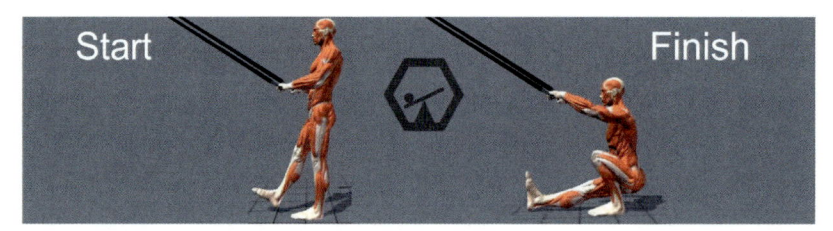

Suspension straps are inherently less stable than a fixed post or bar so you won't be able to put quite as much weight into your hands. Your squatting leg will have to work harder to handle the extra load as well as controlling your position in space. Note the bent arms in the starting position so you don't get pulled forward as you squat down.

Suspension assistance offers a lot of adjustability. The first way is through changing the anchor points in relation to your centerline. The wider your anchor points are the more stable you will be. Moving the anchor points closer together will make the squat more difficult. You can also use the centerline element by moving your hands closer or wider apart as well.

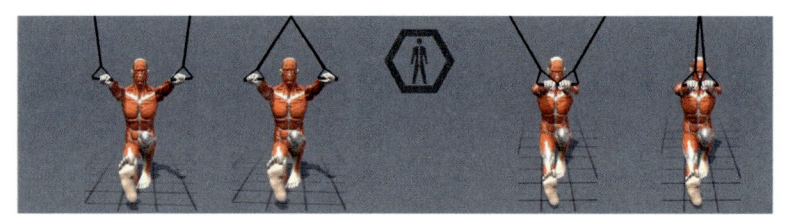

Some examples of how you can use the centerline element with both your arms and the suspension trainer to adjust the support you have for suspension squats.

You can also use the angle to gravity element by leaning yourself back a bit against the trainer. This causes your leg to work a little less against gravity, so you don't have to work quite as hard. Pulling yourself forward with your squatting leg will remove weight on the trainer and place it more on your squatting leg.

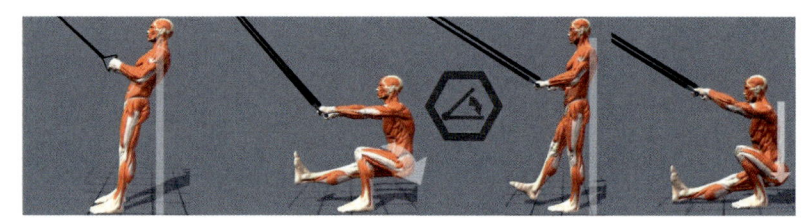

Leaning back slightly is another way you can place more weight in your arms and less on your squatting leg.

Lower body assistance single leg squats

Just like with two leg squats, you can use lower body support to progress and regress single leg squats. Both of these variations require more hip strength to control your body position because you no longer have your upper body to balance yourself.

Box assist

Single leg box squats are one of the most popular single leg variations, and it's the one most people start with when they try squatting without upper body assistance.

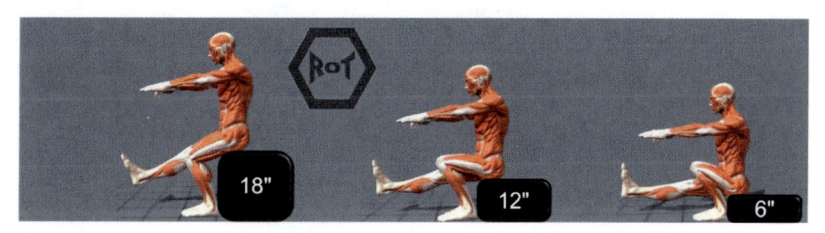

You can progress single leg box squats just as you would two leg squats with lower boxes providing more range and difficulty than higher ones. Again, you can also progress by "kissing" your hips to the box instead of sitting on it and letting your hips rest on it.

Adjusting the intensity is simple. The lower you squat the harder this move is. Another progression you can make is to let your hips "kiss" the seat without putting any weight on them as opposed to sitting and resting for a moment.

Also, be mindful of the tendency to lurch or throw yourself forward when coming out of the bottom position. Use the pulling muscles in your squatting leg to shift your weight forward rather than excessively leaning forward to stand up.

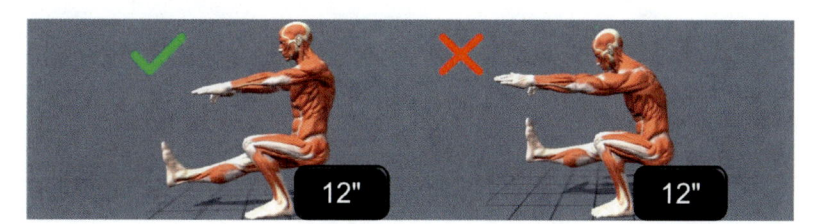

Minimizing the forward lean can go a long way toward improving control and stability in the working hip.

Ball/block assist

This variation uses a block or a medicine ball that you place your hands on at the bottom of the squat. This technique requires a lot of strength and control through most of the range of motion until the most difficult portion at the bottom where your arms can catch you to provide stability and help you get out of the bottom position.

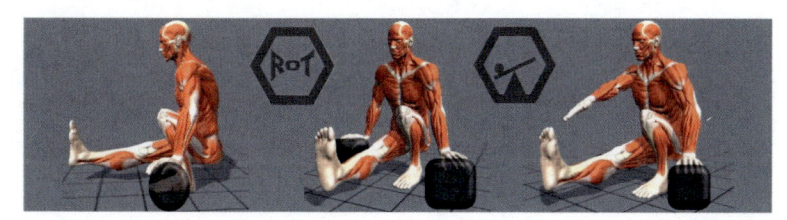

Block assisted squats use a sturdy object to catch you at the bottom of a squat. You can adjust the difficulty by using a smaller object or by placing it more forward or alongside your hips. You can also use just one hand for assistance instead of two.

Elevated assist

One of the biggest challenges with a single leg squat is controlling the front leg and keeping it high enough above the floor. One of the easiest ways around this is to practice on an elevated surface so your front leg can drop down.

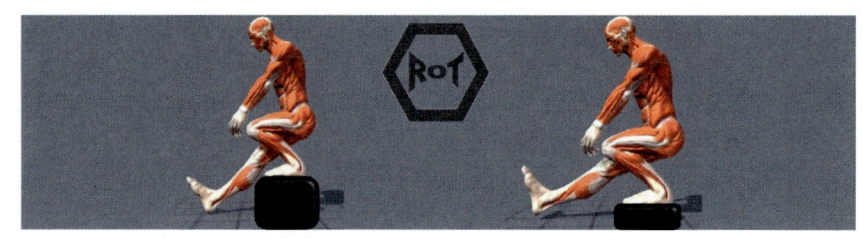

Squatting on an elevated surface allows your non-squatting leg to drop down lower while also not requiring your hips to drop below being parallel to your squatting knee.

Progression of this exercise is similar to the box squat where using a lower ledge is more difficult because you need to pick your leg up higher.

Picking up your non-squatting leg is about more than just hip strength and hamstring flexibility. It's also about hip strength and flexibility of your squatting leg so your hips can drop down low enough to allow the other leg to lift up. You can also do single leg squats on an incline or with an elevated heel to make the exercise easier especially in the bottom position.

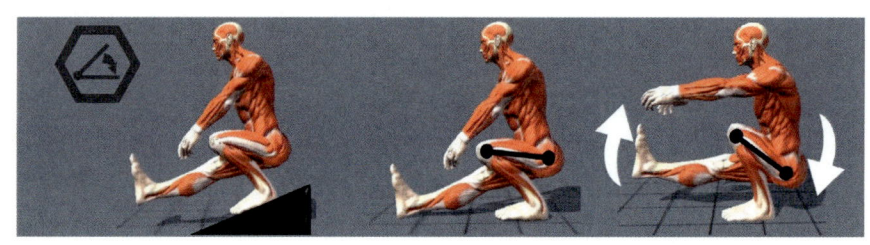

Incline single leg squats assist you the same way they do when doing them with two legs. Squatting your hips lower allows you to pick up your non-squatting leg higher off the floor.

Foot assist

The foot assisted squat uses the non-squatting leg to assist in balance and control. You can place your foot on a rolling object like a ball or a suspension trainer. You can also use towels or slide discs on hard floor surfaces. You'll probably find placing your foot on a lower surface, like a towel, will be easier than a higher position like a suspension trainer.

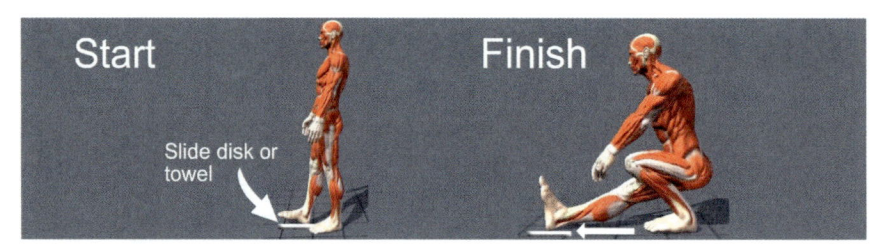

Keeping your non-squatting leg on a sliding towel or disk can provide you some stability by keeping two feet in contact with the floor but it won't help you move much against gravity due to the leverage of a straight leg.

Arm position progressions for single leg squats

You can make single leg squats harder by changing the placement of your arms. One way you can do this is to use the centerline element by clasping your hands together in front of you. This removes some of the stability you gain from your upper body and forces your squatting leg to work harder. Once your hands are together, you can use the weight shifting element to pull them closer to your chest. Really advanced squatters can even place their hands on top of their head or even behind their back.

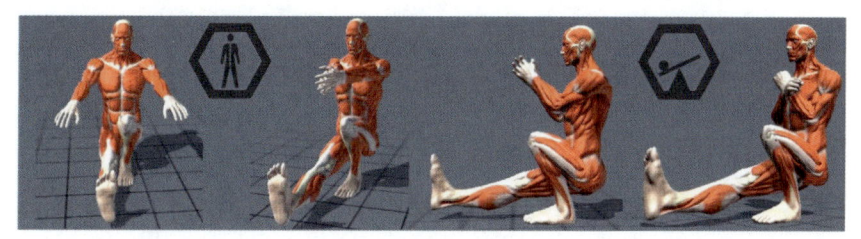

Bringing your hands closer together uses the centerline element to remove stability which makes your squatting leg work harder. Pulling your hands closer to your chest shifts your weight back toward the hip which again makes it more difficult to squat.

Shrimp squats

Shrimp squats are a fun single leg squat where you hold your non-squatting leg behind you instead of sticking it out in front. This makes the squatting legwork super hard because you no longer have the leverage from your front leg to pull you forward. This is why it's common to lean forward a bit and extend your arm in front of you.

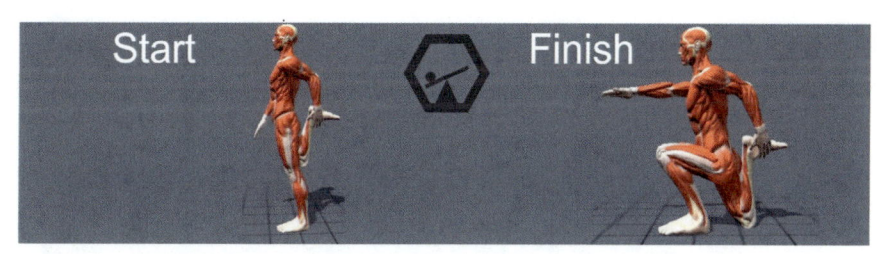

The shrimp squat places your non-squatting leg and one arm behind you. This uses the weight shift element to bring more weight behind you rather than counterbalancing and assisting your squatting leg like in a traditional pistol squat.

A unique aspect of the shrimp squat is how the back leg acts as a range of motion limiter sort of like the box squat. There are a couple of ways around this "limitation" though if you are strong enough to progress beyond it. The most popular is the use of an elevated platform. Standard single leg squats on an elevation don't require as much strength and mobility but the opposite is the case with shrimp squats. These "jumbo shrimp squats" are much more difficult and require more strength and flexibility.

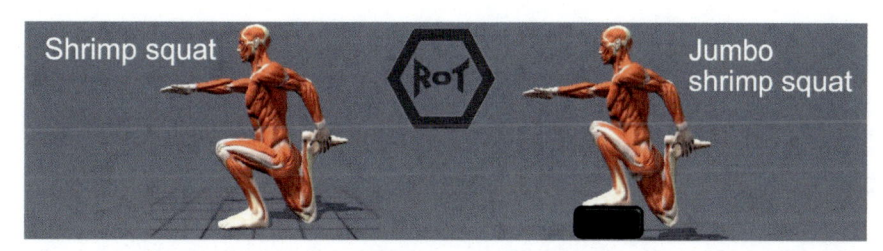

Jumbo shrimp squats use the range of tension element by squatting on an elevated surface so your back knee can drop below the level of your working leg.

Flamingo squats

Another fun variation is what I call the "flamingo squat." This move involves folding your non-squatting leg under you as you squat down. This technique requires a lot of muscle control and strength especially since the tendency is to use the non-squatting leg for assistance even through small movements. Being locked in like this can help you dial in your technique and hip stability which can improve other leg exercises as well.

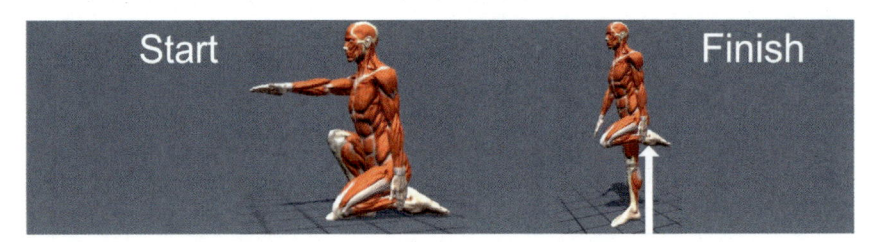

The flamingo squat keeps one leg and arm locked in place so you're forced to squat with a strict technique. It's a good squat diagnostic tool to point out weaknesses.

Keep in mind that you can adjust the difficulty of shrimp and flamingo squats through using the same upper and lower body progressions you use on all other squat variations. Sturdy posts and suspension trainers are particularly helpful for dialing in the tension control for these squats.

Accessory Moves For The Squat Chain

While lunges and squats can work every muscle in your squat chain, some additional exercises can help you focus on a few weak links.

Calf raises

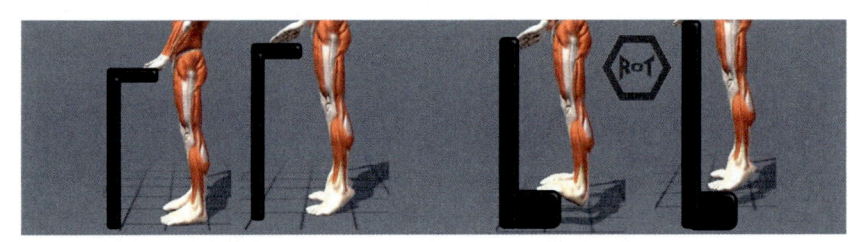

Calf raises are simple, just stand up on the ball of your foot. You can do them flat on the floor or on an elevated surface to increase your range of tension. Upper body support is optional but it does help with stability. Just make sure you don't get in the habit of leaning your weight on your hands.

Calf raises are a great way to beef up those lower legs while adding stability to your ankle and foot. They are simple enough to do, but like all calisthenics, the devil is in the details. Here are a few things to keep in mind when doing the following calf raise variation.

This is still a full leg and hip exercise. Even though you're mostly moving at your ankle joint try to keep your entire squat chain tense. This especially goes for your quads, glutes, and hamstrings.

Keep your knees and hips locked in place. Every movement in any joint other than your ankle will "leak" tension from your calves.

Try not to lean onto a supporting surface like a countertop or chair. Drive as much of your full weight into the balls of your feet. Walls are a good place to put your hands because they offer some support for balance but do not assist in the lift.

Avoid short choppy motions. Keep your movements smooth and relatively slow with about 1 second down, 1-second pause and 1 second up with a 1-second pause at the top.

Calf raises are more about rolling on the ball of the foot rather than clenching your toes. Keep your toes relaxed and press into the ball of your foot to maximize the range of motion and tension.

Be mindful if your feet like to roll slightly outward toward the top of each rep. This is a natural way to make calf raises easier. Keep your feet pointing straight down at the top of each rep.

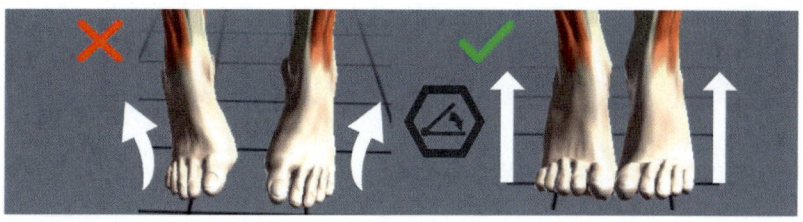

Moving your heels straight up will make your body move more directly against gravity as opposed to letting your feet turn out.

The most basic calf raise is to do them on the floor with your feet shoulder-width apart. Be sure to keep your weight on the ball of your foot at the bottom of each rep. Let your heels "kiss" the ground but don't let your weight rest on them.

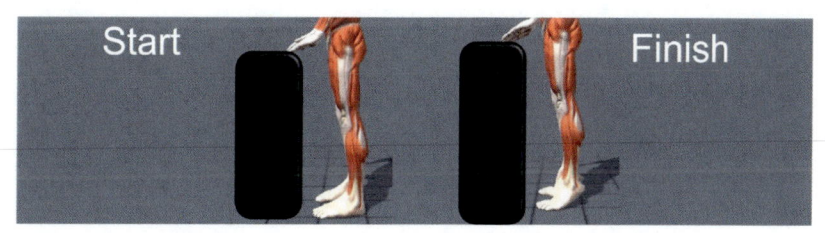

The most basic calf raise is done just standing up on the ball of your foot and then gently touching your heels to the floor. This version is a good technique to improve tension control and stability.

You can progress calf raises with the ROT, centerline, weight shift and weight elements. You can bring your feet together for one progression and then shift your weight onto one leg or the other.

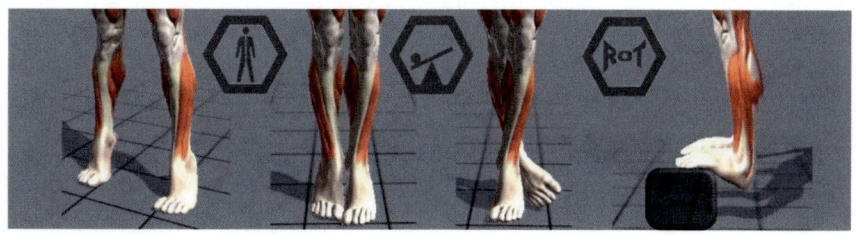

You can progress your calf training with several elements. Move from a wider stance to a close stance by using the centerline element or you can shift your weight onto one foot through the weight shift element. All calf raise variations can be done either flat or on a step which can increase your range of tension.

It's popular to do calf raises on a ledge or step so your heels can drop down below the level of your ball of the foot. Be sure to keep tension in your muscles at the bottom of each rep when you do this. It's easy to improve your range of motion by relaxing your muscles so you can go deeper. Keep those calves tense!

Also be super mindful of your true range of motion. I've seen far too many guys do calf raises on a ledge but their heels never drop below the level of their toes. This isn't bad, but it fools you into thinking you're going deeper than you really are. I've always liked using a calf block that's only 2-3 inches off the floor so I can feel my heels touchdown. That way, I know I'm getting a consistent range of tension on each rep.

Lastly, be prudent with adding weight to your calf raises. If you follow the progressions and tips above you shouldn't need a lot of extra weight when doing controlled single leg calf raises on a block with your whole leg tense. In many cases, 10-20# should be more than enough.

Hip exercises

They say you're only as strong as your legs, but your legs are only as strong as your hips. In some ways, your hips are like the shoulders of your lower body. Every bit of tension in your lower body is directly related to the strength and stability of your hips. Sadly, weak and unstable hips are a plague in modern fitness and hold many athletes back while increasing the risk of injury. You don't have to suffer the same fate because these simple exercises will do wonders to strengthen your hips.

These basic hip exercises work several qualities that are essential to building strong and functional hips. They improve flexibility, muscle control, stability and raw lifting power making them far more versatile than any weight machine or static hip stretch.

Leg raises

The most basic hip exercise involves lifting your leg up to your front, side, and back while standing. The easiest place to start is to hold onto something sturdy while lifting one of your legs. This technique is often done in a fast dynamic motion, but you'll want to perform it in a slow movement so you use the strength of your hips instead of momentum to lift your leg.

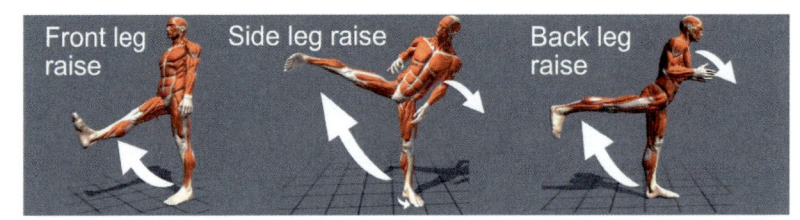

Front leg raises are done by simply lifting one leg in front of you while standing upright. Side leg raises involve both lifting your leg to the side while slightly tilting your torso in the opposite direction. Note the slightly out-turned supporting foot to decrease twisting stress on the supporting knee. Back leg raises involve lifting your leg behind you while slightly tilting your torso forward.

While you are lifting one leg, you're actually working both sets of hips at the same time. You're working the hip of the leg you're lifting to move, but you're also putting tension in the other hip to stabilize and support your body.

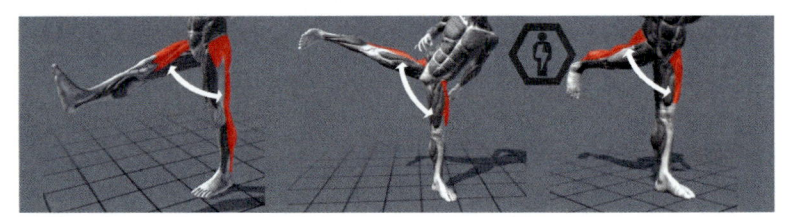

It helps to imagine pulling both legs apart in opposite directions when doing leg raises. This ensures both hips are working, one to lift your leg and the other to stabilize the supporting leg.

Leg raise progression is achieved in several ways. You can improve the extension of both legs by locking out the knees to make the exercise more strict. Second, the range of tension is always a good objective as you work to gain every bit of range of tension. Third, you can use more or less support with your upper body which shifts more weighted support to your working leg. A fully locked and unsupported leg raise requires a lot more hip strength than most athletes will ever need. Lastly, you can always progress using the time element by both doing more reps and increasing the amount of time you can hold your leg up for.

Hip sweeps

Lifting your legs to the 4 points of the compass can be effective, but your hips need to be strong in all 360 degrees of motion. This is why I recommend an exercise I call hip sweeps which work your hips to the front, side and back and every degree in between.

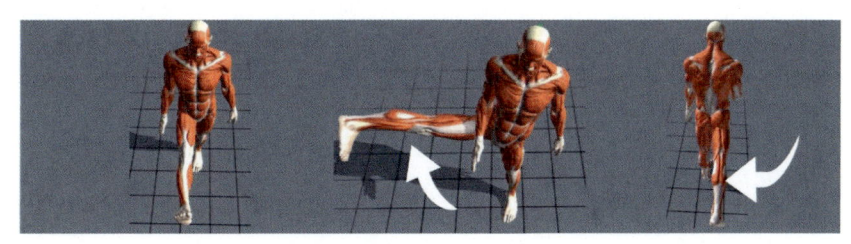

Hip sweeps start in the front leg raise position. From there, you swing your leg out to the side and continue to sweep your foot around your back. Note how your toes point up in the front, forward at the side and down when behind you. From there, you can bring your leg down and rest or reverse the direction and swing your leg back to the front.

Just lift your leg straight out in front of you and sweep it to your side and then behind you in a smooth, controlled motion. Then sweep it back to your front before lowering it straight down. You can also do this in sets and reps without lowering your leg for an extra challenge.

It's perfectly natural for your upper body to tilt and rotate as you move your leg. Trying to keep your torso perfectly upright can impede your range of motion and compromise balance.

Once again, keep tension in the hip of the supporting leg as well as the sweeping leg. You should feel the tension of both hips sweep from front to back in opposition to one another as you move through the exercise.

Points To Ponder

1. Pay close attention to shifts in your weight distribution on your feet. Does your weight fall on your heels at the bottom? How about to the toes? Does your weight shift to the inside or outside of your foot?
2. Look to your knees and any lateral movement they show as you stand up. Ideally, your knees shouldn't "circle" as you squat down or stand up.
3. You can prevent knee circling by pushing your knees outward as you stand up during two leg squats or inward during single leg squats and lunges.
4. While you don't need to keep your back ramrod straight during bodyweight squats, try to limit reaching your arms and shoulder forward excessively at the bottom of a squat. Try to "sit up straight" at the bottom of each rep.
5. Aim to keep your legs together while doing pistol squats and prevent the non-squatting leg from pulling out to the side at the bottom.
6. Work on keeping your arms and torso from moving during each rep. Clasp your hands together or using a squat stick (see chapter 18) to manage upper body movement.
7. Avoid accidental twisting motions in either the upper or lower body to prevent stress on your knees and lower back.
8. Avoid bouncing out of the bottom position especially during single leg squats. Lower yourself down under control, pause briefly and lift up under control.
9. Knee and lower back stress could be a sign of tight hips. Practice regressing your technique and work on opening up the back of your hips as you squat. It helps to imagine trying to stretch the seat of your pants as you squat down.
10. If one leg is noticeably weaker than the other, work to strengthen the weaker leg so it can catch up to the stronger one. Keep the reps the same between both sides even if you need to break up the set on the weaker leg.

11. Try to keep your whole leg involved in the exercise, not just your quads and glutes. Be sure to engage your calves, hips and shin muscles as well.
12. Keep your breathing as smooth as possible. Hard leg training can jack up the heart rate making it feel more like a cardio workout than a strength workout. Inhaling as you lower yourself and exhaling on the way up is a popular way to breath.
13. Watch yourself in a mirror or record yourself on video to observe subtle movements and compensations you may not be aware of.

Chapter 9 Pull Chain

There is a certain mystique to grabbing onto something and pulling yourself up to your hands. The pull-up and other related exercises are the embodiment of raw physical strength and power being applied in a primal, yet graceful, way. Few exercises can match its beauty or effectiveness. That's why learning how to engage and train your pull chain can be one of the most rewarding things you do for your upper body.

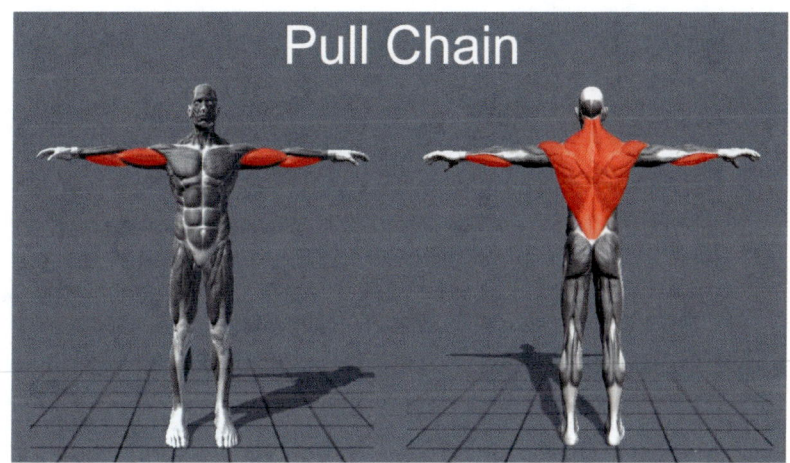

Your pull chain is comprised of all of the muscles in your back including your latissimus dorsi (lats), trapezius and the muscles behind your shoulders. The pull chain also includes all of the muscles in your bicep as well as the flexor muscles in your forearm that help you build a crushing grip.

Not only does pulling yourself upward look cool, but it also has several advantages compared to similar free weight and machine exercises that train your back.

The first advantage is bodyweight pull training won't place your spine at risk. With free weights, you need to bend over to do most rowing exercises. This position makes the lower back the weakest link in your pull chain, and it limits how much tension you can place on the rest of your muscles.

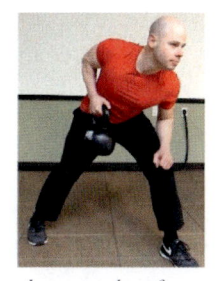

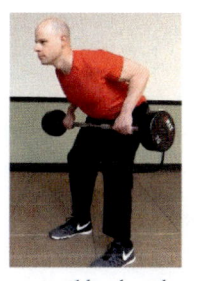

Picking up a weight and pulling it to your torso does wonders for your arms and back as long as you are skilled in keeping your hips and spine stable throughout the set.

Some athletes are uncomfortable with free weights, and they prefer to use weight machines. These devices offer much more support and stability for your spine. The downside to using these tools is they are cumbersome and require a gym membership or an expensive purchase for home use. Even then, the functional aspects of machine training can be questionable. I once witnessed a bodybuilder struggle to hang onto a rope while doing an obstacle course. Even though they were strong in the gym, they couldn't hang onto a climbing rope.

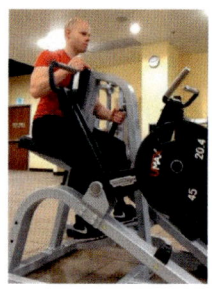

Back machines like this are a great way to work your back, but I do wonder what you're missing out on when the machine supports you so much.

Bodyweight based pull training is pure magic. No other form of training is this safe and effective. It gives you the ability to work every muscle in your pull chain to the absolute limit without any excessive stress on the spine and lower back. These exercises are also very natural. Your body evolved to pull yourself towards your hands. The shape of your hands, the structure of your shoulder, even the way your muscles attach to your back are designed to hang and pull yourself up.

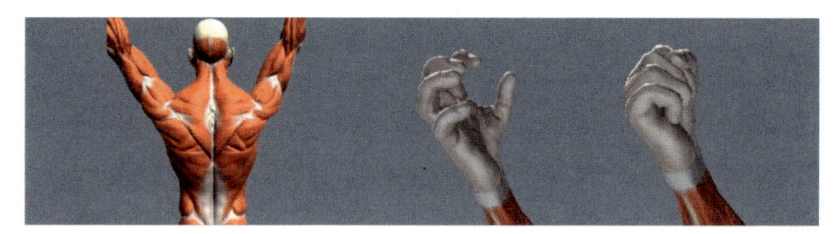

You are quite literally built to hang. Humans evolved while living in the forests and trees and your primal DNA still contains a lot of untapped strength just waiting to be unleashed!

Tap into your primal potential

As a primate, you have an incredible amount of pulling potential. Unfortunately, modern man is no longer swinging on tree branches, so most people never use even a fraction of their potential. Much of this is because we don't hang from an overhead support on a daily basis. Imagine how strong your legs would be if you moved around in a wheelchair all the time. Even if you walked up a few flights of stairs twice a week, your legs wouldn't be nearly as strong as they are now. You now face this same scenario with our upper body in the modern world. Some people find it difficult just to hang from an overhead bar for more than 10 seconds while average athletes can hang for minutes at a time. With even a moderate amount of training, anyone can discover a lot of strength that's lying dormant in their muscles.

The advantages of bodyweight pulls are not limited to beginners. If you're a seasoned pull-up master, I promise you still have a lot of room for progress. Few athletes flirt with advanced pulling techniques like archer and single arm pulls. Even if you can do pull-ups in your sleep, you still have plenty of untapped potential.

What's in a name?

For the sake of simplicity, I refer to all of the exercises in this chapter as members of the pull-up family. The way I see it, any activity where you grab onto an object and pulling yourself towards your hands is a pull-up. You are pulling yourself up. Simple. There's no need to bring other terms into the mix, especially when there's so much debate over what constitutes a pull-up vs. a chin up and a row. Some people claim using an underhand grip is a chin up. Others claim it's a pull-up. As far as I've been able to find, no standard definition was carved into stone eons ago.

Besides, once you become proficient with Chain Training, there won't be much difference in how your muscles are working from one variation to the next anyway. All movements in this chapter should involve putting tension on your entire back, shoulders, biceps, and forearms regardless of what grip or arm position you use.

Turning On Your Pulling Chain

Here are a few techniques you can use to turn on your pulling muscles. The first is to practice a clutching position. Start by making tight fists to activate your grip and forearm muscles. Next, curl your hands toward your shoulders to engage your biceps. Lastly pull your shoulders down and back to turn on the muscles in your back.

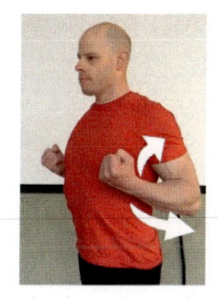

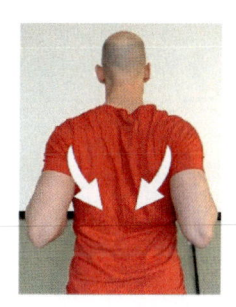

An isometric row or clutch position will help you turn on every muscle in your pull chain.

Another move to practice is what I call an elbow bridge. Lean against a wall or lay on the floor and drive your elbows into your sides while simultaneously pushing into the wall or floor with your elbows. Keep your biceps and forearms tense to keep tension flowing through your arms.

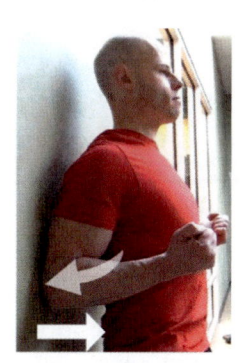

An elbow bridge is where you rest against the wall or floor and press your back away by driving your elbows behind your torso.

Pull back and inward

Like a lot of young bucks, I used to associate the back muscles with width and outward motion when I first started training. This myth grew from seeing guys spreading their lats and the idea that a wide grip pull-up builds a wider back. I thought everything about the back was about going outward, but I actually should have been thinking of the opposite approach.

When you look at an anatomy chart you'll notice that almost every muscle fiber in the back directs tension inward towards the spine.

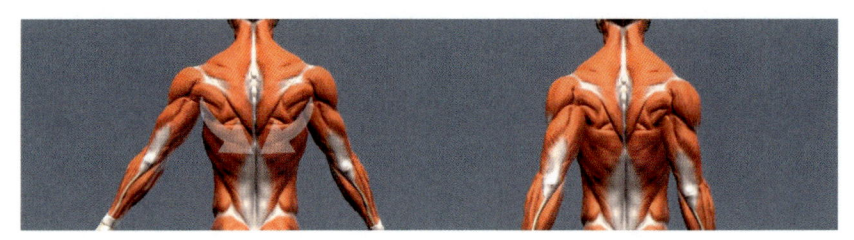

This diagram shows how the muscles in your back work like the muscles in your chest. To optimally engage your back, think about using your muscles to pull your arms inward towards your spine as well as down and back.

Employ arm torque (external rotation)

Pulling moves require a lot of what I call arm torque or external shoulder rotation. Doing this helps you engage your back and arms to pull your shoulders in and down while twisting your hands outward. A good way to practice this is to point your thumbs up in front of you and then turn your thumbs out and down.

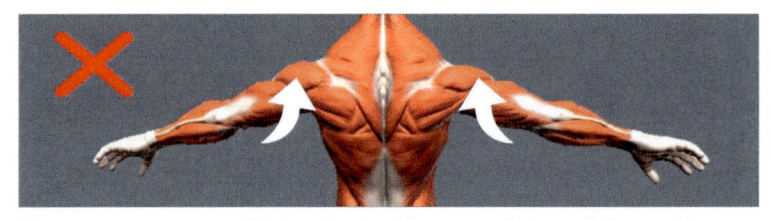

Internal rotation makes your elbows point outward and bring the shoulders up and forward. Doing this can rob your back of tension and shoulder stability.

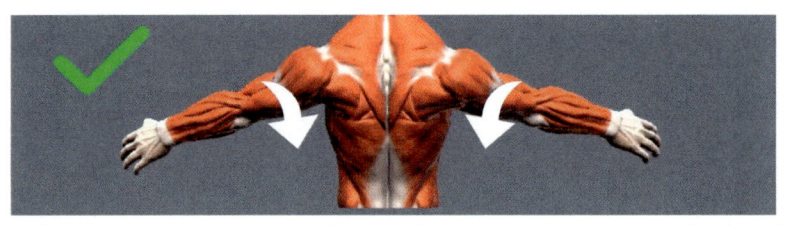

External rotation or "torqueing" brings the elbows inward as the shoulders are pulled down and back. This helps to drive tension into your back and stabilize your shoulders.

Using this arm torque in every pulling chain exercise will counteract the tendency to slouch the shoulders up and forward while flaring the arms outward. Doing this will significantly improve the tension through your pull chain. It will also relieve stress in your joints. One of the most common injuries from bodyweight training is elbow tendinosis caused by heavy pulling without enough back tension and shoulder stability.

Use your shoulders

Over the years, I've noticed many people's pulling strength is handicapped by weak shoulders. More specialty, a lack of tension in the rear deltoid. A lot of athletes can send tension through their lats and upper back. Others can also place plenty of tension in their biceps and forearms. Keeping the back of the shoulders tense connects the tension in the arms and back to create much more strength than using the lats and biceps alone. It's also a lot easier to keep your rear deltoids tense when you torque in your arms.

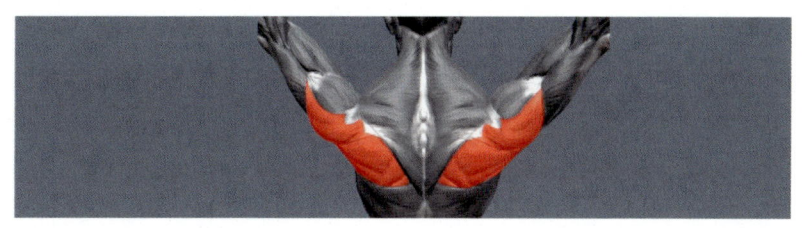

The biceps and lats tend to hold the most tension in pulling moves, but it's the tension behind and underneath the shoulders that connects the two to create the most strength in the pull chain.

Pull Chain Exercises

Pull chain exercises all work the same muscles with some tension variation depending on which joints you move or don't move. It's important to maintain tension in your whole back, shoulder, bicep, and forearm for all pull chain exercises regardless of the variation.

Horizontal Pulling (Rows)

"Rows" are very much a pull-up variation. The biggest difference between vertical and horizontal pulling movements is the range of tension at the shoulder and elbow. Vertical pulling moves start the arm in the overhead position and pull the upper arm down in front of the body. The pulling motion continues until the upper arm is either pressing into the torso or alongside it. Rows use the bottom half of this range of the movement, starting the upper arm in front of the body and pulling it alongside the torso.

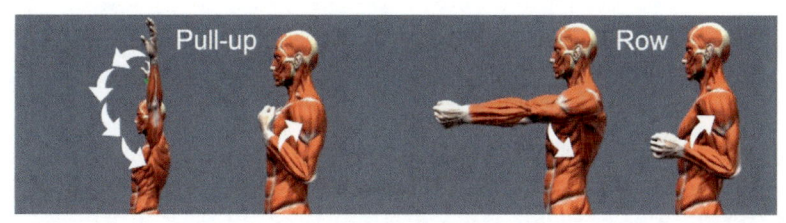

Rows and pull-ups may use a different relationship with gravity, but they both use the same basic muscles to move your arms in the same motions. They both extend the shoulder and flex the elbow so they are not as different as many experts make them out to be.

Some people like to do rows with their elbows out to the side, but I've long found keeping your elbows in tight to the ribs is a more stable position for the shoulder joint. It also makes it easier to place tension in the lats and biceps.

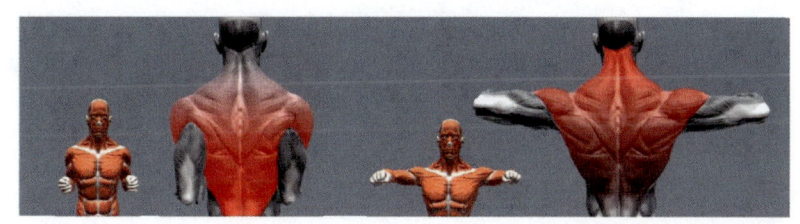

The classic idea is that keeping the arms in tight is better for the lats and lower back while bringing the elbows out to the side places more tension in the middle and upper back. The same idea is proposed for using various hand widths and grips.

The argument for "winging" your arms out to the side is that it helps target your upper back and shoulders a bit more. Usually, feeling more tension in the upper back with your elbows out is due to not using your shoulders and upper back enough when your arms are tucked in.

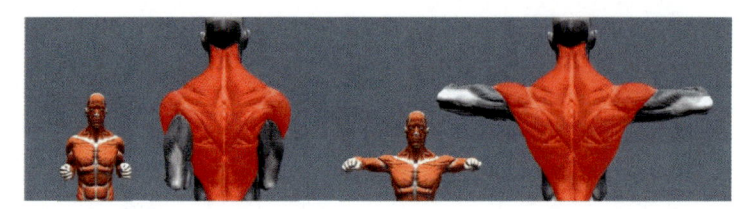

Changes in technique will always slightly alter the "flavor" of an exercise, but the differences should be reduced as your tension skills improve.

I much prefer a relatively close grip when doing rows as the standard way to pull. It's fine to play with a wider grip where your elbows point out to the side, but I think you'll gain more from trying to keep your arms in tight to your body. It's easier on your joints but harder on your muscles. Feel free to experiment with different techniques to see what works best for you. Just always keep in mind that the tension in your muscles is there because your brain is putting it there rather than the use of a particular arm position.

Basic progressions for rows

Rows use both the leverage and body angle elements. Easier row exercises involve pulling on a bar or even a door handle with the body close to upright. Lowering your body closer to the ground places you more against gravity and makes the exercise harder.

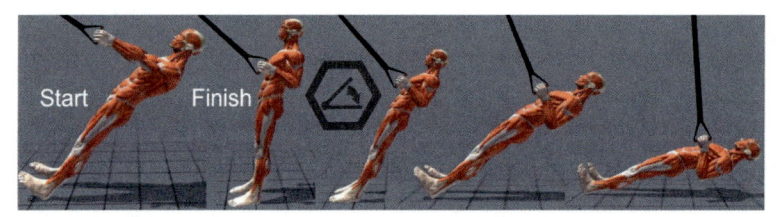

Start by leaning back while holding onto something sturdy. Drive your elbows backward while flexing your elbows. Pause at the top and lower yourself back down under control. The steeper you angle your body the more resistance against gravity you create.

You can also use your legs to make a row more difficult in several ways. First, you can bend or extend your knees to use the extension element to make the exercise more challenging.

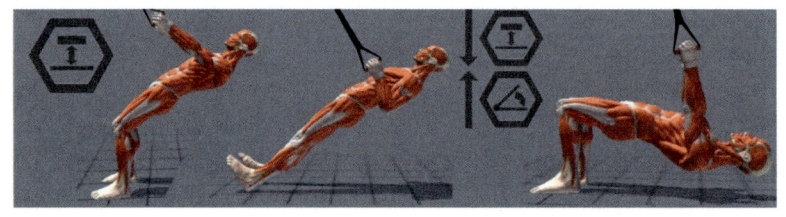

Bending your knees can reduce the resistance through the extension element. It can also help with traction when your feet slide on a slippery floor. "Table rows" are a popular variation that increases the angle to gravity element while reducing the extension element.

Feet elevated row

Rows can be made even harder by placing your feet up on a ledge or box. This position uses the angle to gravity element to bring even more weight onto your hands and makes the exercise more challenging.

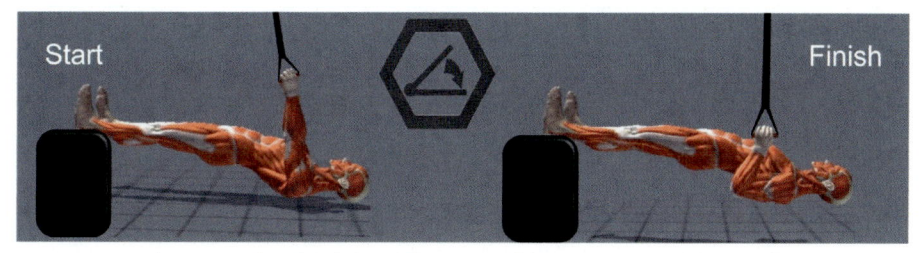

Elevated rows place even more weight on your hands when you have your feet up on a step or ledge. Be sure to grab onto something that is high enough so your arms can fully straighten without hitting your upper back or head on the floor.

Narrow rows

Bringing your arms and hands closer together is a classic bodybuilding technique that uses the centerline element. Weightlifters use a special cable handle when doing narrow rows and you can do the same by placing your hands closer together.

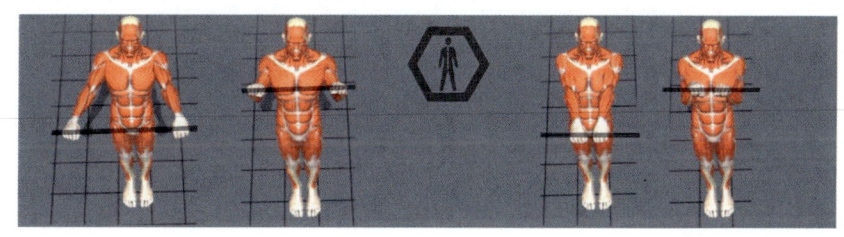

A couple of examples of how using a wide or narrow grip might look for rowing. Bringing the elbows in close to the torso is essential for narrow grip rows.

You can also adjust the width of your stance or the anchor points of your suspension trainer to change the stability of your rows.

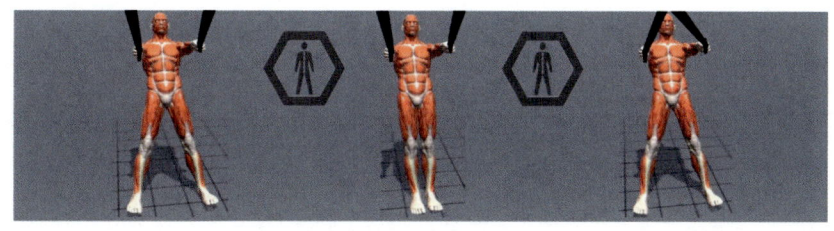

You can use the centerline element to make any row more difficult by using a closer stance or by moving the anchor points of a suspension trainer closer together. Bringing your hands closer will also increase the difficulty.

By moving your feet closer together, you remove some of the stability of the exercise forcing your upper body to compensate by creating more tension.

Single arm assistance rows

Once you're comfortable with narrow rows, you can start to shift your weight onto one arm by extending the other arm out to the side. You can also grab a towel or just hold onto the bar with fewer fingers to place more resistance on the working arm.

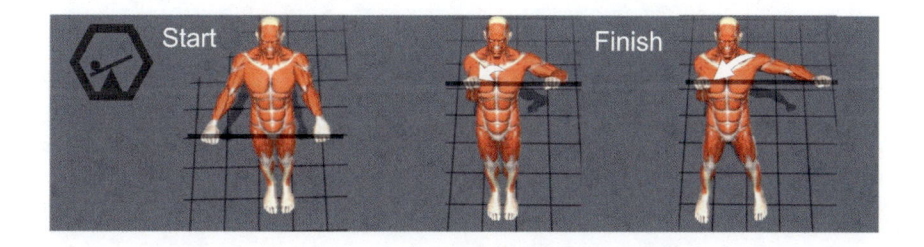

Shifting, or single arm assistance rows involve moving more weight onto one arm while the other arm acts as assistance. Start with your weight equally between both arms and shift to one side as you pull yourself up. Keeping your assistance arm closer to your torso (center) makes the exercise easier and reaching out further, or holding on with less of a grip (right) makes it more difficult.

Single arm rows

Rowing with a single arm requires a lot of tension in your back and even your chest to pull your arm as close to your centerline as possible. The closer you pull to your centerline, the more stable you'll be and it will prevent a lot of torque on your torso. It's also common to use a slight twist in your torso as you pull yourself up to minimize the torque on your body.

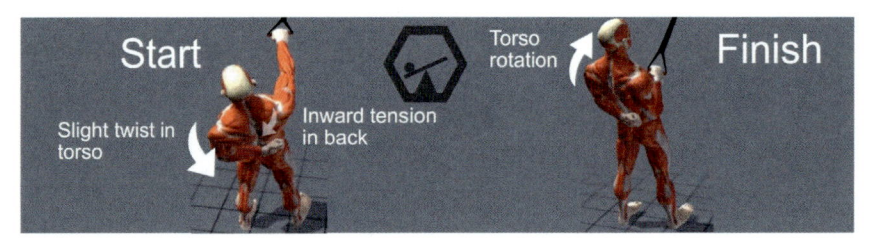

Single arm rows are the full expression of the weight shifting element as you load all of your weight onto one arm while the other is tucked behind your back. As always, experiment with other progressive elements, like your angle to gravity and the width of your stance to make this exercise appropriate for you.

You can use the single arm row with a variety of body angles and stance widths to make it as easy or challenging as you wish.

Full body rows

These two exercises take your feet off the floor so all of your weight is on your hands. It's easier to do these on gymnastics rings or parallel bars so your body can move between your hands.

The first variation involves tucking your knees up to your chest.

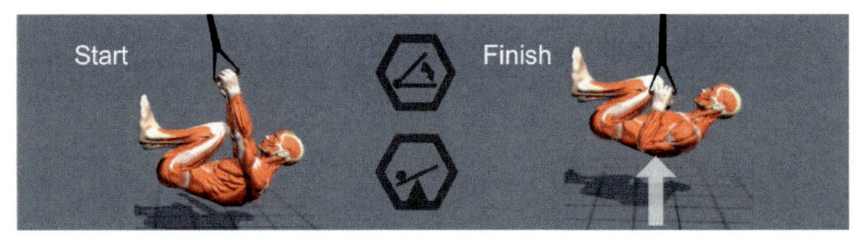

Full body rows use both the weight shift element and the angle to gravity element. The first is because all of your bodyweight is on your hands since your feet are off the floor. Second, You pull yourself directly against the pull of gravity instead of lifting up in a slight arch since you're no longer pivoting on your heels.

You can use the extension element to straighten your body in the air. This position requires significantly more strength just to hold yourself in place let alone pull your body toward your hands.

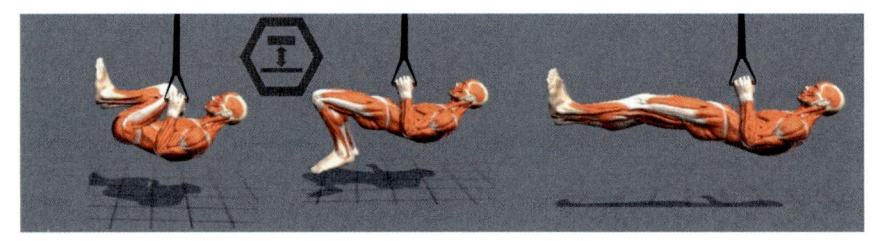

Extending your legs out creates a "rowing lever" and greatly increases the demand on your back to not only pull you up but to also stabilize your body in space.

Vertical Pulling (Pull-Ups)

Vertical pulling exercises use a bigger range of tension than horizontal pulling movements, especially in the shoulder and elbow joints. They also usually need more shoulder mobility and tension control. It's for these reasons that many athletes consider them to be harder than horizontal rows. Some people even write them off as something they can never do. Vertical pulls are not out of reach for most people if you know how to progress and regress them to your appropriate level of difficulty.

Seated pull-ups

Seated pull-ups involve using a low handle to grab onto or raising the floor surface with a chair or plyo-box. They are a great way to start doing vertical pull-ups because your legs can assist your upper body, plus you're only lifting a fraction of your total body weight.

This technique allows you to adjust the resistance a couple of ways. The first is the weight shift element by controlling how much resistance is in either your arms or your legs. The more you push with your legs, the less your pull chain needs to work.

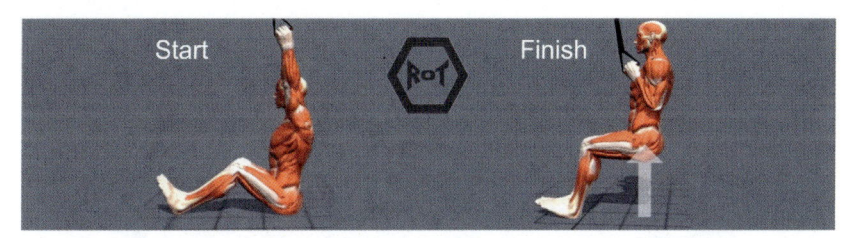

Seated pull-ups are like regular pull-ups but without the weight of your legs. You can even use your legs to help push yourself up.

You can use the extension element to progress this movement in several stages. Straightening your legs in front of you makes the exercise harder, and moving your feet closer makes it easier. You can also progress this move by crossing your legs or using only one leg for assistance.

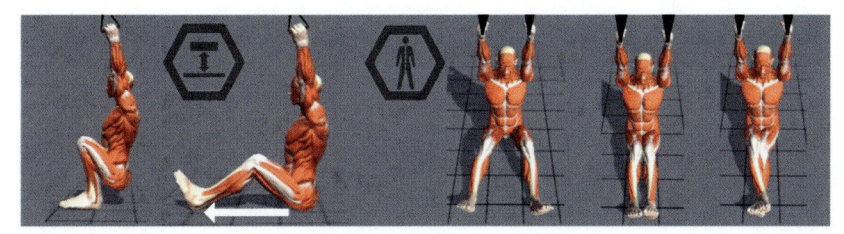

Seated pull-ups can be progressed by extending your legs further out in front which removes the amount of assistance your lower body can give your upper body. Using the centerline element can also remove lower body stability which can also make your upper body work harder.

Another adjustment you can use is the position of your hips. It's easier to pull yourself up if you extend your hips as you lift. It's more difficult to maintain a vertical spine through the full range of motion.

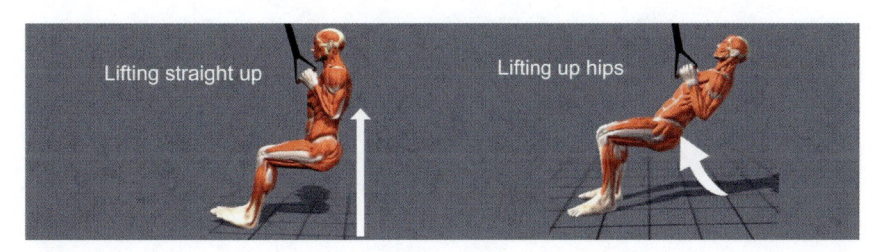

Pressing your feet into the floor will cause your hips to lift and tilt your torso as you pull yourself up. This turns your vertical pull-up into more of a row which will be a little easier on your pull chain muscles.

Lastly, you can adjust the range of tension in your pull chain by changing the height of your handles. Having the handles low will allow you to start each rep with bent arms and less range of tension. Moving the handles higher will require more range as you start with your arms straight.

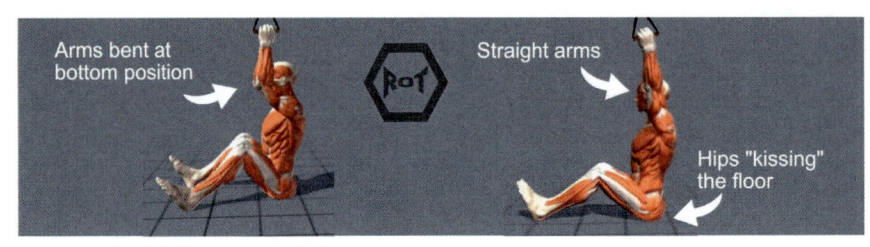

Setting your handles lower can regress the exercise by removing some of the range of tension at the bottom of each rep. Setting them higher will help you start with straight arms and require more range of tension in your pull chain.

Moving your handles even higher will remove more assistance from your lower body until you're pulling up with very little help from your legs.

Jump pulls and negatives

Jumping pull-ups still use your legs for assistance but only for a short period. Once your feet leave the ground you're holding up your full bodyweight which you can then lower back down under control. This is often referred to as doing a "negative" as you're focusing on building strength through the eccentric or "negative" portion of each rep.

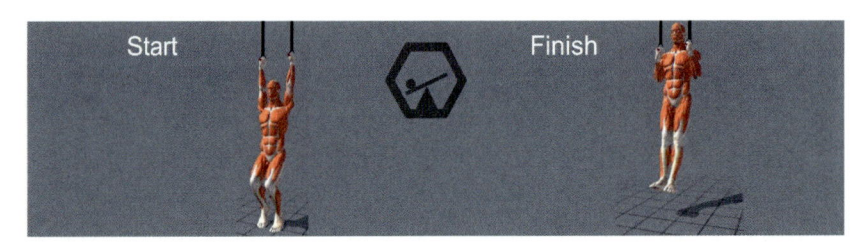

Jumping into the top of the pull-up position quickly transfers your weight from your feet to your hands. From there you can hold for time and slowly lower yourself down under control. This helps your pull chain learn how to handle all of your bodyweight between both arms.

Just as with seated pull-ups you can adjust the difficulty through changing the height of the handles or bar. The higher the bar is, the less assistance you can gain from jumping. You can also use the time element to change how long you're holding yourself up and lowering yourself down slowly or fast.

Full bodyweight pulls

These moves are the classic "pull-up" where you hang your full bodyweight from an overhead support and pull yourself up. This technique progresses the resistance through the weight shifting element since all of your weight is now on your hands.

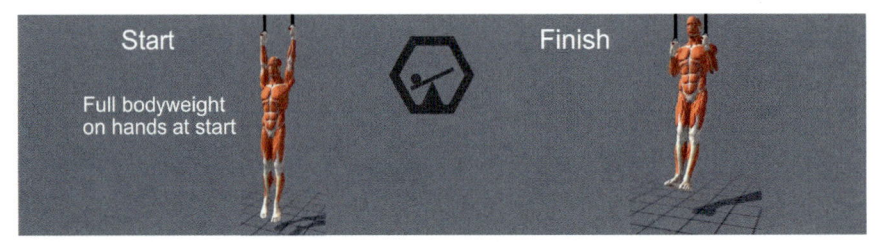

The full pull-up position involves keeping your full body weight on your hands from the bottom hanging position all the way to the top and back down again.

Open and closed shoulders

A lot of your progression with this exercise comes from maximizing your range of tension at both the top and bottom of each rep. A good way to do this is to fully flex your shoulders open at the bottom position so your upper arm is reaching straight up rather than slightly forward. You'll achieve the full range of motion in your shoulders while maintaining tension in your pull chain. This amount of range doesn't have to come through a "dead hang" style pull-up where you relax your arms and shoulders at the bottom of each rep. Remember, this is about range of tension, not just range of motion, so do your best to maintain tension in the pull chain at the bottom of each rep.

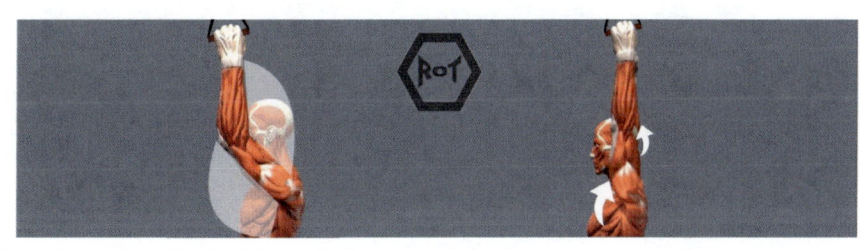

The image on the left shows the angle at the shoulder and elbow joint through a shorter range of tension at the bottom of a pull-up. Working on increasing the range at the bottom of each pull-up involves flexing the shoulder and straightening the elbow more over time to increase the range at both joints.

To optimize your range at the top, imagine pulling your chest to your hands while driving your elbows down and back.

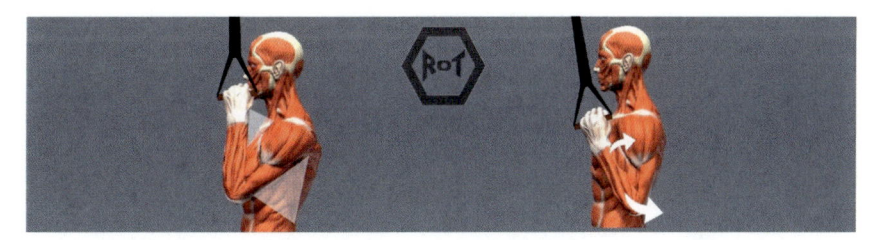

Increasing the range of tension at the top of a pull-up means closing the gaps between your elbows and your side and your forearms and chest. Doing this will flex your elbow and extend your shoulder more to bring your head higher above your hands.

Pay attention to how the tension changes in your muscles through the range of motion. It's common for your back or biceps to relax a little at the top or bottom of each rep. Do your best to proactively tense up all of the muscles in your pull chain for every inch of each rep.

Should you arch your back or not?

Some pull-up aficionados recommend either keeping a straight back or an arched back when pulling up. Both of these techniques have their place, and it's good to play with both to see what's best for you.

Arching your back involves curling your feet up behind you, so your chest is slightly under the bar. Some people find this is an easier pull-up variation to start with and helps them drive tension into their back muscles. The straight back pull-up involves keeping your legs straight and slightly in front of you at the top of each rep.

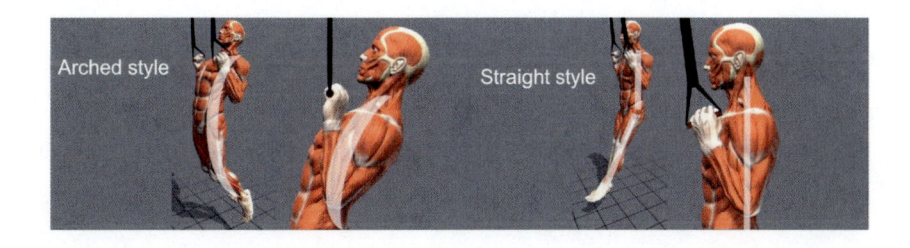

Both techniques are valid ways to build muscle and strength with each having their pros and cons. Arching your back can make it easier to bring more tension to your upper back since the top position can be similar to a row. The straight back technique is sometimes referred to as being a little more strict and traditional. It's also important to master this style of pull-up if you want to explore muscle-ups where you pull yourself up and over your hands.

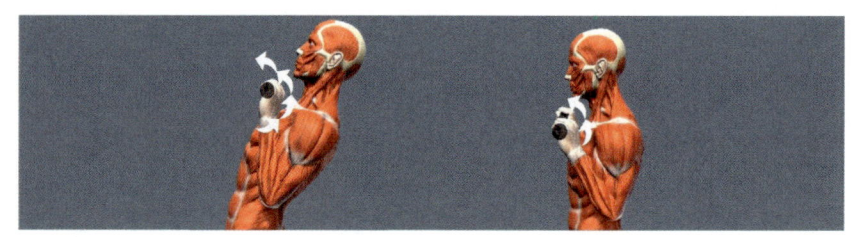

Pulling yourself up and over a bar is easier with a straight back.

Close grip pull-ups

Close pull-ups place your hands progressively closer until your fingers touch. All close work requires a lot of mobility and strength particularly at the top and bottom of each rep. Be patient if your hands and wrists feel tight or stiff and gradually move them closer over time. You can also experiment with a variety of grips. Some athletes feel close grips are easier to do with an underhand or neutral grip with the palms facing each other. This is another advantage to using gymnastics rings or suspension straps since you can rotate your hands to find the angle that works best for you.

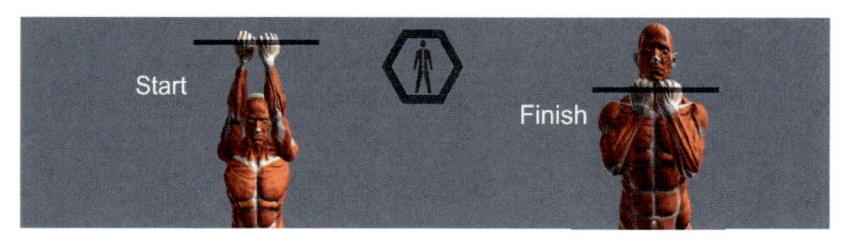

Close grip pull-ups are an art in and of themselves. They require just a little more of all of the qualities the typical pull-up requires including more stability, mobility, and strength.

Towel assist pull-ups

Grabbing a towel removes some of the strength from one arm so you place more weight on the hand that's grabbing the more sturdy handle. It also places one hand slightly lower than the other to create a mechanical disadvantage on the pulling arm.

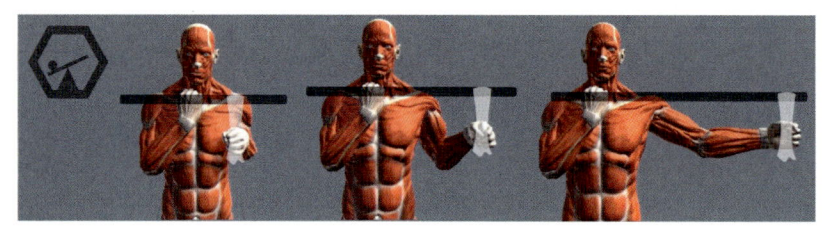

Grabbing on to a towel with one hand brings more weight to the supporting hand that you're using to pull yourself up. This exercise becomes more difficult the further away you place the towel on your centerline.

Start by resuming the same narrow grip you used before and progress the exercise by moving the towel further away from your centerline. Be sure to continue to pull your main working arm to your centerline and avoid balancing out the weight between your two arms.

Finger assist pull-ups

If you don't have a towel, you can always grab onto the bar with a weaker grip to make one arm work harder. The fewer fingers you use to hang on the weaker your assistance grip will be.

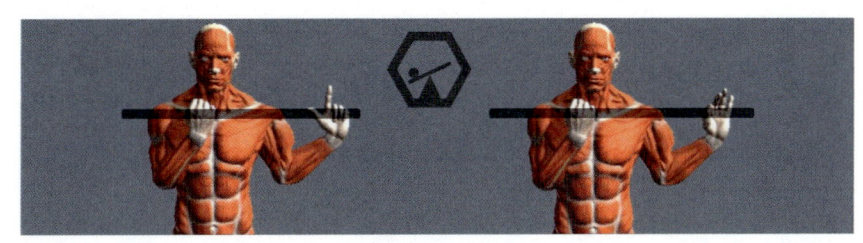

Some examples of shifting more weight onto your primary pulling arm by using a weaker grip on the bar. The fewer fingers you use the more difficult the exercise will be.

Single arm pull-ups

Once you can pull yourself up with minimal assistance, you can move onto pulling yourself up with just one arm. This exercise requires a lot of tension control and strength along your entire pull chain, especially in your grip and shoulder stability.

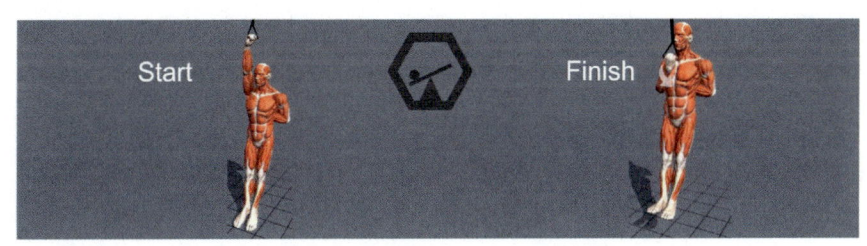

Single arm pull-ups are one heck of a feat of strength. Note the rotation of the hand while pulling it into your chest. If you're using a straight bar you can allow your body to rotate around your hand since it's on a fixed object.

Single arm pulls are not reserved to the super strong. You can do seated pulls to regress how much weight is on your arm by keeping your feet on the ground and assisting you up. You can then progress the seated ground-based pull-ups the same way you would progress two-arm pulls by moving the handles higher.

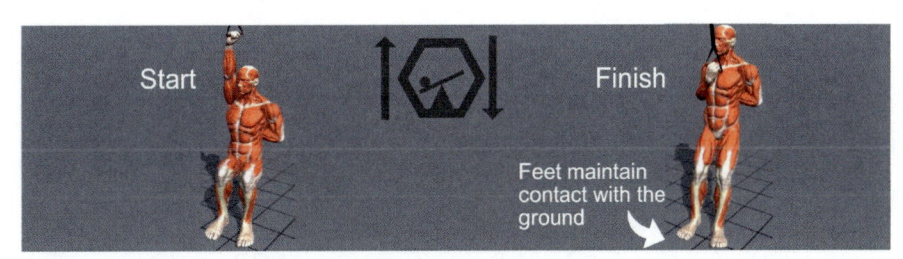

Seated single arm pull-ups progress and regress the weight shift element at the same time. They place more weight on one arm, but also put more weight on your legs so they can assist in pulling yourself up.

Accessory Moves For Pull Chain

Each of these exercises may place more emphasis on various muscles along your pull chain, but they are not isolation exercises. Be sure to concentrate on putting tension on your whole pull chain even if you're only moving one joint.

Curls

Rows and vertical pulling exercises will do far more for your biceps than any curling exercise. Even still, these moves can be fun and satisfying to include as a supplement to your workouts. You can do these on a solid bar or gymnastics rings, but a suspension trainer with rotating handles will work best. You can also use towels for a "hammer curl" variation and work your grip.

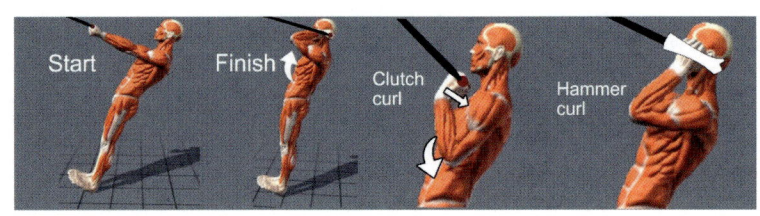

Strap curls are just like rows where you lean back and pull yourself up. You just do it primarily through bending your elbow while keeping your elbow in place instead of pulling it backward. You can also do "clutch" curls where you drop your elbow down while pulling your hand into the top of your chest. Hammer curls use a towel so you can maintain a neutral grip.

Clutch curls can be quite intense and involve driving your elbow down toward your ribs. Pull your hands close to your upper chest in a straight line as if you're clutching something to your chest. Drive your elbows down, but keep them slightly in front of your torso.

Play around with single arm variations as well. Keeping one arm straight with your palm facing down will take one arm out of the exercise while providing just the right amount of assistance for stability.

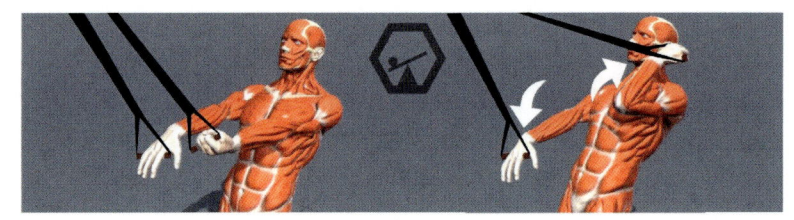

I prefer to still use both arms with single arm curls. I just keep the assistance arm straight and palm down with only light pressure on the handle through the palm. That way, you can lower that hand while the working arm curls up toward your face. Doing this helps to minimize twisting of the torso and makes it easy to switch back and forth between each arm.

Rear flies

I was never a fan of the rear shoulder fly exercise when I was lifting weights. It always felt awkward and hard on the joints when I was using dumbbells and weight machines. I quickly changed my mind when I started doing them on suspension trainers which placed my body in a more comfortable position.

Start by assuming the same position you would for curls and pull your body upright by pulling your arms back. It might help to visualize stretching your arms straight out to your side as you pull yourself up.

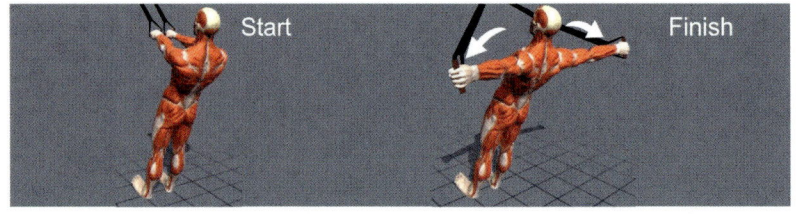

Lean back against the straps with your palms facing down and your arms straight. Smoothly pull the handles apart while keeping your arms straight. Pause a the top without letting the straps go slack and return your hands together in a smooth controlled motion.

It's natural to feel like your arms want to bend a bit and make the exercise easier. It's fine to do this to decrease the resistance if that's what you need. Keep your elbows locked to maximize resistance. It's also helpful to slightly extend your spine to slightly arch your back. Doing this can keep your weight on your heels at the top to the rep and prevent your weight from shifting to your toes which will remove the resistance on your hands.

Straight arm pull

These are a pretty hard move that focuses on the shoulder extension used in most pull chain exercises. Once again, start facing the anchor point and lean back with your hands in front of you. From here, drive your arms down and back while keeping your arms straight.

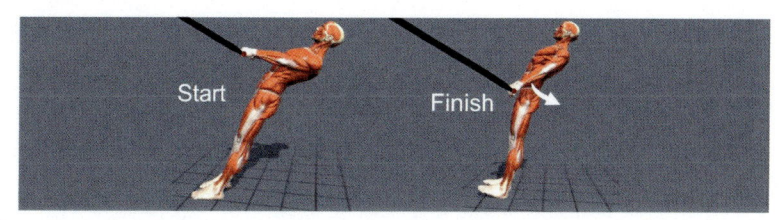

Start with your arms straight in front of you just like when doing a rear fly. Slightly arch your back and keep your arms straight as you pull your hands down by your side. It helps to think of pressing your hands down as you pull yourself up. Pause at the top before you pull yourself onto your toes and lower yourself down under control.

Be sure to only use the range you can move through with resistance. If you pull yourself up too far, you'll stand fully upright and lose the resistance on your arms. Decrease the range of motion if necessary to keep resistance on the muscles.

Levers

Levers are typically an isometric form of the straight arm pull with your feet off the floor. It's like doing straight arm pulls and holding the top position only now you're using your whole body directly against gravity.

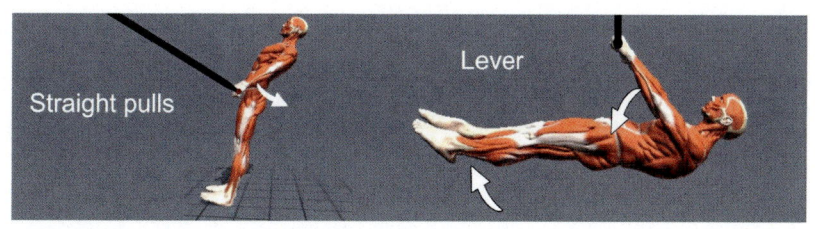

Straight pulls and levers are almost the same exercises. They both use your back muscles to extend the shoulder down while pulling your body upward. That's why straight arm pulls are a good warm-up for lever work.

There are many ways you can adjust the resistance of a lever exercise. First, you can use the extension element through extending your legs.

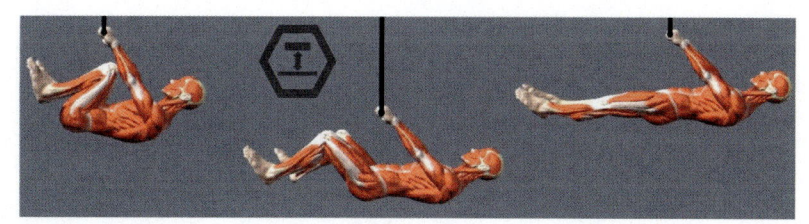

Extending your hips and legs out in front of you is one of the most popular ways to progress your lever training. The further out you extend yourself the more difficult the exercise becomes.

You can also hold your body straight in an inverted position and then angle yourself down until your spine is parallel with the floor which is where you'll have the most resistance.

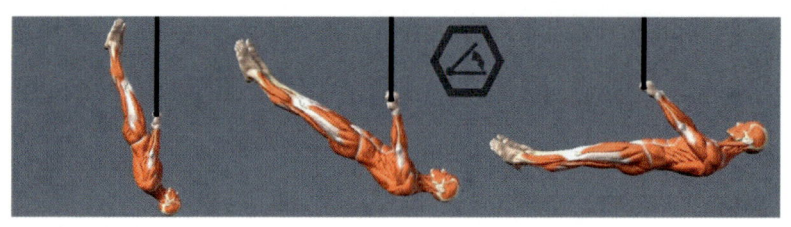

The angle of your body can significantly change the amount of resistance on your pull chain. The closer you bring yourself to being parallel to the floor the more difficult the exercise will be.

Don't forget you can use both the angle and extension elements at the same time by adjusting both the length of your body and your angle to gravity to suit your individual preference for how you do this exercise.

Lastly, you can dynamically do levers by starting off in a hanging position and then pull yourself up without bending your elbows. I Like to call these "straight arm pull-ups" because you're using your arms just as you would with a regular pull-up without bending at the elbow.

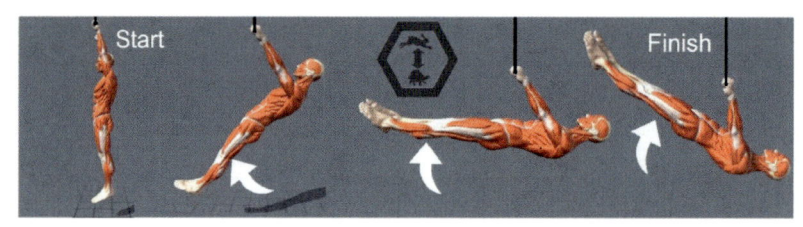

Moving levers or straight arm pull-ups use the speed element to require more tension in the muscles to create movement rather than just holding in place. Don't forget, you can also regress your technique through the extension element by tucking your knees if straight body levers are out of reach.

Towel hangs

I once heard a guy say "it's impossible to do effective pull-ups without lifting straps because your grip will always hold you back."

This idea is complete nonsense. Your grip can have at least 2-3 times the strength and endurance than the rest of your pull chain. You should be able to do as many rows or pull-ups as you can and still continue hanging for a long time afterward. However, a weak grip is an issue for many people and it can hold you back. These exercises will ensure you develop the iron grip you need.

Towel hangs are a pretty simple technique. Just loop a towel over a bar, grab hold and hang. Just remember this is still a pull chain exercise. Even though it might focus on your grip and forearms still apply tension through your entire pull chain.

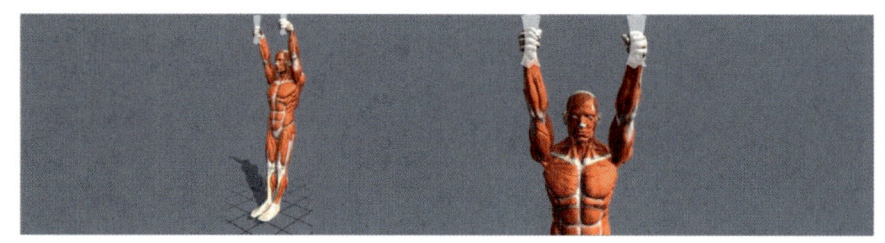

The best way to build your grip is to challenge it by holding onto things that are hard to hang onto. Towels naturally work the whole hand including the thumb while also strengthening the wrist and pull chain muscles.

Some people find this move can be a little hard on the fingers. Don't worry, as this discomfort will fade as your hands become conditioned to the exercise. Also, don't forget that some of your grip muscles work the pinching motion in your palm. I recommend grasping the towel with your palm first and then wrap your fingers around to complete the hold.

You can progress your towel hangs in different ways. You can use thicker towels or double up the towels you are using to create a thicker grip. You can also employ the same progressions used in pulling exercises like using a narrow grip or shifting weight to one side to make it work harder. Any of the progressive elements that work for pull chain exercises will work for towel hangs.

Lastly, feel free to experiment with using towels while doing rows and pull-ups to challenge your grip during your pull workout. Be sure not to use exercises that put you at risk of losing your grip and falling. Start with easy variations and work up from there.

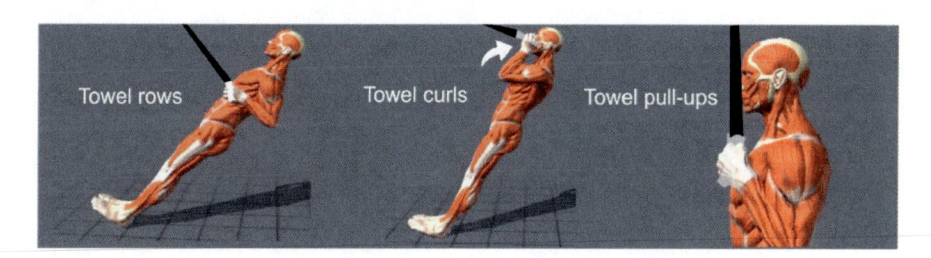

Points To Ponder

1. Pay attention to differences in weight distribution between your right and left arm and keep your weight as equal as you can unless you're purposely shifting it to one arm.
2. Pull your shoulders back while doing vertical pulling exercises to bring more tension to your back and reduce stress on your elbows.
3. Maintain control of your legs when hanging. Try not to let them kick forward and flail around in an uncontrolled manner. Crossing your ankles or pressing your feet together can help.
4. Allow your hips to hinge during vertical pull exercise to maintain an upright torso instead of keeping your legs in line with your torso. This can prevent stress on your elbow.
5. Pull your head up between your hands during vertical pulls to reduce backward motion. Doing this reduces stress on the elbows and doesn't require as much of an angle in your lower body.
6. Keep your hips and hamstrings tense while doing rows to prevent your core from moving and creating momentum.
7. Work on driving your elbows back behind you to engage your back muscles more, especially during vertical pulling movements.
8. Improve your tension control at the bottom and top of each rep. It's common for many athletes to bounce out of the bottom and rush out of the top to get more reps in.
9. Squeeze your arms in close to your sides when using close and shoulder width grips. This will engage your back muscles more and relieve stress on your elbows.
10. When in doubt, work on your range of tension. Lower yourself as much as you can while maintaining tension in your back and arms and pull yourself up until your chest reaches your hands.
11. Play with squeezing your hands harder while pulling to increase the tension in your forearms and improving tension control in your arms.

Chapter 10 Push Chain

Oh boy, it's time for everyone's favorite muscle group, the push chain! So crank up your favorite playlist and get ready for one hell of a pump in your chest, shoulders, and triceps. Things are about to get seriously primal.

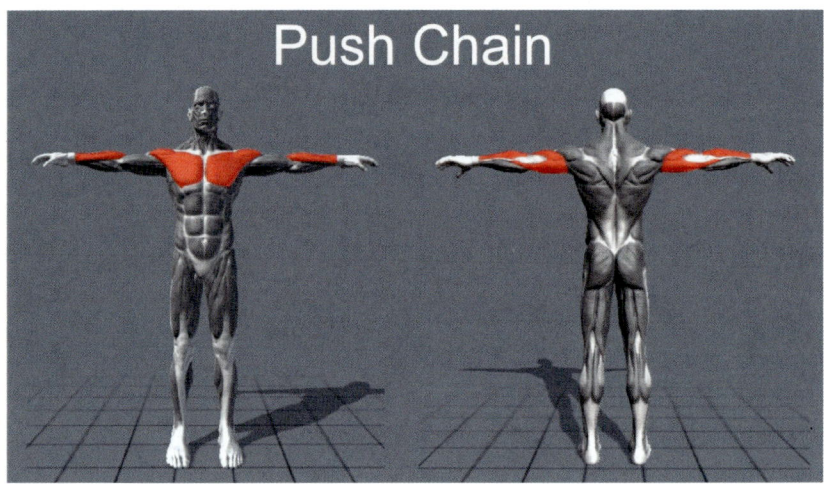

Your push chain is comprised of the primary muscles that push your hands away from your torso. These include the deltoids, triceps, pectorals and even the finger extensors in your forearm.

Push-ups are the most common push chain exercise in calisthenics. Strangely enough, they are also one of the most avoided movements by mainstream exercise enthusiasts. Some believe the push-up is too easy and not suitable for building real muscle and strength. Other's avoid the exercise because they believe it's too difficult and uncomfortable.

The solution to both situations is to understand how to adjust the difficulty of the push-up to fit your current level of fitness. That way, it's not too hard or too easy but just right for you. This chapter will teach you how to do just that and more, but before doing that, you'll need to practice placing tension in your push chain muscles.

The Most Important Part Of The Push-Up

Ironically, the foundation to good push chain tension comes from many of the muscles in your pulling chain. Your back muscles are exceedingly important when it comes to working your push chain, especially with bodyweight training. In the weightlifting world, you can use benches and padded seats to support your body in place. With calisthenics, you don't have any of these supportive devices, so you need to use the tension in your back and core instead. Like all muscle groups, your push chain can only work hard in a stable and supported environment. It needs something to work against, and if your back is looser than an identity thieves ethics, you'll struggle to get much from your push training.

Developing this support is where all of those bridges and pulling movements come in. It takes skill and coordination to control the tension in your back as you push your hands away from your torso. It's like patting your head and rubbing your belly at the same time. It's easy with practice, but you need to become proficient at it before you can get much from your push-up training.

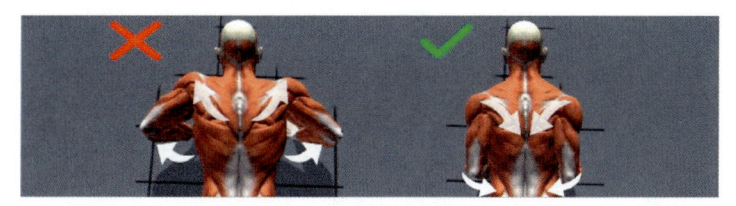

Back tension plays a crucial role in supporting your shoulders and push chain muscles.

So even though you're pushing against your hands keep some of your concentration on your back. Keep your shoulders pulled down and back. Also, make sure you're keeping the back of your shoulders tense to help stabilize your arms. Lastly, your back and chest muscles work together to create a holistic pattern of tension that strengthens your whole upper body. Creating this type of tension is the key to building more muscle and strength while keeping stress away from your joints.

Turning On Your Push Chain

The most basic way to practice push chain tension is by proactively tensing your chest, triceps, and shoulders while your arms are straight. You can do this by pressing into a ledge or countertop. Holding yourself up on a set of dip bars or suspension straps is also a very effective way to practice your push chain tension.

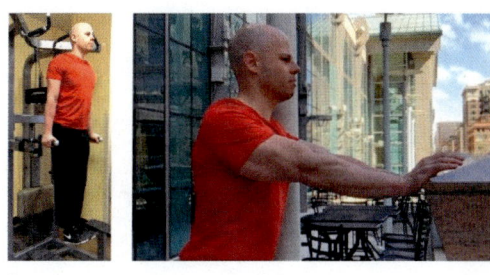

Pushing your hands into a ledge or countertop is a simple way to practice tension control along your push chain.

You may also find it helpful to practice keeping your muscles tense with your hands close to your torso. I find holding the bottom of a push-up position can be helpful for improving tension in the back and triceps.

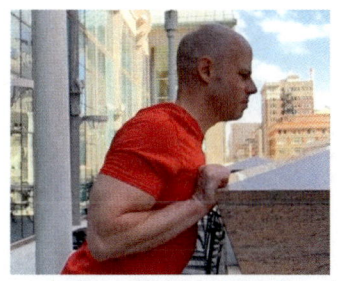

The tension in the back and triceps tends to decrease at the bottom of a push-up. Practicing an isometric hold at the bottom position will reduce the decrease in tension.

Overhead Reach

Some pressing moves involve extending your arms overhead which can feel very different from pressing your hands forward or down. This is why I recommend practicing some overhead reaching on a daily basis. Doing this helps improve tension control with your hand overhead while giving yourself a nice stretch in your back.

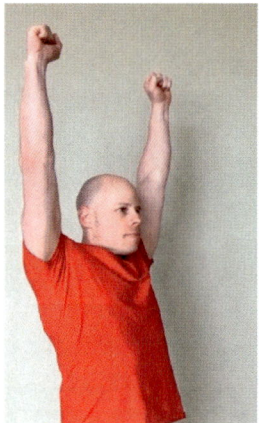

GOOOAAAALLLLL! I practice overhead reaching every day to improve tension in my shoulders while stretching out my lats.

Push-Ups

The humble push-up, or horizontal press, is the gold standard of push chain exercises. It's characterized by pushing your hands away from your chest as opposed to down toward your feet or above your head. You can progress this move many different ways to suit any fitness level.

Incline presses

This technique uses the angle to gravity element to adjust the resistance on your body. The more upright your body is, the easier the exercise becomes. The more you lower yourself to the ground the more difficult it is.

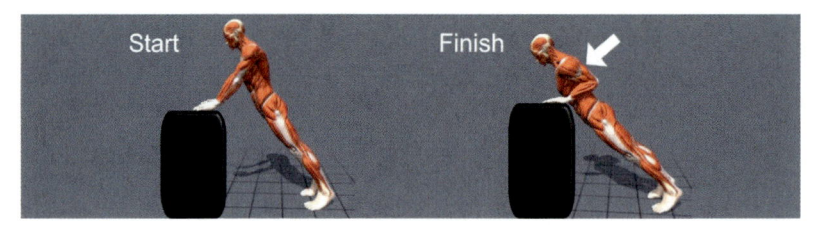

Incline presses are done against a sturdy object like a park bench or countertop.

Incline push-ups are a helpful tool for getting your body used to the movement. It's also good to use them as a sort of tuning shop to work on technical points like improving back tension or shoulder position. It's much easier to work on improving technique with a low level of resistance than trying to improve with a greater degree of resistance.

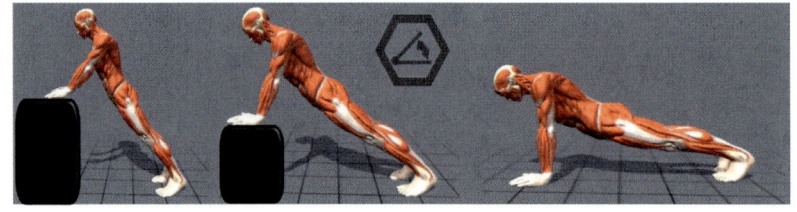

Incline push-ups are a good way to progress toward floor push-ups. Pressing against lower objects increases the resistance due to your angle to gravity.

Knee push-ups

Knee push-ups use the extension element to remove resistance on your arms. They also make the exercise easier on your core and shoulders.

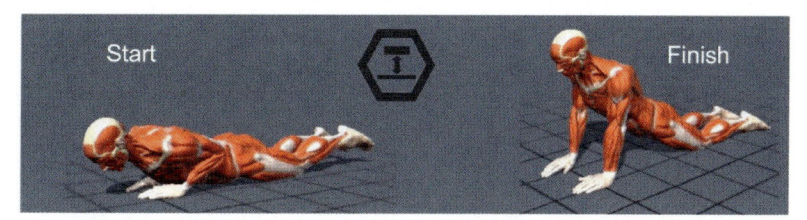

Knee push-ups are a perfectly legitimate push chain exercise. Like incline push-ups, they can be a useful tool for warming up, drop sets and technical practice even for the strongest athletes.

Some people find that going from the knees to the toes is a big jump. You can achieve a mid-level of resistance by placing one knee on the floor, and keeping the other leg straight.

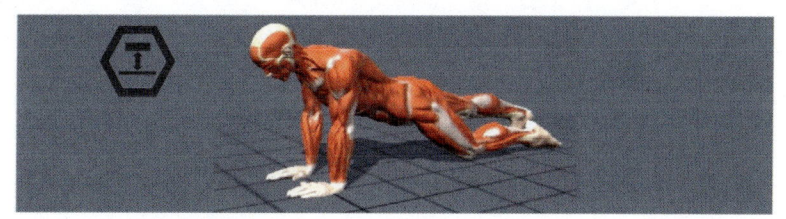

Keeping one knee down with the other leg straight is a good step to use between knee and toe push-ups. Be sure to complete the same number of reps on each side to keep a balanced workout.

You can also mix knee push-ups and push-ups on your toes. Just stay on your knees as you press off the floor, straighten your legs at the top and lower yourself to the floor while on your toes.

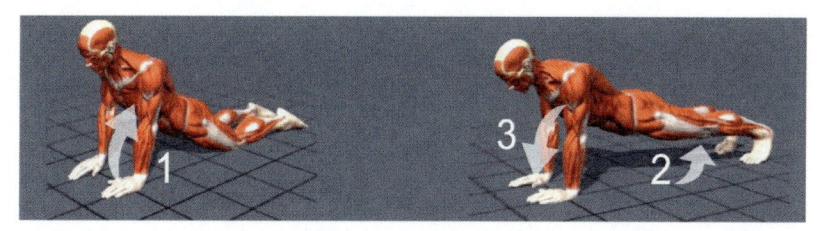

Doing push-up negatives is a simple way to get used to pressing your full bodyweight. First press up on your knees. At the top extend your knees into the full-length push-up position. From there, lower yourself down to the floor in a smooth and controlled motion. Place your knees back on the floor and repeat.

Close push-ups

These are often called triceps or diamond push-ups and involve pressing with your hands together to use the centerline element. The closer your hands get, the more range of tension, muscle control, strength and mobility you will need. Keep in mind that you don't need to jump all the way to a close push-up from a wider hand position. You can work inwards over time to condition your joints and technique.

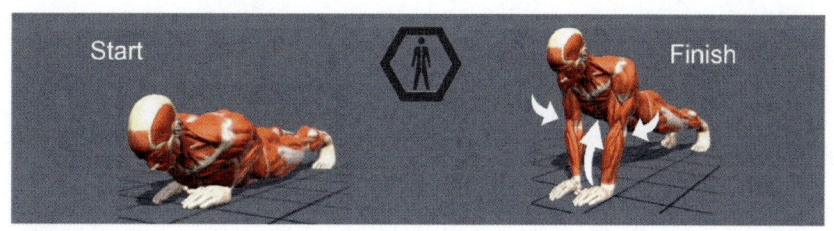

Press up against the floor while driving your elbows in to prevent them from "winging" out to the side. Pause at the top and lower yourself back down in a controlled motion.

Don't worry if you feel this movement mostly in the triceps at first. This emphasis happens when your triceps are the weak link in the push chain compared to your chest and shoulder muscles. Consistent practice of close push-ups will make your triceps stronger, and you'll spread tension throughout your entire push chain in time.

Close push-ups are the key to building exceptional muscle and strength for a couple of reasons. The first is more advanced push-ups use both hands underneath your chest rather than out to the side. Trying to do archer or single arm pushups with your hand out to the side creates a lot of torque and stress on the shoulder, spine, and hips. The closer you push your hand to your centerline the less stress you'll place on your joints while it also makes your muscles work harder.

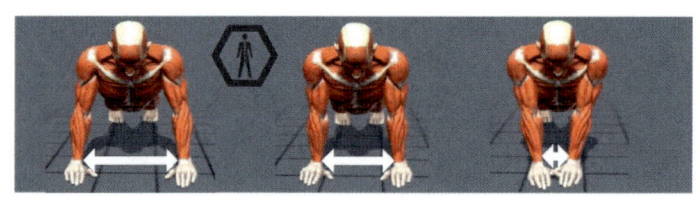

You can progressively move your hands closer together over time. This helps your muscles and joints get used to the close hand position over several workouts.

The second advantage of the close push-up is how it teaches you to pull your arm inward through using both your back and chest muscles. It's a little easier to keep your back tense when your hands are closer together.

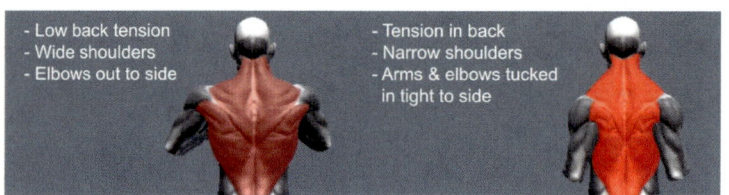

Close push-ups are a great tool for learning how to maintain a tight back and elbow position while doing push-ups. Learning this builds a solid foundation for more advanced push chain exercises.

Third, using a close hand position does a lot to improve your elbow position. One of the most subtle points of an effective push-up is learning how to bend your elbow back towards your hips. This motion reduces stress on the wrists and shoulders while improving tension in your chest and triceps.

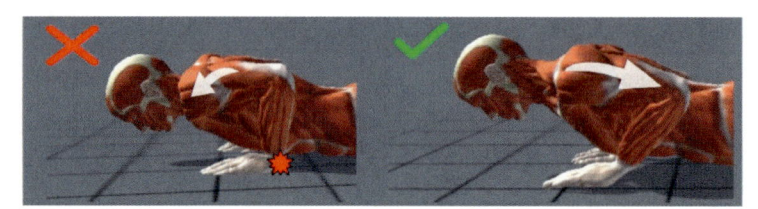

Pulling the shoulders and elbow back during push-ups prevents the shoulders from shrugging forward. This helps relieve stress on the shoulder and wrist joint while bringing more strength building tension to the push chain.

It's easier to do push-ups with your forearm vertical, so your elbow stays over your wrist. This technique is a lot easier to do with a wider hand position, but it's very hard on the joints when your hands are close together.

Unilateral push-ups

These moves use the weight shifting element to place more resistance on one arm at a time. They are "easy" variations of a one arm push-up where one arm is pressing, and the other is assisting in the exercise.

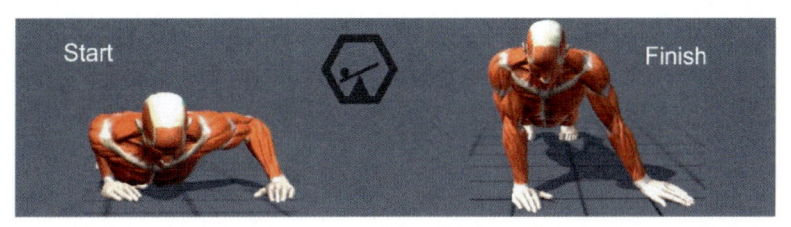

Unilateral push-ups use the weight shifting element to place more of your body weight onto one arm. The other arm now provides assistance to your primary pressing arm.

Progressing this technique is simple. The more you extend or remove support from your assistance arm the more resistance you'll place in your pressing arm. The most common example of unilateral push-ups is "archer" push-ups where you just stick your assistance arm out to your side like in the image above. It's also common to use a few simple tools to add some variety and different types of challenge. Let's explore some of them here.

Medicine ball push-ups

This technique involves using a small medicine ball, or a similar sports ball, to remove support from the assistance arm. This exercise becomes more difficult the further you place the ball away from your center line.

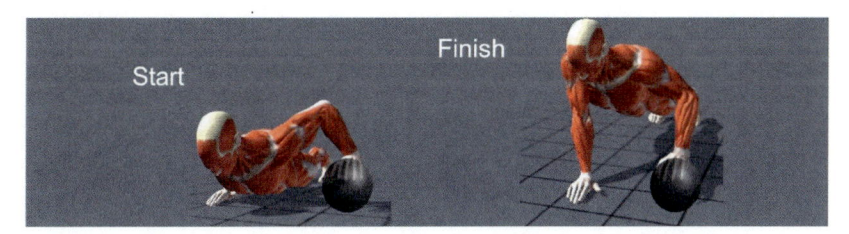

Begin in the bottom position with slightly more weight on your pressing arm. Push into the floor and extend your pressing arm fully. It's normal for the assistance arm on the ball to not fully extend since it's on an elevated surface. Pause at the top and lower yourself back toward the floor under control. You may wish to only lower yourself slightly below your assistance hand if you find it difficult to bring your chest all the way to the floor.

You can experiment with how low you lower yourself down when your assistance arm is elevated. In general, you may want to only lower your chest to the height of your assistance arm when it's close to your torso. Doing so will prevent you from excessive twisting at the bottom of each rep. You'll probably find this doesn't happen as much as your assistance arm extends from your center line.

I like using a ball on the assistance arm because you can adjust the resistance depending on where your hand is on the ball. Placing your palm directly on top allows you to push directly into the floor. Pivoting your hand to the front or back takes away some of the support forcing more tension into the pressing arm.

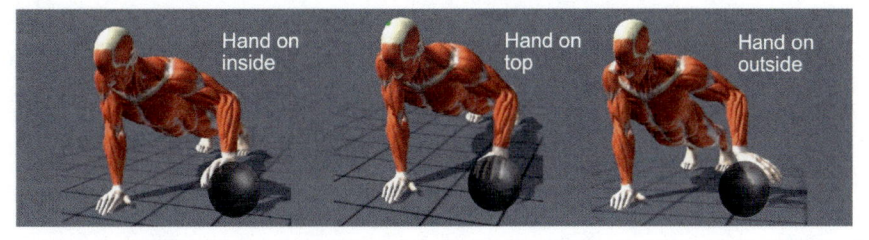

You can change the pressure on your assistance arm by positioning your hand to the front, or side of the medicine ball.

You can also apply a bit of internal or external pressure by placing your hand on the side that is closer or further to you. If you press your palm into the side away from you, you'll create a bit of inward tension. Pushing into the side closer to you allows you to press more weight onto your pressing arm.

You can also roll the ball slightly to change your hand position in the middle of a set. You might start out with your hand at an angle and then position the ball, so you press downward to make the exercise easier.

Suspension strap assistance push-ups

These are a lot harder than they look. Like a medicine ball, a suspended strap or rope will remove stability and make it harder to press off of the working arm. This technique is usually adjusted by how far your support arm is from your centerline.

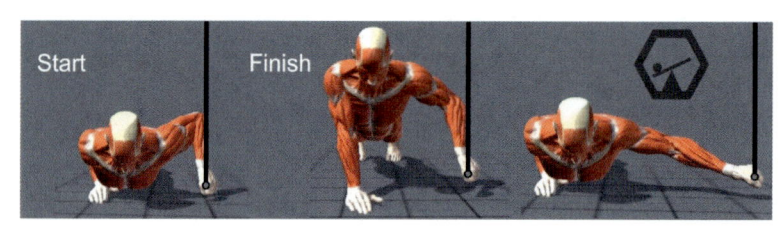

A common example of using a single suspension strap with unilateral push-ups. This example involves extending your assistance arm out to the side as you lower yourself down. You can also keep your assistance arm in close to your body to reduce the workload on your pressing arm.

Suspension straps have the advantage of applying some horizontal resistance or assistance depending on how vertical they are. Gravity is always trying to pull them into an upright position so you can use this to progress or regress unilateral pushups. Moving your body a little closer to the strap will angle the strap outward and put some inward pressure on your arms. Moving further away makes the strap tilt the other way and will pull your hands apart forcing more activation in the chest and back.

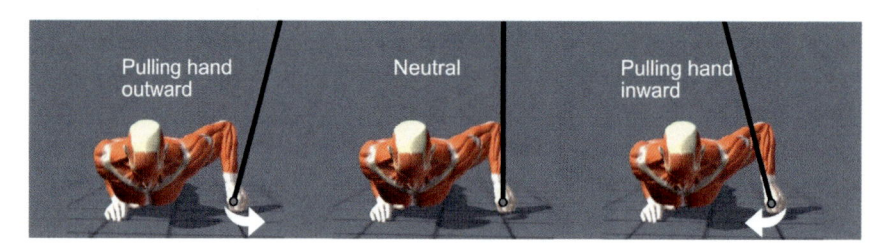

A suspension strap can provide horizontal assistance or resistance depending on where you place your body in relation to the anchor point.

Another advantage of the suspension straps is they give you the ability to move one arm out to the side and pull it back in again as you complete each rep. Whereas a medicine ball only allows a few inches of movement, straps give you the freedom to move your support arm all the way in and all the way out on each rep.

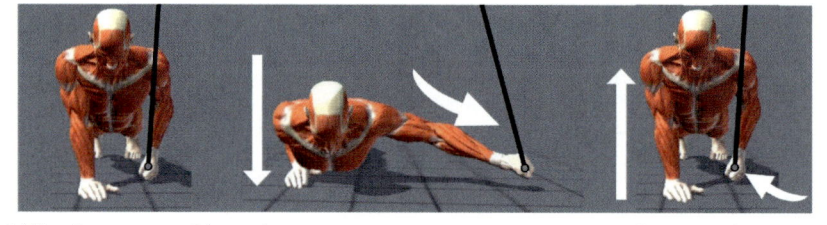

Moving the strap in the middle of a rep can add or subtract pressure on your assistance arm during each rep.

Moving your assistance arm in and out on each rep makes the exercise easier. The more time your support arm spends outward on each rep, the more difficult the exercise is.

Slider push-ups

Sliders are a more stable alternative to straps and medicine balls, but they do offer some degree of mobility. One of the advantages of using a slider is it gives you feedback about the weight distribution between your two arms. The more weight you have on the assistance arm, the more difficult it will be to move your hand. When you shift your weight more onto your pressing arm, you'll find it's easier to move the slider.

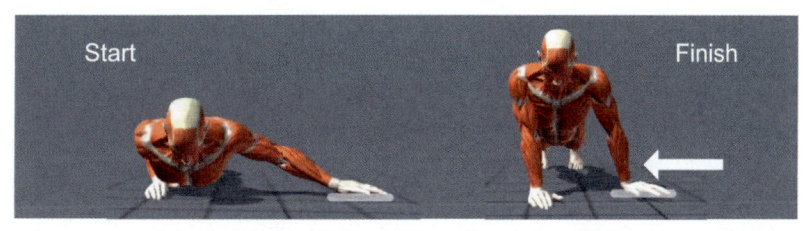

Friction can teach you a lot about your weight distribution during unilateral push-ups. Sliding your assistance arm on a towel or paper plate often works best.

You can use many everyday objects as sliders. Towels work well on hard surfaces like tile and wood. Paper plates work well for carpet and concrete.

Finger support push-ups

You can also remove support from the assistance arm by limiting the contact your hand has on the floor. You can press with your fist or fingertips. You can also reduce how many fingers are pushing into the floor for a greater challenge.

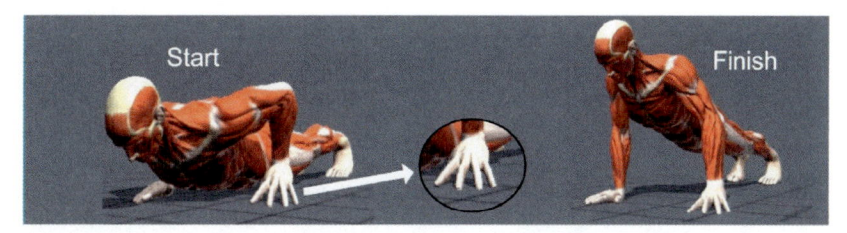

It's easy to add or remove support from your assistance arm just by changing how much of your hand is on the floor. A flat palm is easiest while pressing into your fingertips will be more difficult. Taking a few fingers off the floor will make it even harder still.

Vertical support push-ups

So far we've covered removing support by extending one arm out to the side. There are two more ways you can reduce support from an assistance arm. One is to extend your assistance arm out above your head, and the other is to extend it down close to your legs.

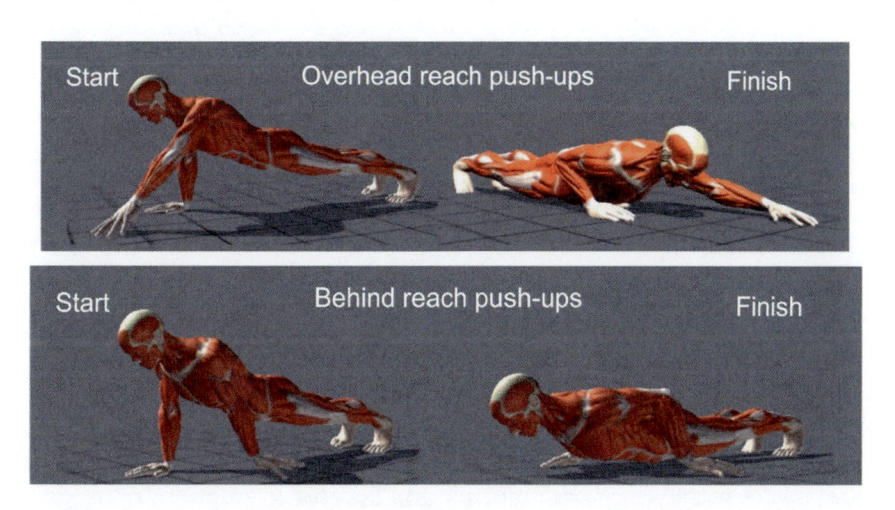

Both overhead and behind reaching push-ups will shift more weight onto your pressing arm while keeping your center of gravity close to your centerline since your assistance arm doesn't extend out to your side.

You can apply these approaches with any of the tools I mentioned before.

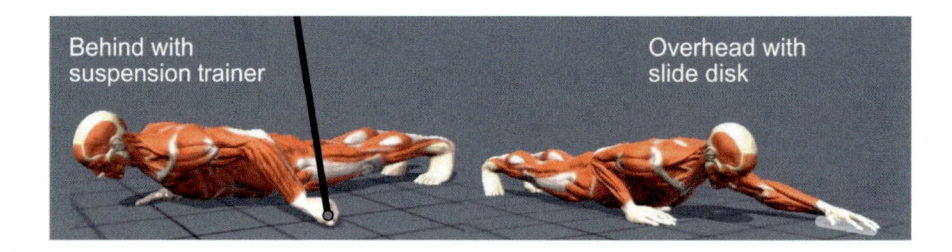

Single arm push-up

Single arm push-ups bring images of ultimate power to mind. They require a lot of muscle control, strength, and technical skill. Despite their elite status, you can progress and regress single arm push-ups to make them accessible to almost anyone.

Incline single arm push-up

I like to use an incline to introduce the single arm pushup. Using an incline not only removes some of the resistance against gravity, but it also reduces the torque on the torso. Just as with two arm push-ups, the more upright you are, the easier this exercise is.

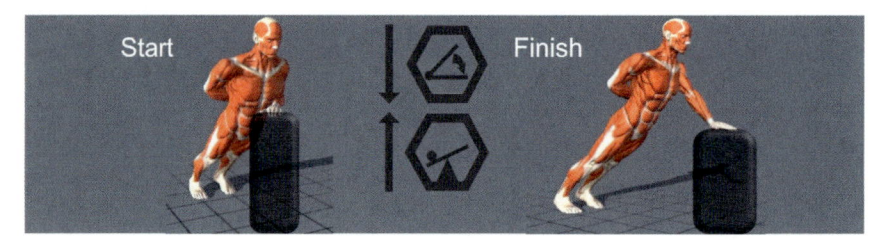

Incline single arm push-ups regress the angle to gravity element while progressing the weight shifting element so you can practice single arm pressing.

You can also play with this variation on a suspension trainer. Doing them with a single suspension handle can teach you a lot about keeping your shoulder blade and elbow in close to your torso. This is due to the natural torque the suspension strap creates by wrapping around your arm. The extra torque on the upper body is also why a relatively wide stance is used with this technique.

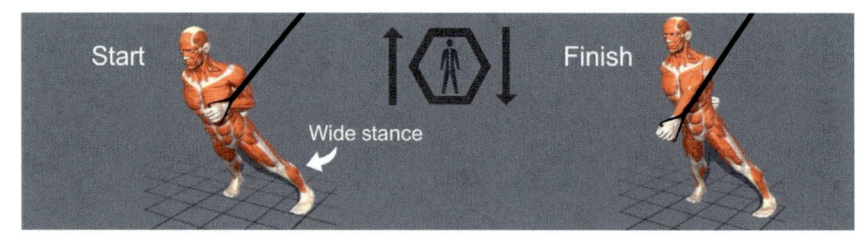

Single suspension strap push-ups progress your upper body centerline control. It's also common to use a wide stance to improve stability thus regressing the centerline element for the lower body.

Adjusting stance width

The width of your feet is another way you can use the centerline element to progress these exercises. Using a wider stance gives you more stability and control. Using a narrow stance requires your upper body to work harder to stabilize your position in space. You can make your push-ups even less stable by crossing your ankles, so you only have one foot on the floor.

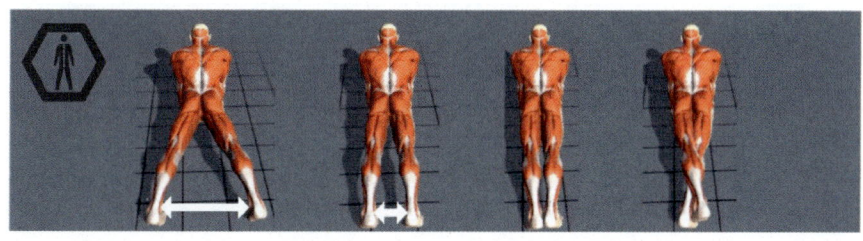

A wider stance provides more stability and makes your push-ups easier. The more narrow your stance the more your upper body will have to work to stabilize your torso.

Once again, you can apply this to a wide range of techniques including incline, single arm, assistance and close hand push-ups.

Dips

I have a funny story regarding dips. When I was 14, I was just starting to work out, and I was doing push-ups every day that summer. I thought I was in good shape until a friend introduced me to a cool new sport called bouldering. It was a simple sport where all I needed to do was get to the top of a large rock.

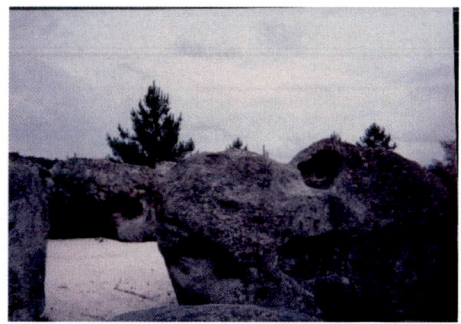

These van-size rocks where the first gym I ever joined when I was 14 and they are still some of the best pieces of equipment I've used.

The first time I made it up a rock I pulled myself onto the peak like some prehistoric creature crawling from the sea. Once on top, I stood up in triumph, only to be scorned by my friend. "That's not how you get on top; you can't touch the rock with anything but your hands and feet!" He then showed me the proper way by pressing himself up over the ledge by pushing his hands downward. He was then able to get his feet up onto the rock and stand up.

Throughout the afternoon I was able to make it to the top of a few boulders where I pressed myself up over the ledge in the proper fashion. The work didn't feel very hard, but I woke up the next morning feeling like my chest and triceps were saturated with battery acid.

It wasn't until I started practicing dips that I was able to figure out why I had such an extreme reaction to the bouldering. It turns out that even though my push-ups were a great exercise, the dip is in a league all its own. It requires a lot of strength, control, and mobility just to do a single rep. It is the squat of upper body exercises. Ever since then, the dip has been one of my favorite exercises.

Dip tips

Some people criticize the dip as being bad for the joints. Like all moves, dips are perfectly fine as long as you don't have any pre-existing injuries or conditions. Outside of any existing issues, pain and discomfort are almost always a sign that something is off in your technique and tension control. Chances are if there's an issue with your dip there's a similar problem with your push-ups. Here are a few points to keep in mind when doing dips.

Keep your shoulders down and back

Many dip problems come from a lack of tension in the back. Back tension is used to keep your shoulder blades from popping up and forward as you descend with both push-ups and dips. It's a good idea to warm up with some isometric holds at the top and bottom positions of a dip to dial in your back tension so your shoulders are stable before doing reps.

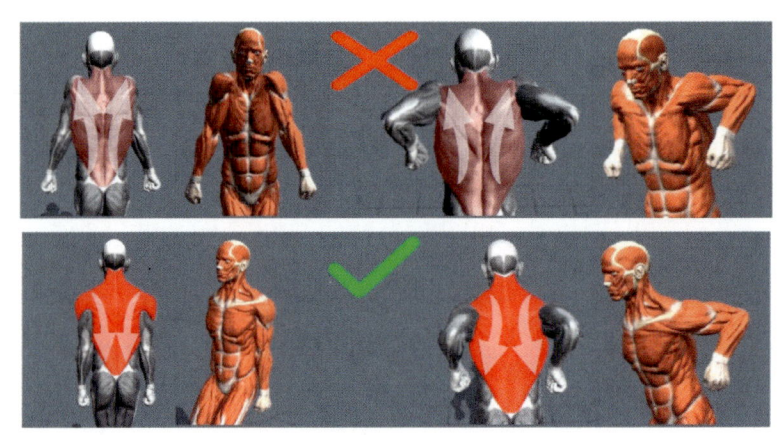

Maintaining tension in the back prevents the shoulders from popping up and forward. This not only reduces the stress on the shoulder joints but also drives much more tension into your push chain muscles.

Don't let your elbows flare out to the side

The other issue is allowing your elbows to "wing out" to the side too much. While some outward motion may be unavoidable due to the width of the bars you're using, try to squeeze your arms in toward your centerline throughout each rep.

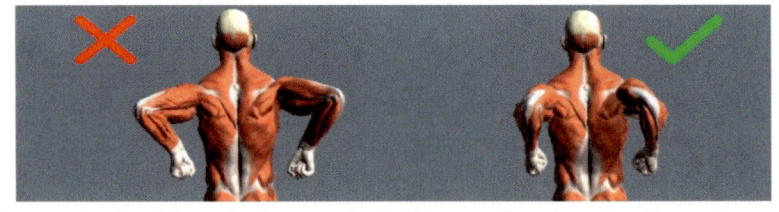

Both figures have roughly the same hand width yet the figure on the left has significantly wider elbows. Keeping your elbows the same width of your hands also reduces joint stress while helping you place more tension in your push chain muscles.

Push your elbows back

Bending your elbows back as you drop down can prevent you from leaning too far foward and ease stress on the shoulders.

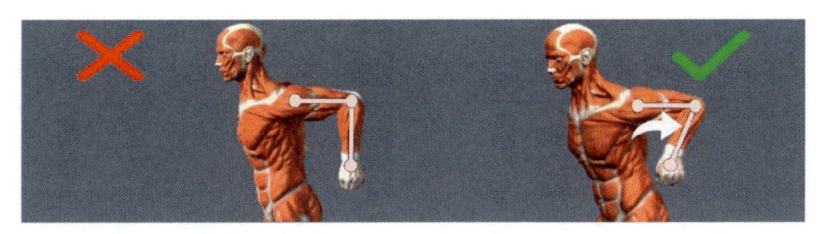

Just like with push-ups driving your elbow back, even slightly, can prevent joint stress and improve muscle tension.

Use the progression that's right for you

The common dip may not be a good fit for many athletes who need either easier or more advanced variations of the exercise to fit their level of strength. If dips are giving you an issue, you may just need to use an easier variation like the ones here.

Leg assist dips

Just like with pull-ups, you can use your legs to regress the resistance of dips. The more pressure you place in your legs, the easier it is for your arms to work. You can progress this by moving your legs behind you so you're pressing more on the tips of your toes. You can also cross your legs and then progress to single leg assistance.

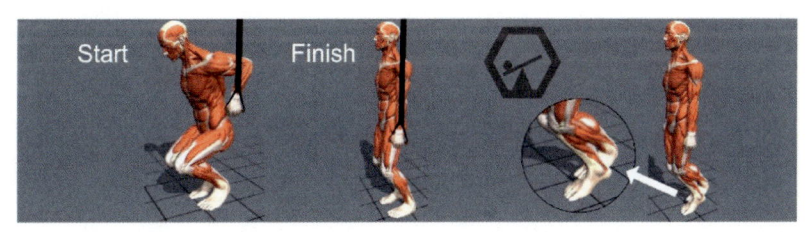

You can regress dips through the weight shift element by placing your feet on the floor or on an elevated platform like a plyo-box or chair. You can also adjust the height of your suspension handles so they are closer to the floor.

These are a great technique to fine tune your tension control skills. I still play with these to work on shoulder position and muscle control even though I can do plenty of dips with full bodyweight. They are also good for warming up and as a drop set after doing dips with your full bodyweight.

Where should your legs go?

Leg placement is something you can play with to suit what's best for your body and your environment. I like to pick up my legs sort of like retracting a landing gear on an airplane. This keeps my center of gravity close to my hips and prevents a lot of swinging back and forth.

If the dip bars are high enough, you can hang your legs straight down. Doing this can help you know if you're moving in a vertical motion. You'll create a pendulum effect if your weight moves too far forward at the bottom of each rep.

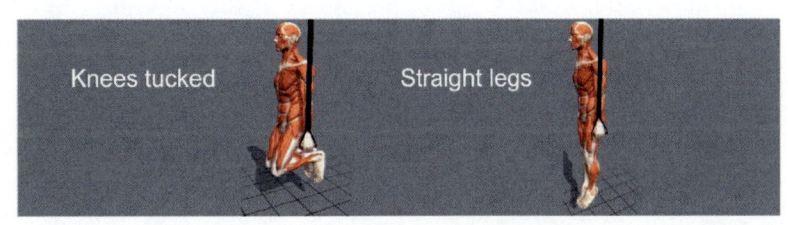

Keeping your legs straight or tucking your legs up helps you keep your body vertical without excessive forward leaning or rocking.

In general, I don't recommend letting the legs hang back as this has a tendency to cause the upper body to move forward a lot at the bottom of each rep. This isn't necessarily bad or wrong, but it can place more stress on the shoulders while robbing you of the vertical movement against gravity.

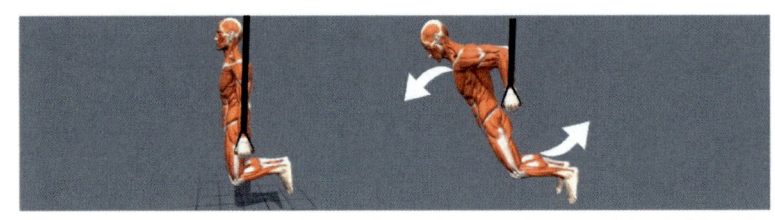

Keeping your legs behind you tends to make your upper body rock forward as your legs reach back. I find this can be a less effective technique compared to moving your body more vertically.

Whatever you do with your legs, be sure to keep some tension in your core and lower body to improve control over body position.

Torso angle

Some coaches teach that altering the angle of the torso during dips can influence where you place tension in your muscles. Leaning forward places emphasis on the chest while keeping upright works the triceps more. I say if you want more tension in your chest or triceps then just focus on controlling your tension and put it in those muscles. You can get a lot more tension in a muscle on a consistent basis by improving your tension control skills rather than messing around with funky angles.

I encourage you to use the technique that you feel the most comfortable using. I like to have a slight forward tilt as I descend in the dip and I extend myself fully upright at the top of each rep. Experiment and see what feels best for you.

Leaning excessively forward may also be a sign of stiff shoulders. Try holding a bench dip position while keeping your spine vertical to stretch out your shoulders. This will help stretch the front of your shoulders and improve mobility.

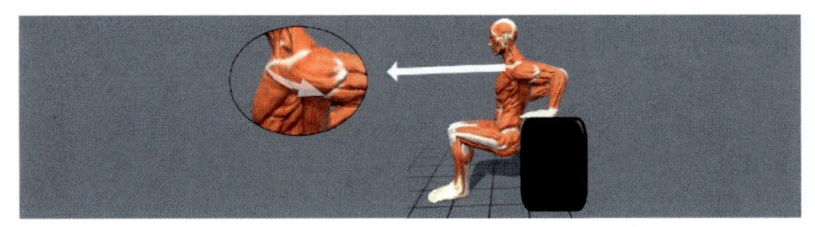

An isometric bench dip is a good way to stretch the front of the shoulder. Press your hands into a surface that's about waist high and lower your hips straight down so they stay close to your hands. Keep your weight on your feet while pushing into your hands at the same time. Remember to pull your elbows toward each other rather than let them flare out to the side. Hold for 15-30 seconds.

Strap/ ring dips

Doing dips on suspension straps or gymnastics rings is a fun yet humbling challenge. The lack of stability requires a lot more tension in your muscles with each rep. If you're concentration breaks for even a second, you'll instantly know it by the movement of the straps.

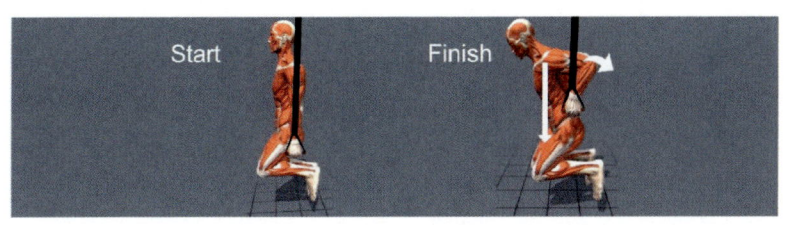

Dips on rings or suspension straps can challenge every aspect of your push chain including your strength, mobility, and stability.

Strap dips also give a tactile cue about where your elbow is during the dip. It's much easier to imagine leading backward with your elbow when you push your elbows behind the straps on each rep.

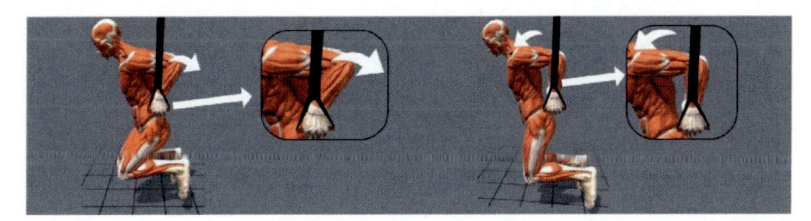

The vertical strap can provide tactile feedback about your elbow position and movement during dips. Keeping your forearm in line with the strap means your torso needs to move forward as you descend. Moving your elbow behind the strap allows your torso to move downward.

The straps also keep you honest about how much inward tension you're generating in your back. When your arms flare out to the side they rub against the straps which lets you know you need more tension in your back.

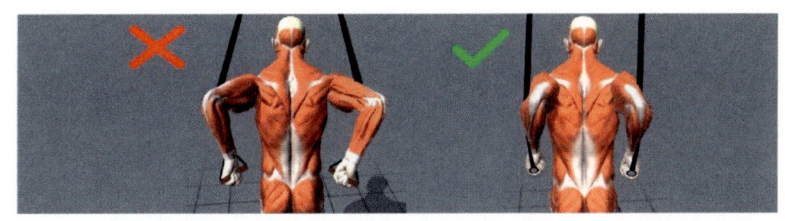

Straps provide tactile feedback on the width of your elbows while doing dips. You'll feel your arms press and rub into the straps when your arms are too wide. Pulling your arms in will improve the quality of your dips while reducing abrasive rubbing against the straps.

Another benefit of strap dips is they give you the freedom to adjust the height and width of the handles to best suit your needs. This adjustment comes in handy for leg assisted dips or full dips without having to jump up into position. Throw in the fact that rings and suspension straps are essentially portable calisthenics gyms and you can see why they are one of my favorite piece of equipment. I'll be sharing some of my favorite DIY suspension trainers later on.

Single bar dips

Doing dips on a single bar is a real challenge because the bar prevents you from lowering your torso between your hands. This position requires a lot of tension control in your arms and back to avoid excessive rounding of your shoulders and outward flair of your elbows. It's also a challenging position for your triceps. You'll need to allow your legs to reach forward as you descend to maintain balance.

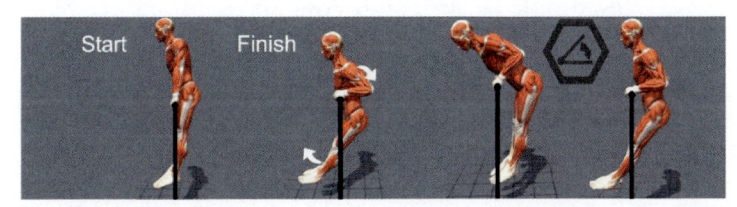

Straight bar dips are always a challenge since your torso is always behind the bar. You can tilt your body to adjust the resistance through the angle to gravity element. The more upright your torso is the more difficult the exercise becomes.

Ledge dips

I used to work in a building that had an elevated loading dock for trucks. I liked to do dips off the edge of the dock because the wall prevented my feet from moving forward like they would on a straight bar dip. I also found a lot of value in placing my hands flat on the floor of the dock as opposed to holding onto a bar.

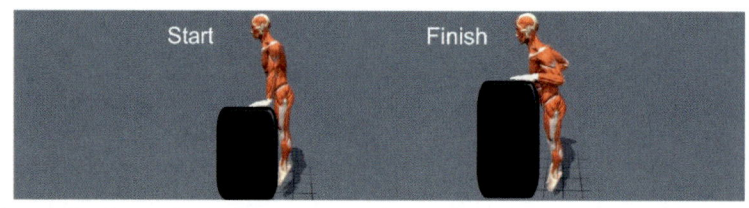

Ledge dips don't allow your legs to flex forward to balance your weight on your hands. This forces all of your weight to remain behind your hands which creates a lot of resistance on your push chain. Start at the top of the ledge with your legs hanging straight down. Lower yourself off the ledge in a slow and controlled motion being careful not to catch the front of your body on the ledge or wall. It's normal for the toes of your shoes to rub against the wall. Pause at the bottom and press yourself back up over the ledge.

Be sure you're not using a ledge that's too high off the ground so you can easily land on your feet after your last rep. Also, watch out for sharp edges or exposed nails on the surface your feet are sliding on. You wouldn't want to drag your legs up against anything sharp.

Handstands

Handstands are some of the most impressive bodyweight exercises in the calisthenics universe. They are also very potent for building a strong muscular physique. Unfortunately, they can be a little intimidating for some folks, like me, who feel uncomfortable being upside down. The following techniques can help you feel more comfortable with pressing yourself into an inverted position.

Wall bracing

This exercise can help you feel more comfortable with tilting your body upside down. Start with your hands on the floor and your legs facing a sturdy wall. Lift your hips and place one foot on the wall behind you. Brace yourself by pushing one leg into the wall and then place your other leg on the wall.

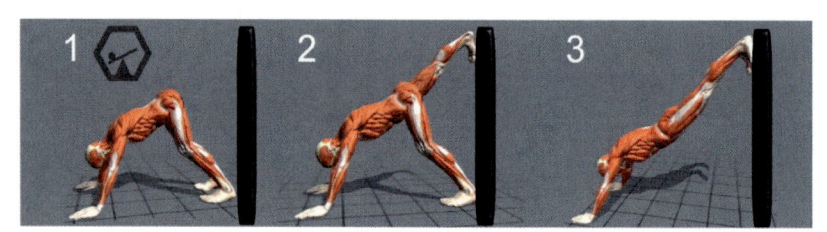

Wall bracing uses the weight shift element by shifting your weight onto your hands. Start about 3 feet from a sturdy wall and lift your hips up while keeping your arm straight (1). Reach one leg up to the wall behind you and push it into the wall by pressing your hands into the floor (2). Once you're braced bring your other foot up on the wall and hold that position for time (3). Be sure to step back down on the floor in a controlled motion so you don't slide down the wall and crash your feet into the floor.

Progressing this move is as simple as adjusting your angle to gravity by placing your legs higher up on the wall. The higher you place your legs, the more weight you'll load onto your arms.

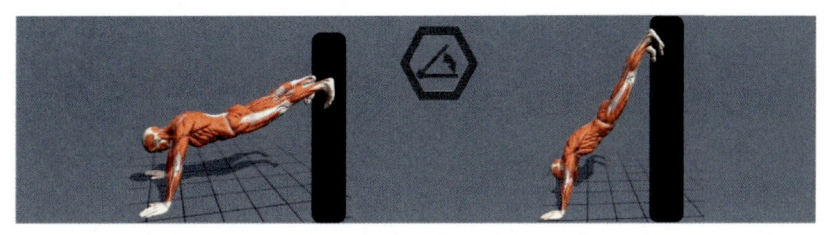

The higher you place your feet on the wall the more your upper body will work due to the angle to gravity element. Note that your hands will also have to be closer to the wall the higher you place your feet.

Perform this exercise as an isometric hold, but avoid going to failure and holding yourself up as long as possible. Always bring your feet back to the floor under control before your arms become too tired to hold you up. Crashing down on top of your head is not a good way to finish a workout.

Wall Walking

Walking up the wall requires you to shift your weight onto one arm while "stepping" with the other. It also allows you to get yourself into a steeper angle than you might achieve with wall bracing.

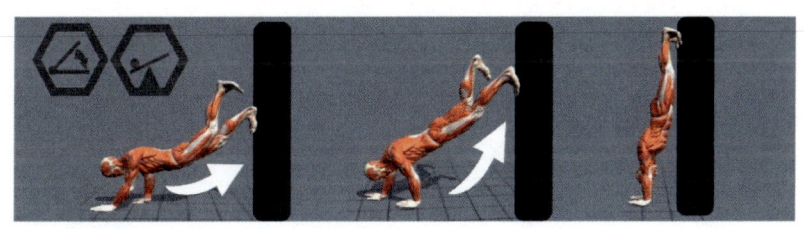

Wall walking uses both the weight shift and angle to gravity elements. This is because you're shifting your weight from one arm to the other as you walk yourself up into a vertical position against gravity.

Just as with wall bracing, the higher you go, the more of your weight you'll place on your arms. Walking up also requires a lot more shoulder control since you need to balance on one arm at a time.

You'll want to deliberately step with both your legs and arms as you move up and down the wall. Don't let your legs slide down as you walk down with your arms. Try your best to walk in smooth and deliberate steps. The same fatigue rule as with wall bracing applies here as well. It's fine to walk up and hang out for a while in an inverted position. Always make sure you have plenty of energy to walk back down in a smooth and controlled motion.

Speaking of safety, be sure to keep your breathing deep and relaxed at all times. Holding your breath in an inverted position can be dangerous. Lastly always allow your feet to come back to the floor in a controlled motion. Slamming your feet back onto the floor can be very hard on your feet and can increase your risk of injury.

Kick-Up Handstands

Kick-up handstands involve facing the opposite direction of wall bracing and walk-up handstands. In some ways, kicking up into a handstand is a bit safer because you can quickly return your feet to the ground after each set.

Kicking up is usually done by pushing one foot off the floor while keeping the other one straight to provide some upward momentum.

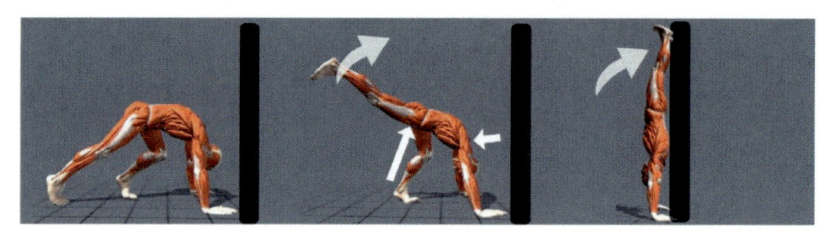

Kick up handstands use one leg (right) to swing up onto the wall while the other (left) remains bent to push off the floor. Start with your hands about 6-12 inches away from the wall. As you kick with one leg and push off with the other keep your upper back tense to flex your shoulders. Press up into the handstand with your shoulders and upper back while lightly leaning on the wall. When you're done, be sure to bend your legs so your feet gently come back to the ground rather than falling hard to the floor. As with all calisthenics, grace and control are the cornerstones of good technique.

Remember the P.T.R strategy with handstand work. Make sure your arms, chest, shoulders, and back are tense before kicking up. Doing so will make getting into a handstand much easier and safer.

Handstand push-ups

Holding a handstand position as an isometric will certainly help you build muscle and strength. Remember, tension is tension even if you're not moving. With that said, doing reps allows you to use the speed and ROT elements to generate more muscle tension.

I've found it's a lot easier to start with a short range of motion at first and build your range over time.

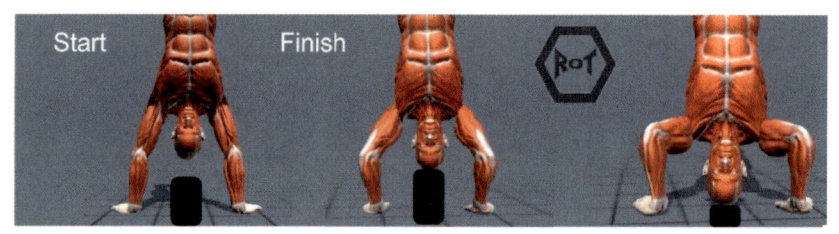

Handstand push-ups don't have to be done to the floor. Gently lowering the top of your head to an object, like a yoga block, allows you to progress or regress your range of tension depending on how low the block is. Be sure to always "kiss" your head to the block rather than hit it.

Progression is simple. The closer you lower yourself to the floor, the more range of tension you create making the exercise more difficult.

Handstand push-ups typically involve letting the elbows flare out to the side a lot. Flaring elbows makes the exercise easier, but can place more stress on your joints. It's good to torque your arms in as much as you can. Think of squeezing your elbows in toward each other. This inward motion will make the exercise harder, but it will also be a lot more effective. You'll also notice this will make it easier to create stability in your back and chest.

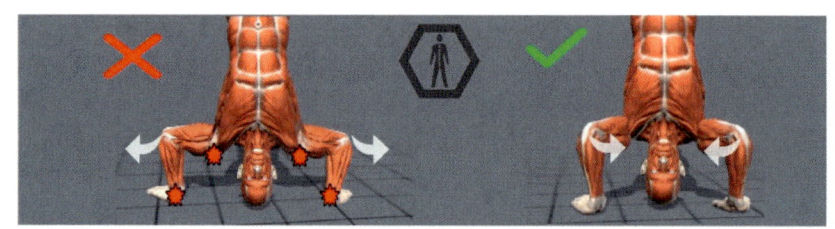

Keeping your upper back tense and driving your elbows inward will prevent excess stress on your wrist and shoulder joints. It will also make the exercise more difficult since you're progressing the center line element so regress your range of tension if necessary.

Handstands are a great shoulder exercise but don't forget about the rest of your push chain plus your back and core. A solid handstand also requires a lot of forearm tension and hand strength to "claw" the floor. I like to imagine pressing into the ground with each of my fingertips as hard as I can. Keeping tension in your hands will improve stability even if you're doing handstands against the wall. The tension in your lower arm is also helpful when doing pushups and will ease the stress on your wrists.

Keep your traps turned on

Shrugs with heavy weights are not the only way to build up your upper traps. Putting tension in your upper back will improve shoulder stability while bulking up that mountain range on the top of your torso. If you don't feel your upper traps working it could be because your elbows are flaring out to the side too much. Pull them in a bit, and your upper back should light right up.

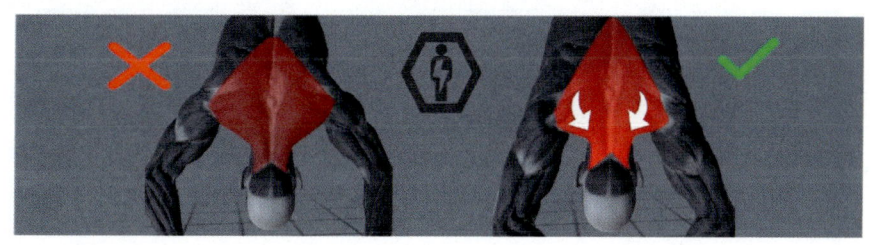

Keeping tension in your upper back through driving your shoulders toward your ears improves handstand stability and upper back strength.

Narrow handstand push-ups

Just as with horizontal pushing moves, you can progress handstand push-ups by using the centerline element to bring your hands and elbows closer together.

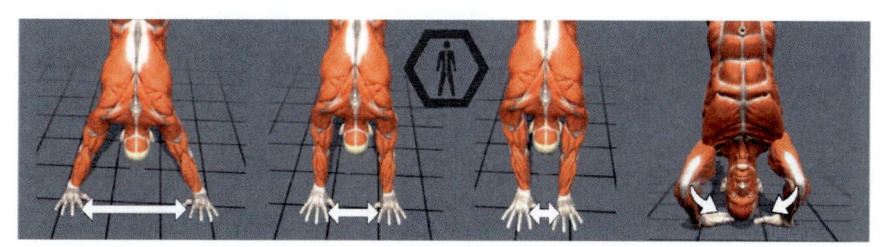

Narrow handstands use the centerline element to increase the difficulty of both isometric handstands and handstand push-ups. Be sure to also drive your elbows inward as well.

Unilateral handstand push-ups

This technical variation move is where you'll use the weight shifting element to place more resistance on one arm over the other. You can start with using a fist on the floor with one arm, or even your fingertips to "weaken" your assistance arm to force the pressing arms to work harder.

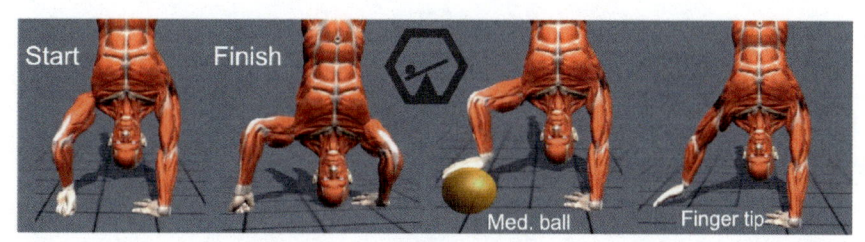

Unilateral handstand push-ups use the same basic techniques as unilateral push-ups. Placing your assistance arm at a mechanical disadvantage forces more weight onto your pressing arm. You may even use the same tools like medicine balls, sliders and finger pressing.

Feel free to experiment with the width of your feet while doing unilateral handstand work. The wider your feet are the more stable you'll be.

One arm handstand push-up

The single arm handstand push-up is a serious strength exercise. It requires a lot of strength, as well as shoulder stability and core control. It's common to use a corner while doing this to help stabilize your body.

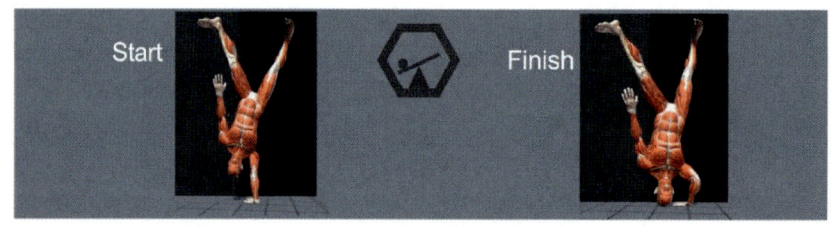

Single arm handstands and handstand push-ups require a lot of strength and stability. Doing them in a corner can help with your stability and control so your pressing arm can work more efficiently. Setting up is done by kicking up into a standard handstand and shifting your weight onto one arm while bracing with your back, core and leg muscles.

To balance or not to balance?

Sooner or later you'll have to decide if you want to pursue handstands against the wall or do them freestanding. Both variations work very well for building muscle and strength. After all, you'll have to create more tension in your muscles when you remove an external support like the wall. The lack of support is why freestanding moves are more challenging and require more muscle tension. When doing handstands against a wall, you have more support, so you don't have to use as much muscle tension to perform the exercise. That's why you'll be able to do more reps or hold for a longer period of time. Working on the wall can also make it easier to work with advanced techniques. You'll have to regress to easier handstand variations if you want to use for free-standing work. Either way, you'll still build muscle and strength so use the variation that best appeals to you and your goals.

What About Your Upper Chest?

One of the most common questions I receive is how to work the upper chest with bodyweight training? A popular solution is to do push-ups with your feet up on a ledge to achieve a similar motion as an incline bench press.

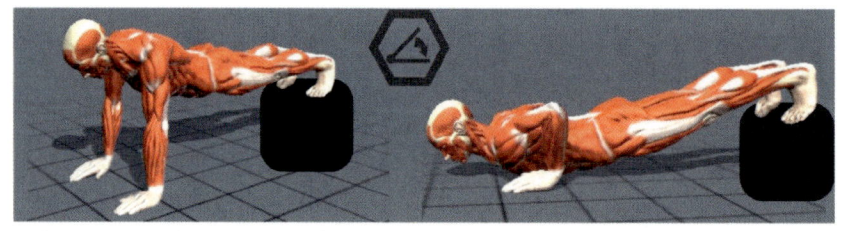

The "incline push-up" is a classic way to change your angle to gravity so your upper chest is slightly lower to the ground. This is one of the most common ways calisthenics athletes try to isolate their upper chest muscles.

While this is certainly a viable technique, let me show you something that may make such incline work unnecessary in the first place.

Advanced press work, especially single arm pressing, requires a lot of tension in the entire chest from top to bottom. Your chest muscles must always work hard to keep your arm close to your torso throughout the rep. This continuous adduction causes tension to flow through your full pectorals.

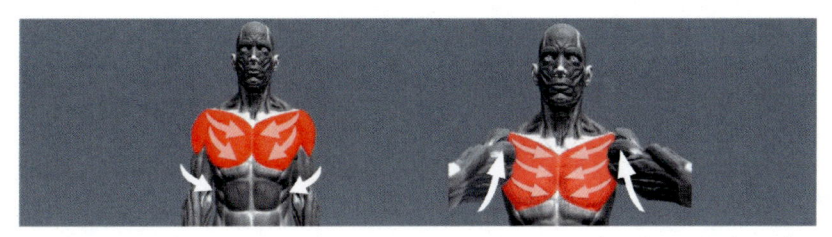

Using the chest muscles to maintain arm adduction through a pressing motion creates a lot of tension throughout your entire pectoral muscles.

The use of the chest to create adduction as a form of stabilization is what makes progressive push-ups and dips such a powerful way to build up the chest. These moves involve a little bit of upper arm adduction, but the chest is heavily worked to create stability first and mobility second. This type of approach creates not only complete activation of your entire chest but it also prevents excessive stress on your shoulders.

The other common pressing technique is to let the elbows flare out to the side rather than close to the torso. This style of pressing is sometimes used with push-ups but it's much more common in weightlifting methods especially when it comes to the bench press motion.

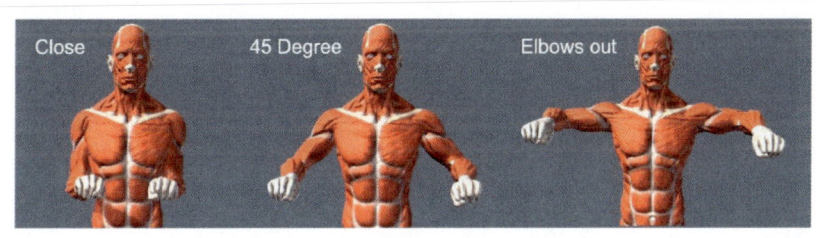

Common upper arm positions for pressing motions. Keeping the arms in tight uses the chest for stability first and mobility second. Flaring the arms out to the side uses the chest for mobility first and stability second. The 45-degree angle is a happy compromise for many athletes.

Pressing with the elbows out to the side changes the job your chest muscles perform during a pressing motion. Now, instead of using your pecs for stability they are being used to create (rather than maintain) adduction of your upper arm to press your hands away from your torso. The theory behind this is your chest will get a better workout if it uses adduction for mobility rather than just stability. There is certainly some merit to this strategy as I used to use it for years myself, but it comes with some significant disadvantages.

The first disadvantage is the leverage created on the shoulder joint. Abducting your upper arm away from your torso can create a lot of stress on your shoulder. Martial artists have understood this idea for centuries and use techniques that involve adducting an opponent's arm to cause harm.

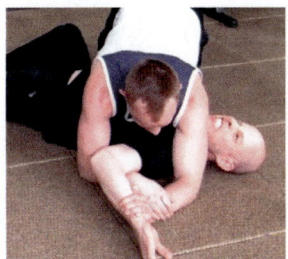

My friend uses my outstretched arm to demonstrate a classic arm-bar technique.

The second cost to this position is working with the arm out to the side may create some emphasis on where you place tension in your chest muscle.

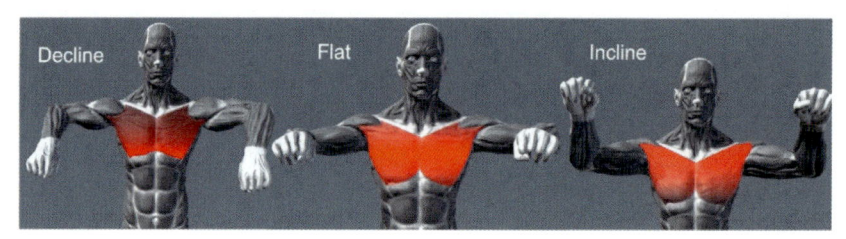

All press motions work your chest as a whole, but press angle theory is based on the idea that pressing at various angles can emphasize certain areas. Most of this is based on the idea that flaring your arms out to the side may create this emphasis while also turning down the tension in other areas of the chest.

While flaring your arms may very well create an emphasis in one area of your chest, it also means you lose tension in other areas. This fragmented training makes pressing at various angles necessary to cover all of your bases.

The ultimate solution isn't to find a bodyweight exercise that mimics the incline press. Instead, the answer is to pull your arms into your sides, so you return to using your chest for stability. Doing this causes you to flood your entire chest with tension while creating a more stable environment for your shoulders.

By all means, play with some incline work. It can be a fun challenge but do your best to turn on your whole chest with all push-up and dip variations. You'll probably find you won't need any additional incline work to build a thick chest from top to bottom.

Accessory Moves for Push Chain

The primary pushing moves in this chapter are all you need to build your chest, shoulders, triceps and more. However, there are a few moves that can be fun to use. As with all push chain exercises, be sure to place tension in the chest, shoulder and triceps as well as your back with each of these exercises.

Triceps extensions

These are one of my favorite moves to place emphasis on the triceps. They are still a type of push-up only now you're primarily moving through straightening your elbow while your shoulder remains stable. There are many variations of this exercise and here are a few of my favorites.

Floor triceps extension

You can do triceps extensions on the floor in a similar fashion to the push-up. Start off placing your full forearm on the floor, so both your hand and elbow are touching the ground. From there, press your hands into the floor and push yourself up while straightening your elbow. You can progress this exercise just as you would progress any other push-up variation.

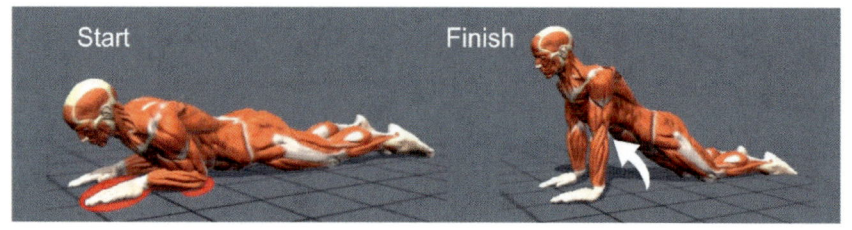

The floor triceps press is most often done on the knees since you're using less muscle and therefore strength than a traditional push-up. Start at the bottom position on the floor with your elbows on the ground as well as your hands. Press your hands into the floor and lift your

elbow off the floor to extend your arm as you press yourself up. Pause at the top and lower your elbow to the floor in a controlled matter. For safety, be sure to lower your elbow back to the floor and let it "kiss" the ground rather than hit it.

Another way you can progress is to place your hands on a ball or block so your elbows can drop below the level of your hands.

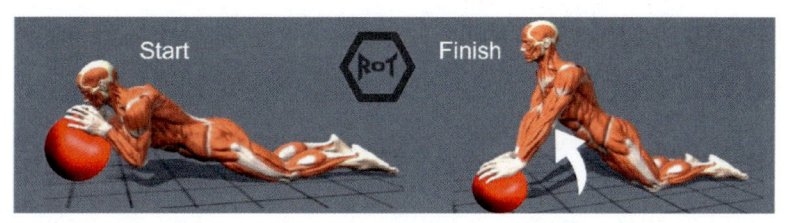

Doing elbow extensions on a medicine ball or block can give you a greater range of tension since your elbows can drop below the level of your hands.

Strap triceps extensions

Suspension straps are a great tool to use for triceps extensions. They don't require getting on the floor, and you can progress the resistance by stepping back a few inches to use the angle to gravity element.

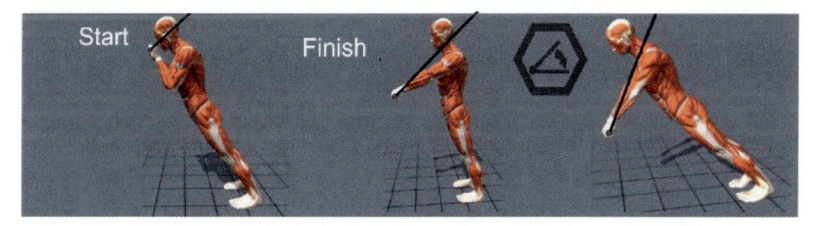

Suspension strap triceps extensions are simple and effective. You can quickly adjust the difficulty through the angle to gravity element.

Chest Flies

Chest flies use the upper arm in the same fashion I mentioned earlier where you point your arms out to the side. It's for this reason that you'll want to use these chest flies with moderate resistance to protect your shoulder while ensuring you have plenty of supportive tension in your back.

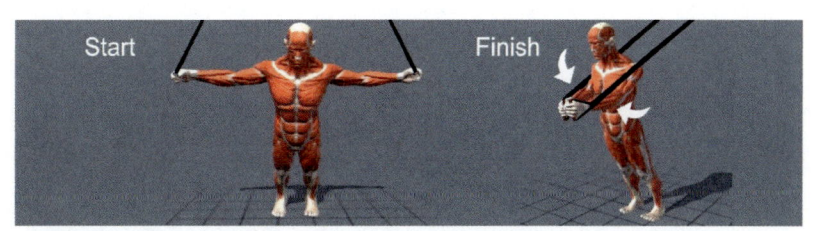

Start with your arms out to the side so you know how much resistance to use in your weakest position. Keep your back tense and your shoulders down to prevent your elbows from rotating forward. Keep your body tense as you press yourself up by bringing your hands together. Pause and lower yourself back down in a controlled motion.

Some people like to do super wide pushups which mimic the chest fly activation in your chest. You don't get much range of motion with this move, but that's okay. It will still light your chest up even if you're holding this position as an isometric exercise.

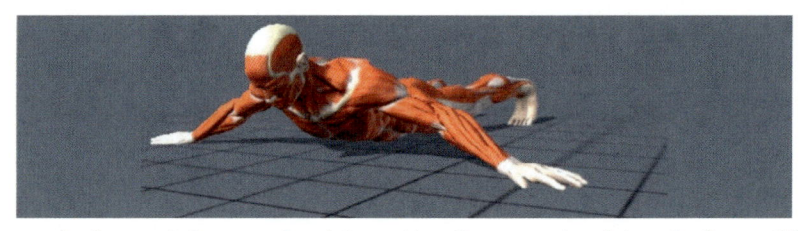

Start with your torso resting on the floor and place your hands in position. Press your hands into the floor to lift your torso a couple of inches and hold. Be sure to gently lower yourself back to the floor rather than crash down.

Y-flies

This exercise does the job of 4 separate dumbbell shoulder exercises. It works the shoulders like front raises, lateral raises, rear flies and upright rows all at once. It's also easier on your shoulder joints

Set up is easy. Just lean slightly back on a pair of suspension straps that are anchored together. Arch your back slightly and pull your arms up and out without bending your elbows. Think of extending your arms up like you're making the "Y' in the YMCA dance. Be sure to keep your upper traps tense for a complete shoulder and upper back exercise.

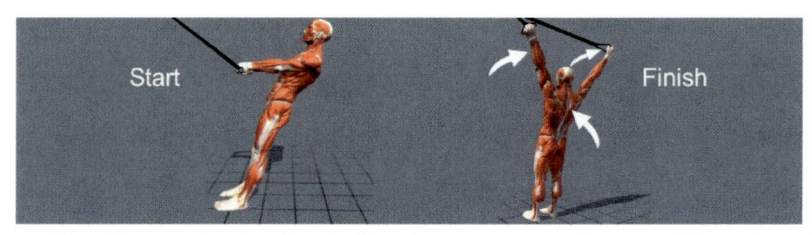

Y-flies are a great supplemental shoulder exercise. Just lean back against some suspension straps like you're going to do a set of curls or rear deltoid flys. Slightly arch your back and pull your arms up and slightly out so you resemble an uppercase Y. Be sure to slightly shrug your shoulders up to get some extra tension in your upper traps. Pause at the top and bring your arms back together and in front of you in a controlled motion.

Fingertip pressing

Pull chain grip exercises work the lion's share of your hands and forearms, but there's still the extensors in your hand to consider. Fingertip pressing will work your extensors and the other side of your forearm, so you build a robust lower arm, wrist, and hand.

You can apply fingertip presses to any push-up variation you like. All you need to do is spread your hand and press your fingertips into the floor with your palm about an inch off the ground.

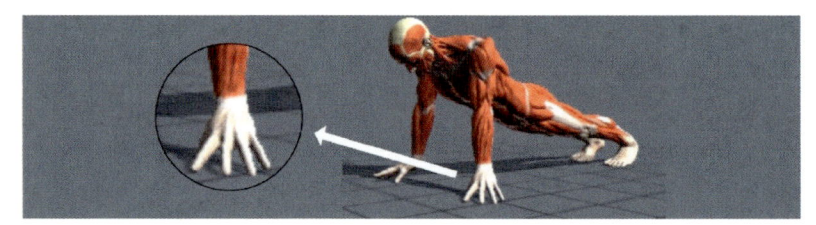

You can turn any pressing exercise into a forearm and hand exercise by spreading your fingers and pressing your fingertips into the floor. You can do this both with your palm on the floor or elevated for an extra challenge.

Imagine pressing your fingers outward and tensing the back of your hand and fingers. Some people even start off with just keeping their palm on the floor and pressing into their fingertips to get the idea. They'll then progress to variations with the palm raised off the floor.

Just like with pulling grip work, you can practice this move as an isometric or a dynamic move. You can do fingertip push-ups for reps, or just press into your fingertips and hold a plank position for time.

Points To Ponder

1. Most pushing exercises require a lot of tension in the back to stabilize your shoulder and elbow. This is why it pays to keep at least a little tension in your lats and traps.
2. Watch for elbow "circling" as you press up. Try to squeeze your elbows inward as you press to place more tension in your pushing chain.
3. Pay attention to the tension control in your flexion chain during push-ups. This especially goes for tension in your abs to prevent your lower back from sagging.
4. Play with the direction you point your fingers during close push-ups. Some prefer to point their fingers inward at a 45-degree angle while others point more forward.
5. Look out for "tenting" your hands during push-ups. This happens when you place more weight on the outside of your palms causing the inside of your hand to pop up like a tent off the floor. Squeezing your elbows in while pressing into the inside of your hands will prevent this.
6. Experiment with scapular movement during push-ups. In general, push your shoulder blades apart at the top of each rep and pull them back and together at the bottom.
7. Watch out for rounding your shoulders forward toward the bottom of push-ups and dips. Instead, feel like you're pulling your shoulders away from your ears.
8. Try not to reach forward with your chin. Keep your neck in a neutral position or look up slightly during push-ups.
9. Pay attention to the tension in your upper back, abs, and glutes while doing handstands. Full body control is important for stability even while doing handstands against a wall.
10. Practice pausing at the bottom for a full second to improve tension control especially during dips.
11. Avoid bouncing out of the bottom position and push-up smoothly rather than in a sudden jerky motion.

Chapter 11 Flexion Chain

I started the exercise section of this book with the extension chain because I believe it's one of the most important, yet neglected, areas of the body. As we head toward the end of this section it's high time to do the opposite and address one of the most overused, and abused muscle groups; the flexion chain.

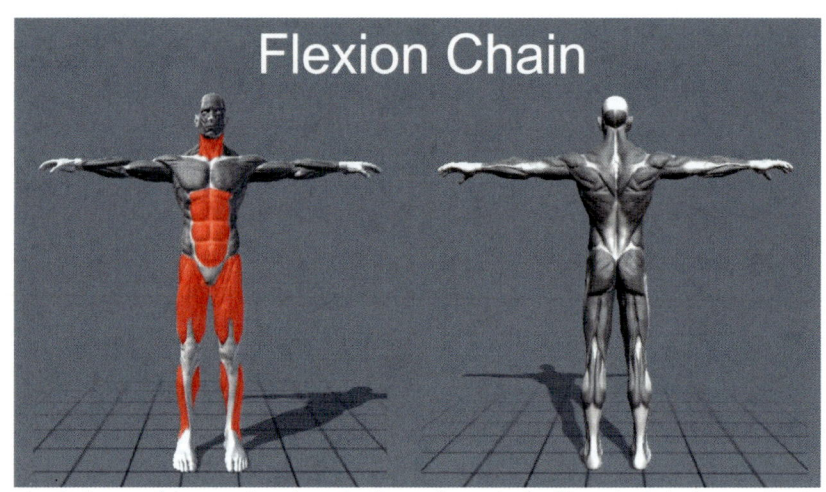

Your flexion chain is comprised of most of the muscles along the front of your body. These include the muscles in your shins, quads, hip flexors, abdominals and even the muscles on the front of your neck.

Not that the flexion chain isn't important, it is. I fully agree with experts who claim the "core" is a key muscle group for health and performance. I've just long felt the desire for a strong core, and the instructions on how to achieve it were separated a long time ago. Maybe it's because the pursuit of a strong midsection became more about aesthetics than function. Perhaps there's just too much light-weight information out there about how to achieve a six-pack in 4 weeks or something. Whatever the case, one thing is certain. While a strong core is aggressively pursued, modern abdominal training has been disappointing people for a long time.

3 Flaws In Modern Abdominal Training

Effective core training is hardly rocket science, but modern ab training methods fall victim to the following three trends.

#1 Pick relatively easy exercises

Effective abdominal training isn't different than training any other muscle group. You want to place a progressive amount of tension in your abs for an increasing amount of time. Unfortunately, many ab training methods make use of light-weight exercises that fail to put enough tension on the muscle to be very effective.

#2 Train for many reps and sets for high volume

Doing exercises with low amounts of tension goes hand in hand with using a lot of volume. Being able to do hundreds of crunches or holding a plank for long stretches of time will not make you very strong. It just eats up a lot of time and effort while offering little in return.

#3 Use a wide variety of exercises

Few muscle groups are more fragmented than the core and abs. There are exercises for the upper abs, lower abs, and the middle abs. Even your oblique muscles on the side of your belly require separate exercises. This high degree of fragmentation has given rise to the popularity of using many different abdominal exercises that eat up your time and energy.

These three flaws in modern abdominal training are the reason why many people feel they need entire core workouts and 300-page books with complicated routines. It's all an attempt to compensate for the lack of muscle tension that's required to train your abs sufficiently. The good news is you can escape these ineffective methods by practicing old-school core training techniques.

Old School Abs

Effective core training is simple and efficient. You don't need a lot of different exercises nor do you have to spend hours in the gym plowing through endless reps and sets. Expensive fancy equipment is also not required. All you need to do is flood the front half of your body with a lot of tension to work the muscles in your abs, hips, and legs.

As with all muscle chains, the key is to flow your muscle tension along the full chain. While many of these exercises are considered abdominal movements your abs are just one link in the full chain. Bringing some tension through your hips, quads and shin muscles will help you gain more from the exercises in this chapter.

Turning On Your Flexion Chain

Seated flexion

Seated flexion is a simple isometric exercise that will improve your abdominal tension control. Sit in a chair with your back straight and your hands on your knees. Press your hands into your knees through flexing your abs and hips. Hold for about 3-5 seconds and then relax. Try not to round your back or move your shoulders.

Seated abdominal flexion is simply using your abs to press your hands into the top of your legs.

Standing flexion

Standing flexion is the same idea as seated flexion only now you're pressing your hands down into a table or countertop. Once again, try to make your hips and even your quads tense so you can engage your entire flexion chain.

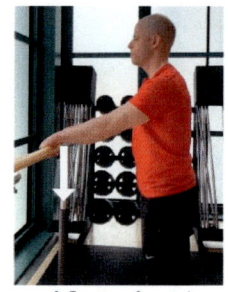

Standing abdominal flexion is the same idea as seated flexion but it's easier to also place tension in your hips and quads.

Cat cow exercise

The classic cat-cow exercise is a dynamic exercise that focuses on spinal movement so you can understand how to increase the range of tension in your abs without too much resistance against gravity.

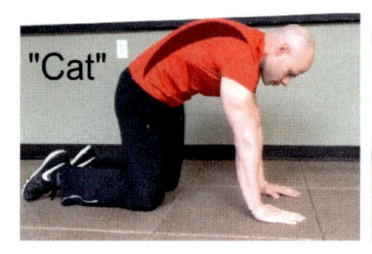

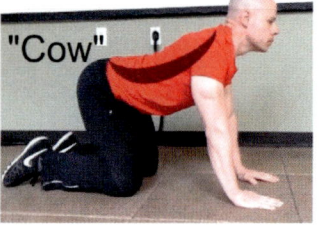

I recommend flexing your abs and hips in the "cat" position first. From there, see if you can maintain the tension in your abs as you extend your spine into the "cow" position. Hold there for a second or two and then return to cat position. Cat-cow is also a great exercise to warm up with before your core workout to wake up your abs and improve tension control.

Shoulder and back tension

As with other muscle chains, your back plays a supportive role for your flexion chain. You'll probably find that keeping your back tense will help bring more tension to your abs especially while doing exercises that involve your upper body.

So even though the following exercises are about working your core, be sure to keep your lats tense and to torque your arms inward to tense the muscles behind your shoulders. This will also help alleviate stress on your lower back.

Isometric Holds

Isometrics are very popular when it comes to core training. Part of this is because it's easier to control the tension in the muscle when you're not moving. The other reason is your abs and core muscles play a supportive role in many athletic activities while most of your mobility comes from your hips.

Hollow body hold

The hollow body hold is a great isometric exercise for honing your muscle tension skills. It's also a helpful way to learn how to use your abs to control the position of your pelvis while allowing your legs to move independently at the hip joint.

Start off with laying on your back and tuck yourself up into a ball position by contracting your abs and hips.

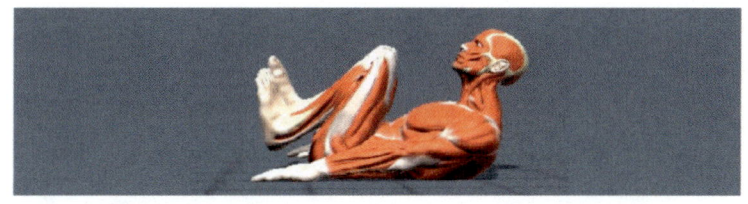

The lying tuck position is one of the easiest position to hold while maintaining tension in your hips and abs. Make sure you keep breathing while holding this position for time.

The next step is to rest your upper back and head on the floor while still keeping your abs tight enough to press your lower back into the floor. Press your hands into the floor to keep your upper body tense. This position will slightly stretch your abdominals, and you'll find it a little harder to maintain tension in the muscle.

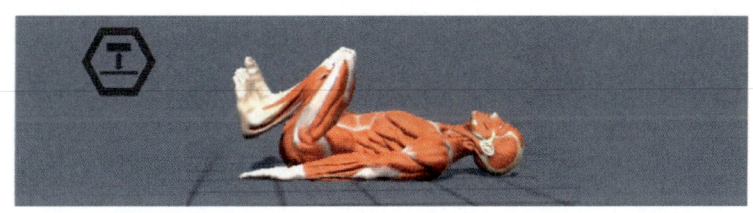

Resting your upper back and head on the floor slightly extends your back. Doing this makes it a little more difficult to maintain tension in your abdominals while also controlling your pelvis so your lower back doesn't lift off the floor.

Once you can lay on the floor, while maintaining your abdominal tension, you can use the extension element with your legs to increase resistance. You can do this by extending at your hip joint, knee joint or both. When you extend at your knees, you straighten your legs to create a longer lever. When you extend your hips you lower your legs to the floor which requires more strength and abdominal control.

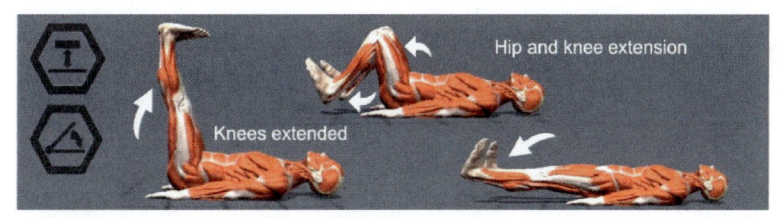

Extending your knees out uses the angle to gravity element while lowering your feet closer to the floor uses the angle to gravity. Both of these elements are used to progress the hollow body hold and challenge your ability to maintain supportive tension along your flexion chain.

Your objective with these exercises is not to merely bring your legs close to the floor or make your legs straighter. It's to use leverage to challenge your ability to pull your pelvis upward with your abs.

Planks

The plank is one of the most popular isometric core exercises. You can do it anywhere, it mimics push-ups, and you can progress them from very easy to insanely difficult.

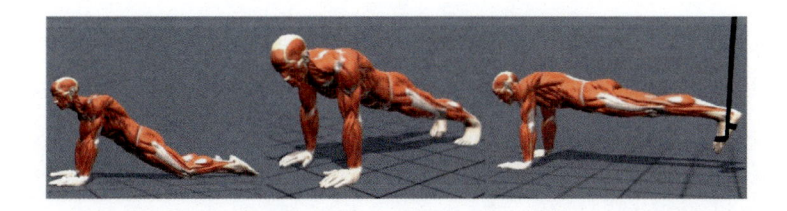

The common plank is one of the best isometric flexion chain exercises. It's easy to set up and offers many progressive variations.

Knee Planks

Knee planks are a good exercise to start with because they are only slightly harder than the cat cow exercise. It's also a good way to get a feel for keeping your abs tense in a plank position while using your core to squeeze the floor together between your arms and legs.

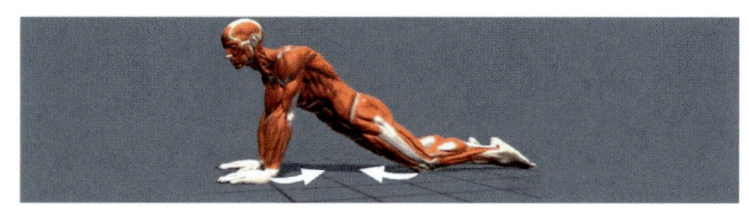

The knee plank is a good exercise to start your flexion Chain Training. Even if it feels easy, it's still a good exercise for improving tension control along your flexion chain and the supportive muscles in your back. It's also a helpful way to get a feel for using your abs to pull the floor together between your upper and lower body just as you do with bridging.

Toe Planks

Toe planks are the typical plank most people think of when they imagine doing a plank. It uses the lever length element to add more resistance to the exercise.

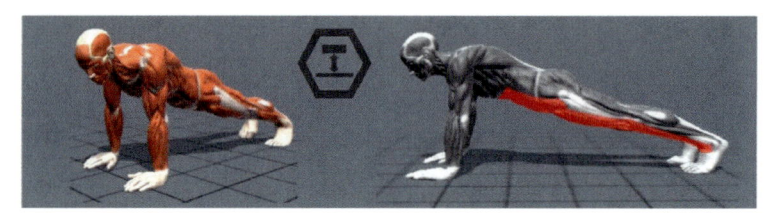

The standard toe plank, or plank, is a great way to dial in the tension along your flexion chain while improving stability in your shoulders, hips and back.

Reach out plank

Once you're comfortable with doing planks on your toes, you can start to reach out with your arms to extend your body and add resistance. The further you reach out the more difficult the exercise becomes.

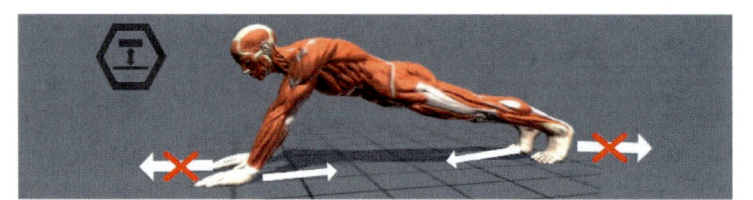

Reach planks continue to use the extension element to progress the resistance on your flexion chain. Be sure you're still trying to press your hands and feet into the floor and together instead of pushing them apart.

Reaching out requires a lot of tension in your back to support your shoulders. The tension is similar to the type used with pull chain exercises like rows and pull-ups, only now you're using your back to prevent shoulder flexion instead of creating shoulder extension.

You can also progress any plank variation through the centerline element depending on where you place your hands and feet. A wider hand or foot placement will be easier due to the wider base of support.

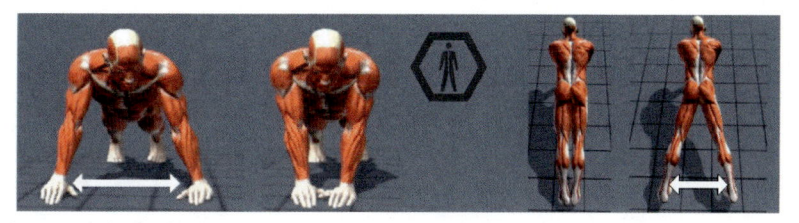

You can use the centerline element with planks the same way you would use it with push-ups. You can adjust the width of your hands, feet or both to reduce your base of support which makes your flexion chain work harder to provide stability.

Slider and strap planks

Removing friction can be a fun way to make your planks more challenging. When your hands and feet are on the floor, friction helps stabilize your body. Removing friction means you eliminate some of the friction between you and the floor so your flexion chain needs to work harder.

You can get a feel for this type of training by placing your feet on a towel or slide disk.

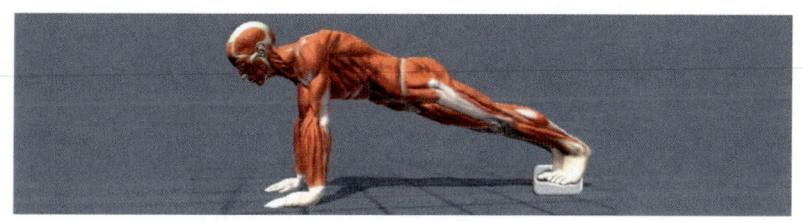

Doing planks with your hands or feet on a semi-slick surface can help you learn how to squeeze the floor together.

Suspension handles can work with both your hands and feet. They remove all friction from half of the plank and make holding yourself up a real challenge.

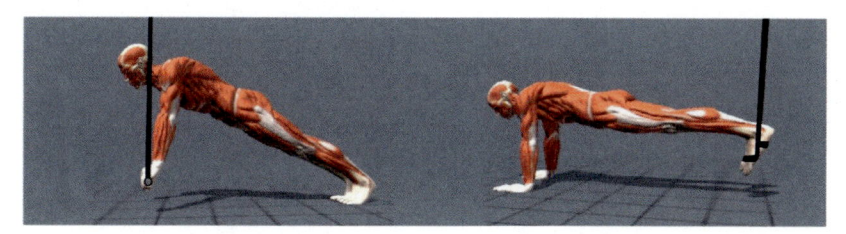

Suspension strap planks can be very humbling, yet telling, as they will expose any weaknesses along your flexion chain and upper body.

Another advantage of using suspension trainers is they can add or remove resistance depending on their relationship to gravity. Since gravity pulls the straps to a vertical position, you can slightly angle the straps outwards to help pull you together.

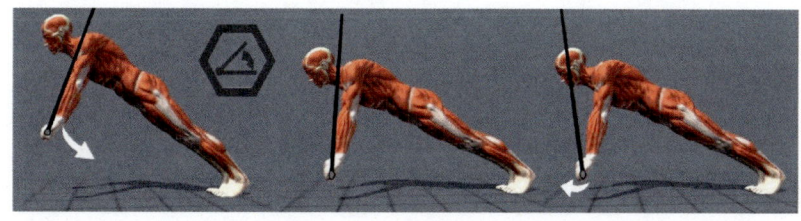

You can use the angle to gravity element to adjust the difficulty of strap planks. Stepping forward reduces your resistance on the handles while the straps want to swing back toward your feet (left). This effectively gives your flexion chain a bit of an assist in keeping the tension between your hands and feet. Moving your feet back reduces this assistance (center). Moving back, even more, causes the straps to pull your hands away from your feet which forces your flexion chain to work harder to prevent yourself from getting stretched out (right).

This strategy also works with using your feet in the suspension straps. Moving backward allows the straps to assist you in pulling yourself together while moving forwards makes you fight the straps.

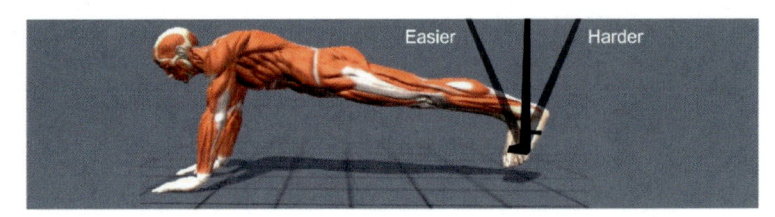

Angling the straps toward your torso uses the suspension trainer to pull your hands toward your feet. This makes the plank easier. Doing the opposite and angling the strap away from your torso will make your flexion chain work harder to support your body in the plank position.

Sit-Ups

The sit-up has fallen out of favor with many experts. While shunning this exercise has reduced the amount of injury and discomfort it's a classic example of tossing aside a perfectly good exercise due to poor execution. Sit-ups are perfectly safe and effective for your flexion chain, provided you avoid these common pitfalls.

The sins of the sit-up

The first sin is not having enough abdominal tension control. Unfortunately, you don't need good tension control, or even much abdominal strength to sit-up from a lying position. There are plenty of other muscles along your flexion chain that force you to sit-upright even if your abs are relatively weak. One of the most notable is the psoas muscle which can act as a hip flexor. This muscle attaches from your femur and runs across your hip and pelvis to attach to your lower back.

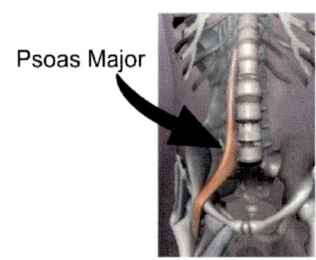

Your Psoas Major muscle runs across your hip and over (although sometimes through) your pelvis to attach to your lumbar spine. It's one of the primary reasons why people can experience low back pain while doing core work.

Your psoas pulls against your lumbar spine as you flex your hip. This is not an issue if your abs have enough tension to balance the stress on your lumbar spine. If you don't have enough tension in your abs, your psoas will create pressure on your lower back.

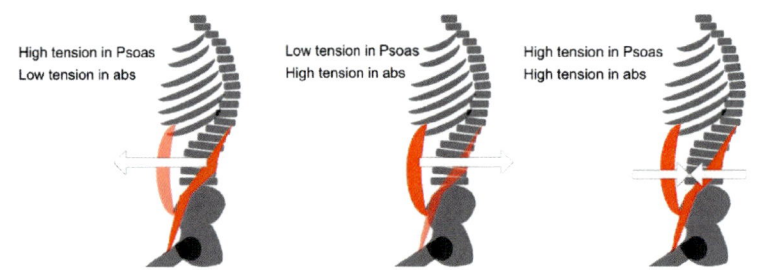

High tension in the psoas can pull your lumbar spine forward which can feel stressful on your lower back (left). Too much tension on just your abs can pull your lumbar spine back which can also be problematic (center). Balanced tension on both the abs and psoas creates balanced pressure in the lumbar spine (right).

Some experts recommend trying to decrease the tension in the psoas or even find a way to turn it off if possible. In theory, this should reduce the stress on the lower back since the psoas isn't pulling on it anymore. Unfortunately, it also means you're creating more fragmented muscle tension along your flexion chain.

I've found that it's counterproductive to turn off your hip flexors, including the psoas. If anything, I recommend getting your hip flexors to activate as much as possible. You want those muscles to work and become stronger. Hip flexion is important in many functional movements like running, kicking and stepping up. So instead of trying to turn your hip flexors off, it's better to learn how to turn your abs on more and make them stronger. You'll restore the healthy balance between your psoas and abdominals which will not only reduce pressure on your lower back but will strengthen both muscles as well.

The next sin is the tendency to lock the legs in place when doing sit-ups. Holding the legs isn't always a bad thing to do, but it's a strategy that's easy to abuse. Preventing movement in the lower body can stress the lower back and hips depending on how you do the exercise. It's especially risky for activities that involve twisting and explosive movements.

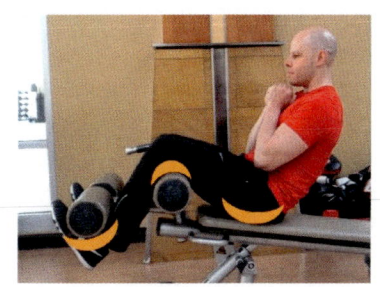

Using a classic sit-up bench locks the ankles, knees, and pelvis in place (orange). Doing this makes it difficult to move your lower body as needed to avoid stress on the lumbar spine. The issue is only compounded with explosive and twisting movements.

The third sin is using far too much volume. Some sit-up routines involve doing many reps, even hundreds of them at a time. People boast about doing 1,000 sit-ups in a day or over the course of a week while ignoring poor form and discomfort in the back.

The real problem isn't sit-ups. Any exercise is going to be unsafe and ineffective when you combine volume and excessive joint stress. The solution isn't to stop doing sit-ups but to learn how to do them safely and effectively.

How to do safe and effective sit-ups

Sit-ups require a lot of strength and control, not just in your abs but your whole body. I recommend starting with mastering slow negative reps first. Begin in the top position of the sit-up with your legs straight out in front of you and exhale while slowly lowering your upper body to the floor. Roll over to your side and return to the start position for the second rep. Doing this will help you fine tune your neural code to do sit-ups in a smooth and controlled fashion.

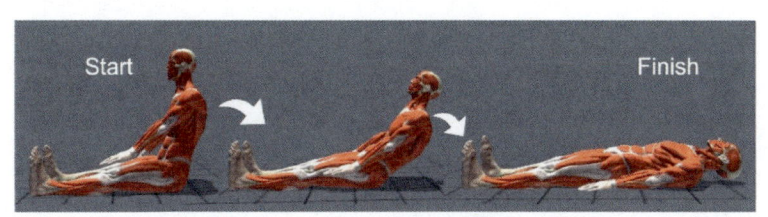

Start seated in an upright position with your legs straight out in front of you. Slowly round your back while lowering your torso down to the floor. Maintain tension in your flexion chain the whole way down and lower yourself in a slow controlled motion. At the bottom, roll over to your side and sit back up to do another rep.

Once you can comfortably control at least eight negative sit-ups, you can work on sitting yourself back up. Be sure to take a breath at the bottom position, tense your flexion chain and exhale as you smoothly lift your torso off the floor. Pause and breathe in at the top before exhaling and lowering yourself back down.

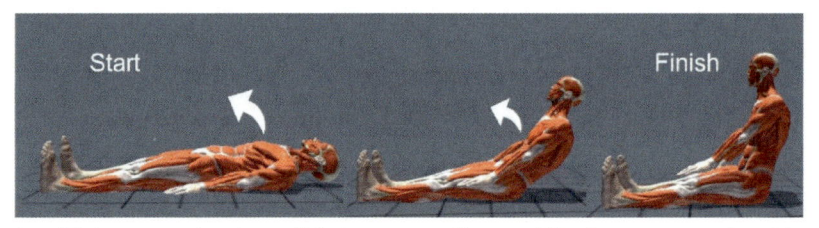

Sitting back up is the opposite of doing a negative sit-up. Exhale as you pull yourself back up to a seated position using your flexion chain.

Try to minimize upper body momentum and focus on lifting yourself up without any jerky movements.

There are a couple of ways you can progress the resistance of the sit-up. One way is to slightly bend your knees to reduce the leverage your legs place on the floor. The more you bend your knees, the harder the exercise will be. It may help to slightly press your heels into the floor to avoid lifting your legs.

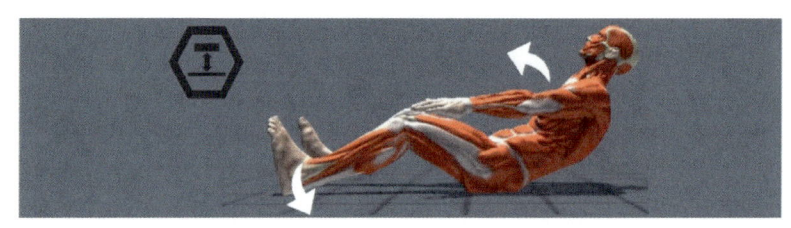

You can use the extension element to make sit-ups more challenging by bending your knees a little. Keeping tension in your hamstrings can help prevent your heels from lifting off the floor.

Another technique is to employ the weight shift element by bringing your arms closer to your torso and even up to your chest. Eventually, you'll become strong enough to do sit-ups with your arms overhead.

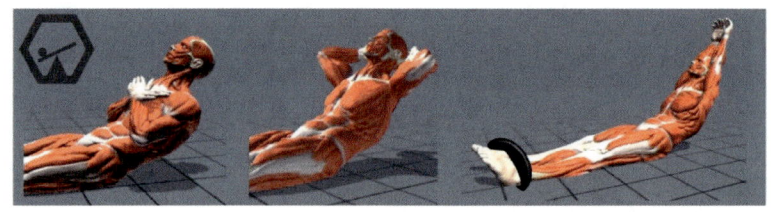

Moving your hands higher shifts your weight away from your feet toward your torso. Eventually reaching overhead with straight arms will give you the most resistance. It's common practice to place a small counterweight on your ankles or feet to avoid tipping over.

Moving your weight more to your torso can make it difficult to keep your legs on the floor. It's a natural consequence of being top heavy. This is one case where holding down your legs can help. The key is to use assistance on your feet, so you only need a little bit of force on your feet. You can do this with a partner to hold down your feet, or you can use a weight like a kettlebell or a sandbag.

Avoid clasping your hands behind your head. Pulling on the back of your head can produce stress on your neck and spine. Besides, the muscles in the front of your neck are part of your flexion chain so don't cheat them from the workload they need to become stronger.

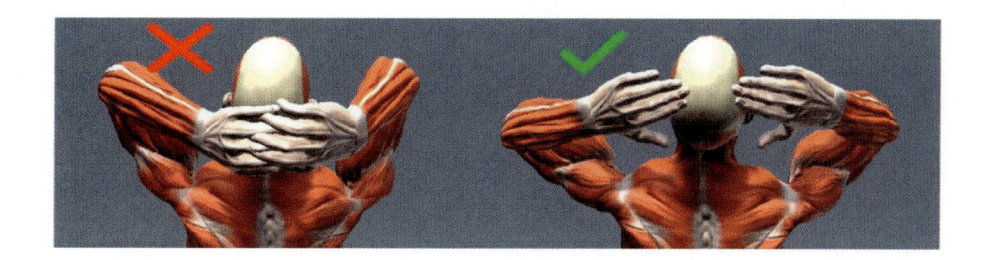

Leg Raises

Leg raises are the Yin to the Yang of sit-ups. Instead of keeping your lower body still while moving your torso, you're now keeping your torso still while moving your lower body.

I prefer leg raises because they allow more freedom of movement for the pelvic bone. Doing sit-ups means your pelvic bone needs to move against the floor which can be difficult and uncomfortable for some people and depending on the surface you're sitting on. Lifting your legs tends to be more ergonomic allowing your pelvis to tilt and move as needed.

You can start doing leg raises by using a little more dynamic motion in the hollow body hold. Instead of holding your legs out in the air, lower your heels to the floor. Allow your heels to "kiss" the floor lightly and then lift your legs back up into a tucked position.

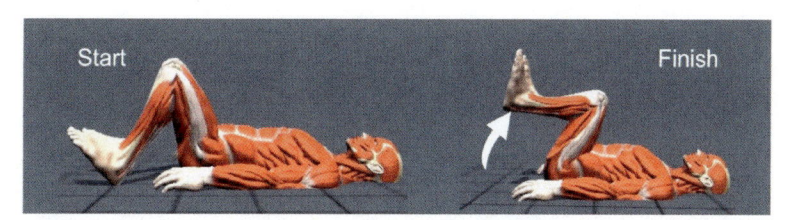

Lying bent knee raises are a good place to start with practicing leg raises. Start with your heels on the floor near your hips. Pull your knees up toward your chest while pushing your hands into the floor. Pause at the top and lower your heels to the floor in a controlled motion.

Progression is accomplished through the extension element. The straighter your legs are the more resistance you'll place on your flexion chain. It's also possible to progress through the range of tension element.

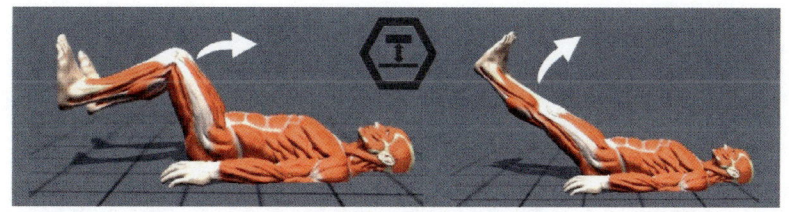

The classic lying leg raise is usually progressed through the extension element by straightening the knees to increase resistance and bending them to reduce it. Keep tension control and range of tension in mind while practicing this exercise.

Hanging leg raises

Hanging offers a few advantages over doing core work on the floor. First, hanging places your body in a vertical position and forces you to lift your legs directly against the pull of gravity.

Second, keeping tension in your back is the foundation of safer and more effective core training. It's a good idea to bring some tension in your back with all core exercises, but it's a lot easier to use your back muscles when hanging from a bar. Back tension provides the stability your abs need to work their hardest. It also helps prevent you from swinging from a hanging position. Lastly, hanging is like squatting; almost everyone can benefit from spending more time hanging.

Hanging with isometric pelvic tilt

This is a great exercise for learning how to keep your pull chain and flexion chain tense at the same time. Start by hanging off the bar and slightly flexing at your hips and abs to pull your legs slightly upward. You can do this exercise for reps or as an isometric where you're holding for time. It's also a good exercise to warm up the mind-muscle connection in your abs before harder hanging core work.

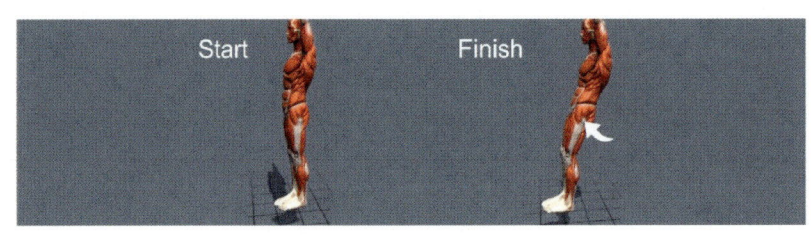

The hanging pelvic tilt is a subtle move but it can do wonders for controlling the tension in your abdominals and learning how to tilt your pelvis while doing hanging leg raises. Be sure to work on improving tension along your pull chain, especially in your upper back, to provide support for your lower body.

Hanging knee raises

Once you can reliably set the tension in your pull and flexion chain, you can play with bent leg raises. Pull your knees up while curling your pelvis up toward your belly. Try to minimize the movement in your upper back.

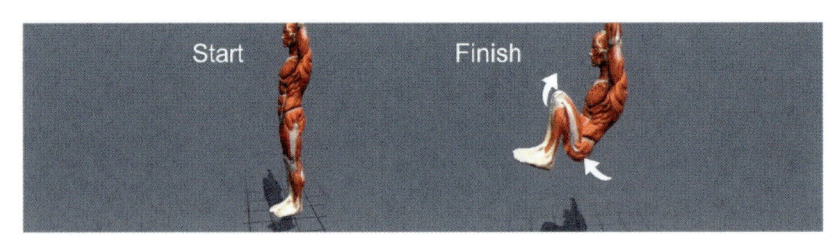

It's helpful to think about picking your feet straight up and then lowering them straight down rather than swinging them back and forth. Pausing at the top to add more time under tension. Be sure you return your feet underneath, or slightly in front of you rather than letting them swing behind you.

From there, you can progress through the extension element by straightening your knees.

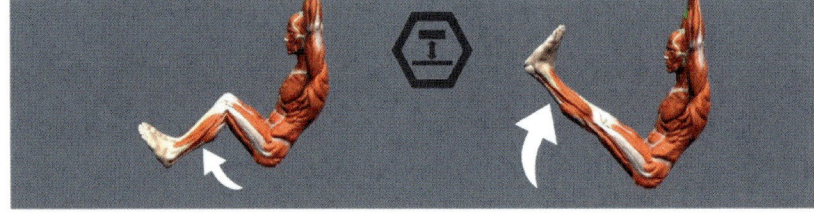

Extending your legs adds resistance to hanging leg raises just as it does to lying leg raises. Don't forget to pay attention to the range of tension as well. Lifting the legs higher will work your flexion chain harder.

Beware the tendency to use momentum and "kick" your legs up into the air. Lifting your legs and hips in a smooth motion with a one-second pause at the top will make a big difference in your time under tension.

Another thing to consider is your leg position at the bottom of each rep. You'll create more resistance if you keep your feet slightly in front of you instead of letting your legs hang straight down or swing behind you.

Twisting leg raises

Leg raises involve the entire front side of your core, but you can slightly rotate your legs to emphasize your oblique's. The same rules of progression apply as with leg raises with extending your legs being the primary mode of progression.

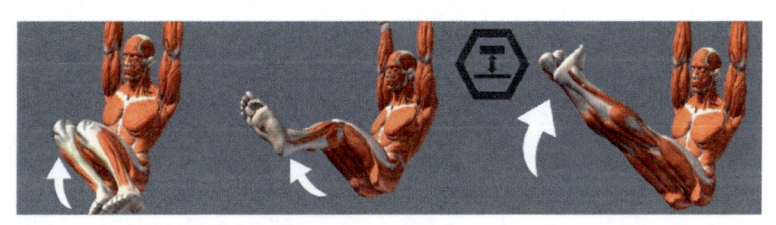

Twisting your legs and pelvis to the side while lifting your legs up is a popular way to bring more resistance to the oblique muscles on the side of your core. Be sure to do the same number of reps on both sides. Once again, the extension element is a common method of progression.

Using the centerline element

Leg raises are usually performed with the feet and knees together, but it's slightly easier to let your legs come apart by an inch or two during the exercise. Pressing your knees and feet together throughout the full range can make it easier to bring more tension to your abs.

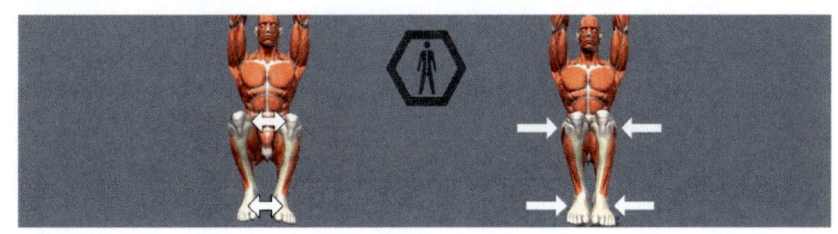

Keeping the feet and knees together may seem like a small detail, but it can make a big difference when it comes to the tension in your flexion chain.

The centerline element can also be used with your upper body. Using a wider grip will give you more upper body stability while a closer grip decreases that stability forcing your back and core to work harder.

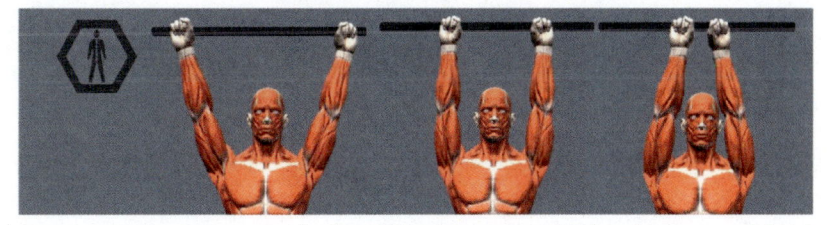

A narrow grip decreases upper body stability forcing your back and core to work harder.

Stretch-outs

Often referred to as rollouts, stretch-outs are essentially dynamic planks where you progress and then regress through the extension element during each rep. The most common variation of this exercise is done on the knees.

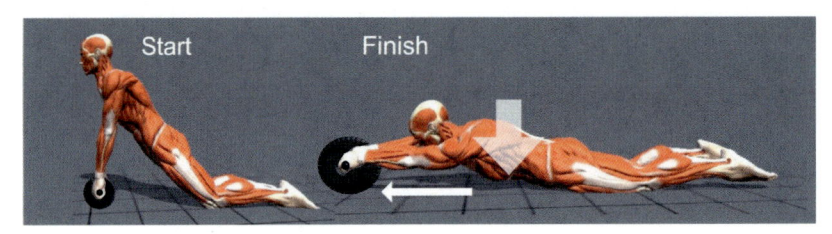

Stretch-outs are commonly done with an ab wheel while kneeling on the floor. Start in a similar position as at the top of knee push-ups with your hands under your shoulders. Roll your hands forward while flexing at your shoulders to lower your torso closer to the floor. Pause at the bottom and return by pulling your arms back under your chest. Try to avoid hinging at your hips so your body maintains a straight line.

Progression is done through the extension element two ways. Reach out further if you are not able to extend far enough to lower your torso all the way to the floor. You can also do them on your toes to extend the length of your body just as you would progress your push-ups by moving from your knees to your toes.

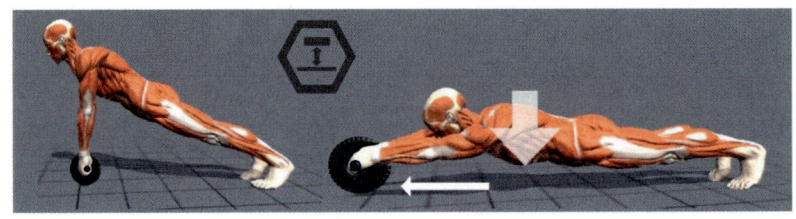

Stretch-outs on your toes requires a lot of strength and stability in your back and flexion chain. Don't worry if you can't reach all the way out. It's perfectly fine to roll your hands forward a couple of inches and return them back under you. The important thing is to maintain tension in your flexion chain to support your body as you extend outward.

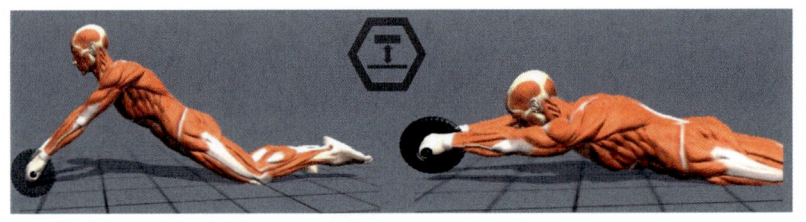

Reaching further out is another way you can progress the resistance of your stretch-outs. Not reaching out as far is a regression I recommend if you start to feel stress on your lower back if your abs are no longer strong enough to support your lumbar spine.

Suspension straps are a very handy tool to use for stretch outs since they use very little friction with the floor so your flexion chain and upper body must work very hard to move and support you.

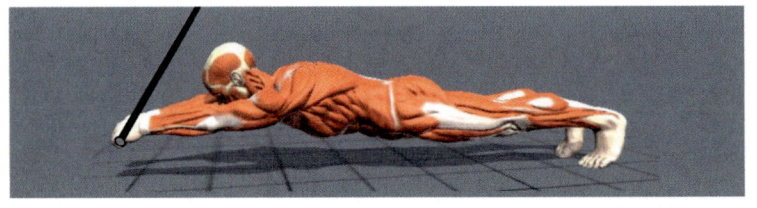

Suspension trainers are a handy tool for stretch-outs since you can use your body position to adjust the resistance of the exercise.

Suspension trainers offer the same adjustable resistance for stretch-outs as they do for push-ups and strap bridges. Moving your feet forward removes resistance while stepping back will add it.

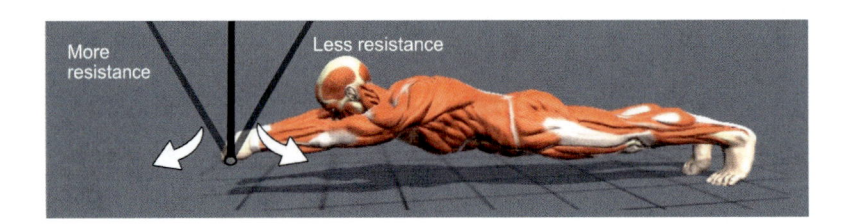

Moving your body forward of the anchor point will reduce the resistance on your flexion chain while stepping back will increase it. This is due to the pendulum affect the trainer has relative to gravity and will either help pull your hands toward your feet or pull them apart.

Accessory Moves for Flexion Chain

Front neck plank

Like your extension chain, your flexion chain extends up into your neck. Working the front of the neck is similar to the back of the neck where you hold an isometric position for time.

I recommend starting easy and not placing too much tension on your neck. Be sure to keep your neck straight and avoid any funny angles or movement. This exercise is probably best as an isometric so you don't place any of the small muscles or nerves in your neck at risk.

Progression is through the angle of gravity and extension elements. You can start by standing against a wall to get the basic idea of how to place tension on your neck. Be sure to keep the rest of your flexion chain tense from your head to your toes.

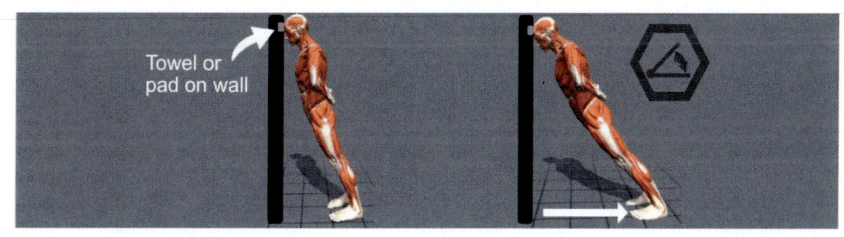

Neck planks are easiest to start with against the wall. Place a towel to rest your head against and lean on the wall using your flexion chain to provide support. You can progress through the angle to gravity element by increasing the distance between the wall and your feet.

From there, you can move onto the floor with your knees bent to bring most of your weight onto your legs. Progression is accomplished through the extension element by straightening your legs to extend your body.

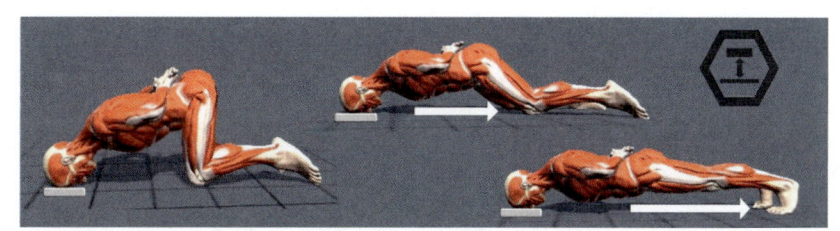

Neck planks on the floor are easier when your knees are closer to your torso. The further you reach out with your knees the more resistance you'll place on your flexion chain eventually moving up on your toes. Keep in mind that these planks are still a flexion chain exercise. They may feel like they focus on your neck muscles but do your best to pull the floor together between your feet and forehead rather than pushing them apart.

Points To Ponder

1. When in doubt, work on improving tension control in the abs. You can always proactively contract your abs tighter.
2. Stress on the lower back is a sign you have too much resistance on your legs and your abs can't stabilize your pelvis. Consider regressing your technique and working on improving tension control in your abs.
3. Work on improving your range of tension especially at the top of each rep during leg raises. Lifting your legs as high as you can is much more difficult than just lifting them high enough to feel your abs working.

4. Fragmented abdominal tension in the abs is not uncommon. If you feel like your upper abs are working harder continue to improve tension control in the lower abs until you can contract your abs equally. Continue to practice full abdominal tension with the cat/cow and hollow body exercises.
5. It's easy to create a lot of momentum during leg raises. Experiment with moving at half the speed you're used to.
6. Put a solid pause at the top and bottom of each rep to improve tension control. This can make a big difference in the difficulty of hanging leg raises.
7. Make your breathing a top priority. Keep your abs tense but your breathing relaxed even if it means taking short and shallow breaths at first.
8. Don't neglect the tension in the rest of your flexion chain. During leg raises keep the muscles in the front of your legs tense.
9. Hanging flexion exercise is just as much a back exercise as a flexion exercise. Keep your back tense just as you would at the bottom of a pull-up.
10. Experiment with keeping light tension in the back of your hips and hamstrings to provide extra resistance and stability in the lower body.
11. If you can, prevent your legs from swinging behind you. Keep your feet either underneath you or slightly forward at the bottom of hanging leg raises.
12. If lifting straight legs is too difficult, but bent knees are too easy, consider lifting up with bent knees and lowering down with straight legs for a compromise.

Chapter 12 The Lateral Chain

The lateral chain isn't the most popular part of the body to exercise in both bodyweight and weightlifting disciplines. Part of the reason could be because you already work most of your lateral muscles through other exercises. Your squat chain works the muscles on the sides of your legs. Your extension and pull chain will cover the side of your back and the muscles on either side of your spine. The push and flexion chain will hit the muscles on the side of your shoulders and core. So the question remains; why would you spend the effort to work these muscles through additional exercises?

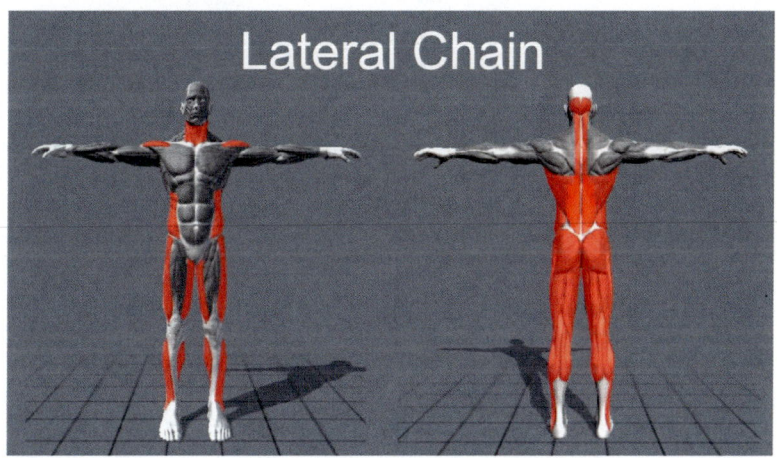

Your lateral chain is made up of the muscles that face either side of your body. These include the muscles along your spine, lats, deltoids, hips, and the muscles that run along the outside and inside of your legs. The muscles along the side of your core and neck are also included and are often the focus of many lateral exercises.

The answer is working your lateral chain isn't about just putting tension in major muscle groups. It's about managing how you use that tension to create a certain type of activity. Yes, all of the other chains will work these muscles, but none of them will work these muscles together as one cohesive unit. It's the ability to neurologically connect the muscles on either side of your body that makes training the lateral Chain valuable.

Turning On your Lateral Chain

Most lateral chain exercises will teach you how to turn on the sides of your body just fine. Even so, I usually find the muscles in the lateral hips are a weak link that could use some extra attention. This weakness can jeopardize your leg strength, core strength, and the strength of your extension chain as well. These muscles are also important for kicking and agility.

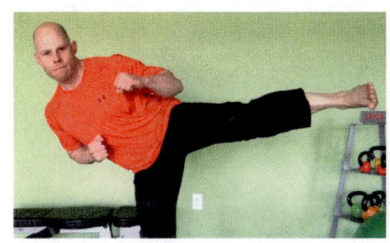

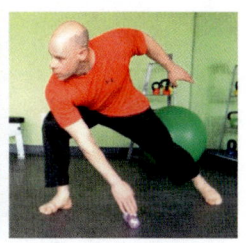

Your lateral chain is seldom used in isolation, but it is involved in every lateral and twisting motion you do from picking your leg up to the side to changing direction while running.

You can practice engaging these muscles by pulling the floor apart in a standing position. Distribute your weight equally between both feet and press your feet outward in an isometric contraction as if trying to pull the floor apart. The same isometric exercise can be applied to the inside of your legs when you try to push your feet together.

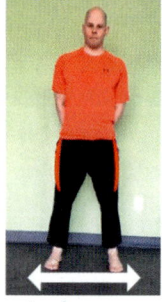

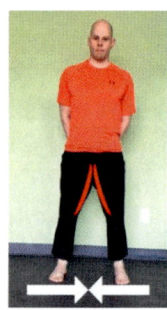

Trying to push the floor apart with your feet is a simple way to practice sending tension into your lateral hips and leg muscles. Pushing the floor together will do the opposite and improve the tension control of your medial leg muscles.

Side Planks

The side plank is a good exercise to start with for both engaging and strengthening your lateral chain. It also teaches you how to incorporate a bit of shoulder stability which is essential for advanced push and pull chain exercises.

You can start doing side planks on your knees and later progress to your feet through the extension element.

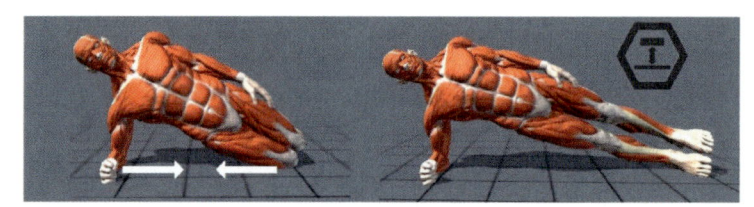

Just like bridges and planks, side planks use the lateral chain to pull the floor together between the two points of contact. You can start with the knee side plank and progress using the extension element by doing them on your feet.

When doing these on your forearm, I recommend slightly shifting your weight forward, so you're not placing too much force directly on your elbow. It's also important to keep your body as straight as possible between your two points of contact to get the most benefit from the exercise.

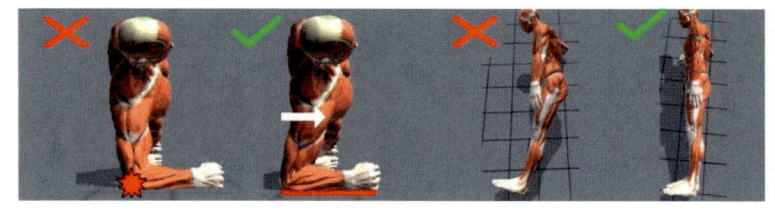

Shifting your shoulder forward slightly can relieve stress on the point of your elbow while distributing pressure along your forearm. Striving for a straight side plank, rather than a curve will not only make you stronger, it will also relieve stress on the joints.

If you're using a straight arm, practice torqueing your arm with the point of your elbow pointing slightly toward your feet. Doing so will improve stability in the shoulder and arm. Remember to keep the back of your shoulder and lats tense to allow the tension to flow down the side of your back.

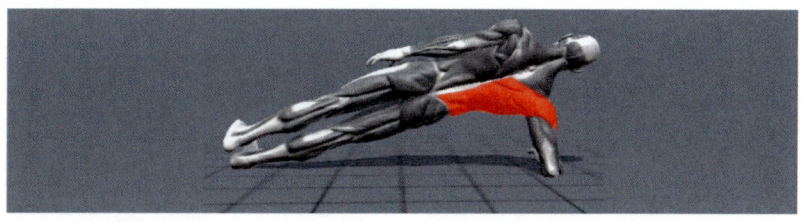

Your lats play a big role in supporting yourself in a plank position. Pulling your shoulder down and back to keep tension in your back will help to stabilize both your core and shoulder.

You can start side planks with your feet spread to establish a more stable base of support. The narrower your feet go, the more tension you'll need to generate to stabilize your body. The end goal is to place one foot on top of the other.

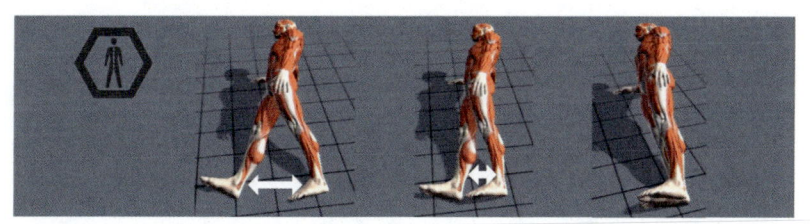

Separating your feet creates a wider base of support for your hips and lateral chain. The closer your feet come together the more difficult the exercise becomes through the centerline element.

Be sure to pull your foot and toes up to create some tension in your lower leg as opposed to letting your toes point away from your body.

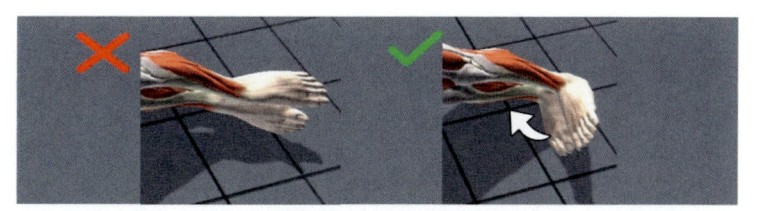

Pulling up your toes while doing side planks can improve stability while maintaining tension in the lateral muscles of the lower leg.

Lifting your top leg is the next level of progression. This technique places a little more emphasis on your lateral hip. In fact, this "starfish plank" is one of the best ways you can work your hips. You can progress the starfish plank through the range of tension element by changing the height of the top leg. The higher you lift your leg, the harder the exercise becomes.

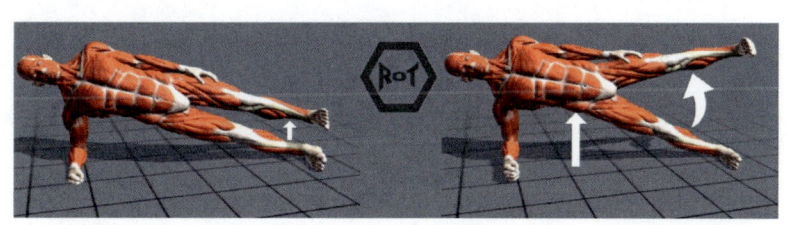

The higher you lift your top leg the more difficult the exercise becomes.

You can also do a similar side plank for the inside of your legs as well. You'll need a step or platform to rest the inside of your top leg against that's about 6-12 inches high. You can also slip your foot into the foot slings on a suspension trainer.

Press down on the inside of your top foot to lift your hips up. Keep your other leg bent at a 90-degree angle. You can alter the resistance of this exercise by keeping your nonworking leg on the floor and use it to assist you up. Progress through applying less pressure in the bottom leg until you can lift it off the floor.

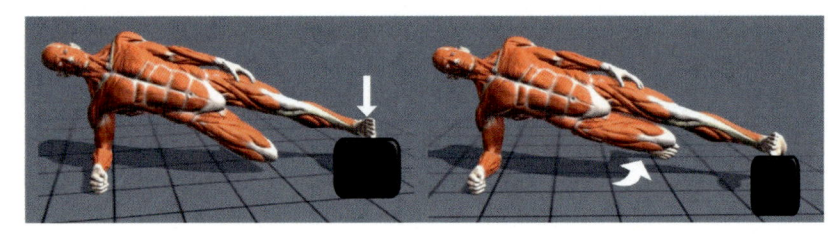

Pressing the inside of your top foot onto an elevated surface will work the inside of your lateral leg muscles very effectively. Keeping the other knee on the floor (left) will make the exercise a little easier. Pulling the bottom leg upward will progress the resistance on the inner thigh of your top leg.

You can bring an incredible amount of resistance to side planks when you do them on a suspension trainer. The unstable nature of the straps requires more tension in your lateral chain plus you can extend your arm out to add even more resistance. You can do these with either your feet or hands suspended.

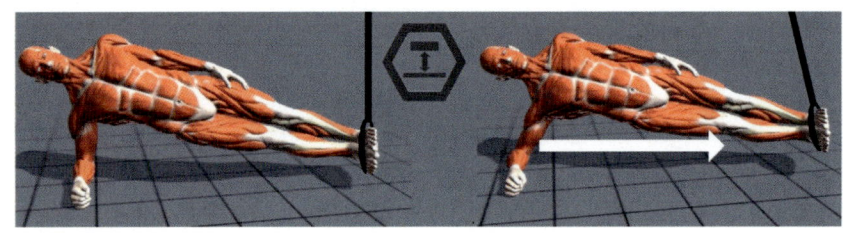

Side planks on suspension straps are one tough challenge for your lateral chain. They remove the friction between your feet and the floor so your lateral chain must work harder to support your body. You can use the extension element to shift your body downward to significantly increase the resistance. As always, the pendulum effect of the suspension trainer is another way you can make the exercise easier or more difficult.

Isometric vs. dynamic movement

Lateral chain exercises are usually isometric techniques where you hold yourself in a static position for time. While isometrics can be enough to strengthen your sides, you can progress the range of tension element by lifting and lowering your hips.

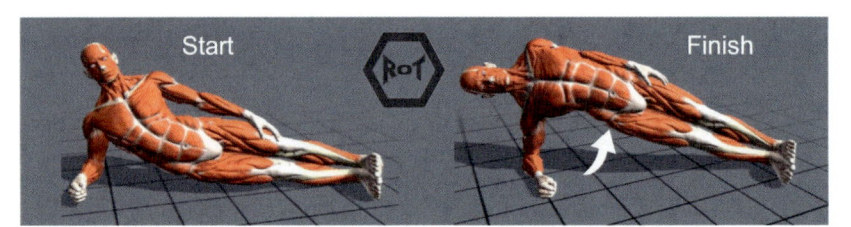

Dynamic side planks are a subtle movement and are not meant to be done in a fast aggressive manner.

Move in a slow and smooth motion while maintaining tension in your lateral chain, particularly in the bottom of each rep.

Human Flags

When I was younger, I witnessed someone doing a clutch flag, and I thought it was one of the most incredible feats of strength. It was like watching someone do a magic trick where my mind didn't quite believe what my eyes were seeing.

Now I know that such a feat is not only possible, but it's well within reach with a little knowledge and a bucket full of determination.

Clutch flags

The first stage of flag training is the series of clutch flags which involve holding a vertical post close to your chest. Start with wrapping the upper arm around the pole, so it sits in your armpit. Your bottom hand is just below your hips so you can drive your elbow into your hip for support.

Once you feel strong enough, drive your hands into the post and gently lift your legs a couple of inches off the ground. This position will help you get used to holding your body up along the vertical post.

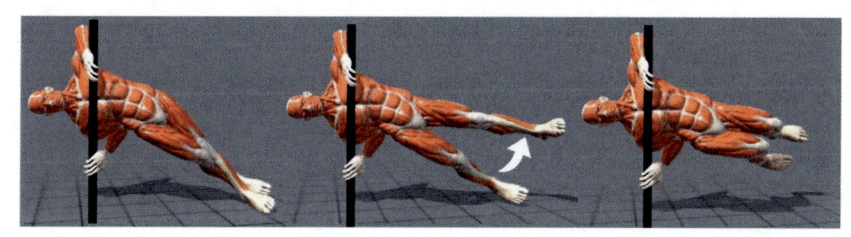

Gradual clutch flag progressions are a good way to start getting used to hanging on a vertical post while using your lateral chain to lift your legs. Note the tilting pelvis toward the floor to make the exercise a little easier. At this stage, the goal is to feel comfortable holding your full weight on a post.

You can progress this move by picking up your top leg just as you would do with the side plank progressions. You can then slowly adjust the amount of weight you are supporting with your legs and your arms until you're feet are completely off the ground.

Once your legs are off the ground, you can play with the two main progression elements of flag work which are the angle to gravity and the extension element. The angle to gravity element is used by bringing your legs closer to perpendicular to the pole. In the case of clutch flags, this is about lifting your legs higher off the ground. The extension element is used through straightening your legs so you reach your feet further away from the post.

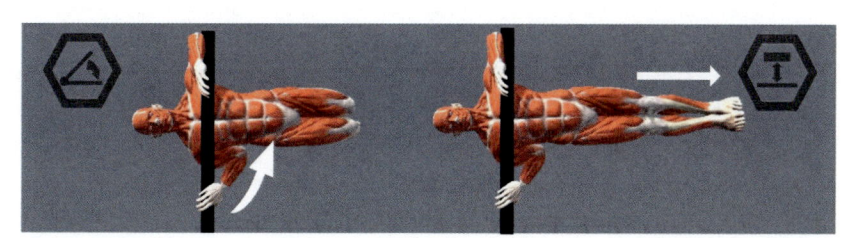

Progression of the clutch flag is accomplished by extending your spine to lift your legs and then extending your knees.

Press flags

This style of flag requires some coordination since they involve extending your whole body away from the post with both arms. The hand on top works in a pulling motion while the arm on the bottom presses you upward.

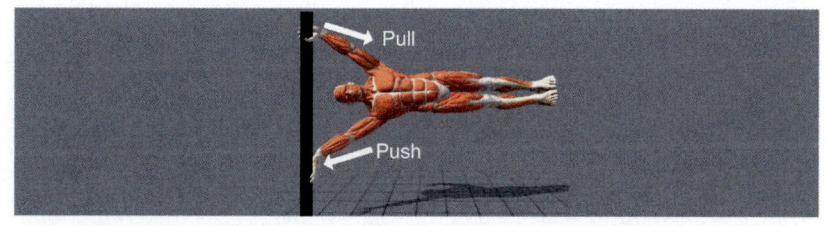

The classic human flag requires both pushing and pulling strength through the upper body to support the position of your torso. Your lateral chain supports your midsection and legs.

45-degree press flags

The easiest way to start out with press flags is to use a pull-up bar with a vertical support. This type of equipment gives you the ability to train the push-pull motion while maintaining a slight angle to gravity. You can then progress through changing your angle to gravity and the length of your body through extending your legs.

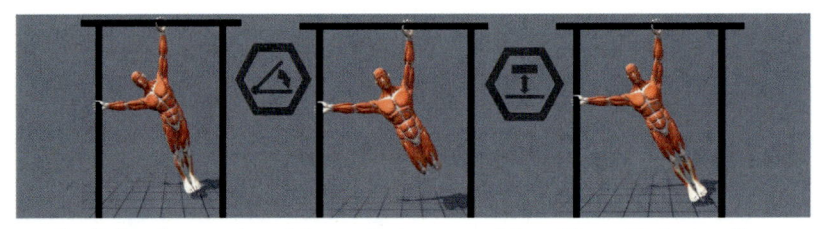

A 45-degree flag helps you get the feeling for pressing with your bottom arm while pulling with the top. You can progress your technique in the same way you can progress the clutch flag with the angle to gravity and extension elements.

Sometimes, you may find an angled support you can hang from like the supports on a swing set at the park. Playground elements like this can make the 45-degree press flag easier to learn and a little more joint friendly.

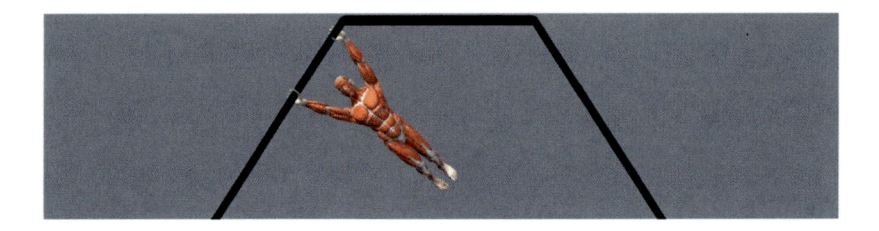

Horizontal press flag

Once you've become comfortable with the 45-degree press flag you can apply the same progressive elements to the full horizontal flag on a vertical post. Keep in mind that progressing your horizontal press flag will not only require more strength in your core but also in your upper body. If you feel like these are not possible because your upper body is not strong enough, work on progressing your push and pull chain exercises for a few weeks and then try these once again.

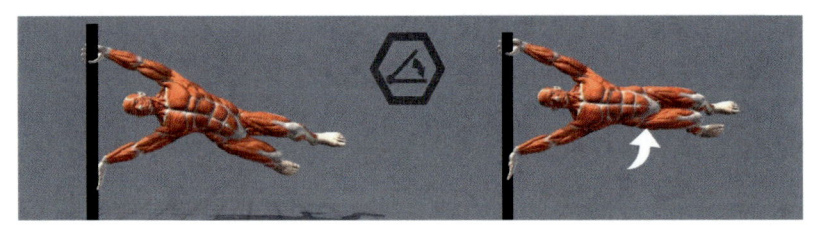

Horizontal flags can be progressed just like clutch flags where you start building enough strength to lift both of your legs off the ground yet you may have an arched torso. From there, you can progress your angle to gravity by picking up your legs higher so your spine is straight and perpendicular to the post.

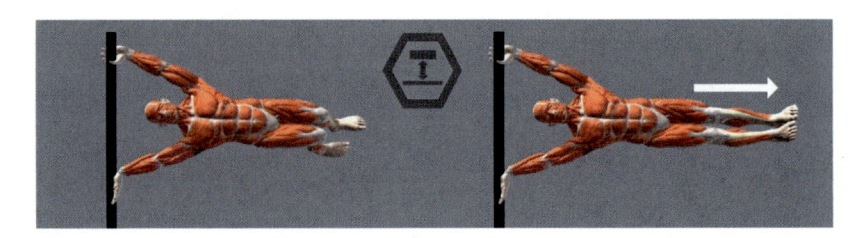

Using the extension element to straighten out your full body length is the pinnacle of isometric flag work. As with all lateral chain work, be sure to work both sides of your body with equal time and resistance.

The isometric horizontal flag is truly an admirable accomplishment and it will certainly ensure your lateral chain is a strong as iron. Just remember there is no top of the mountain as there are always ways you can progress. You can practice dynamic planks where you lift and lower your legs from the ground. Some athletes can do flag push-ups where they bend their arms to bring their head to the post and then extends back out again. You can even combine the two and do one flag push-up followed by a rep of a flag leg raise. Be creative!

Whatever level athlete you are, I highly recommend easing into lateral Chain Training. This chain is notoriously known for including a few weak and stiff links in even advanced athletes. So take a few weeks to start with gentle side planks to work on your neural code to include every muscle along the side of your body. It will pay off in the long run and create a lateral chain without any weak links.

Points To Ponder

1. Flags are just as much an upper body exercise as they are a lateral core move. If your upper body is the weak link, adjust your routine to emphasize vertical pushing and pulling strength a bit more.
2. Be sure to keep your shoulders back and your lats tight while doing side planks and flags to prevent your body from flexing and twisting.
3. Try to keep your neck in line with your spine. If your neck bends or flexes your spine will usually follow and be harder to straighten out.
4. Keep light tension in the front and back of your legs to help control them in space during flags.
5. See if you can spot any differences in how your right and left lateral chains feel and perform. Aim to make your weaker side match your stronger side over time.
6. Aim to keep your breathing smooth and relaxed even when you're applying a lot of tension along the full length of your body.

Chapter 13 Weighted Calisthenics

Weighted, or loaded, calisthenics is a topic that fosters a bit of debate. Some people love strapping extra weight to themselves to add resistance to their exercises. Other's take more of a purist approach and frown upon such a practice.

I've fallen into both camps over the years. I did a lot of weighted bodyweight movements when I first got into calisthenics. Over time, I've gotten away from the practice as my tension skills have improved. It's not because I avoid the dip belt or dumbbell lunges. I just feel like I don't need to do those things as much as I used to. I can generate all of the tension I can handle through technical adjustments.

I wanted to include this chapter for you if you have any interest in smartly pursuing weighted calisthenics. If not, feel free to skip this section.

The Pros And Cons Of Weighted Calisthenics

Like all disciplines in fitness, there are benefits and drawbacks to adding extra weight to bodyweight exercise. Let's explore the potential benefits first.

The biggest advantage is adding extra weight can make an exercise more challenging with relative ease. You don't need to improve your skills or develop other qualities like stability or mobility. You just add, or subtract, weight from your own bodyweight and continue to practice your technique as you normally would.

The other supposed advantage is some people find weighted calisthenics easier to quantify. While you can quantify progressive bodyweight training, weights are easy to measure in pounds or kilograms.

Lastly, sometimes getting stronger can make advanced progressive techniques a little easier to do. If you're struggling with archer push-ups or narrow pull-ups, doing an easier technique with some added weight might help.

These advantages alone make them a tempting option for people who want to progress their training when strength and building muscle are their primary goals. Now let's check out some of the disadvantages of weighted calisthenics.

The first downside mirrors the advantage I mentioned. You can make an exercise harder without having to improve your technical skills. The drawback is you can make an exercise harder without having to improve your technical skills. Weighted calisthenics can improve your strength, but you miss out on the other benefits like joint mobility and stability.

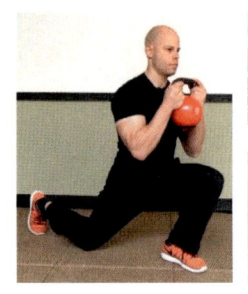

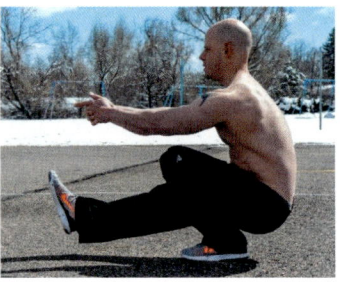

Adding weight to a relatively easy exercise, like lunges, can provide more resistance without having to develop the technical skills required by more advanced techniques. This can be good or bad depending on your point of view.

The second disadvantage is the need for equipment. Basic progressive calisthenics does not require much more than a place to hang. Weighted calisthenics requires dip belts, weights, vests, and chains which can compromise the freedom and flexibility of bodyweight training.

The third disadvantage is it can become tempting to focus on numbers while neglecting the quality of your exercise. It's easy to start cutting corners in your technique while chasing after more weight and reps.

The Smart Way To Use Weighted Calisthenics

The key to smart loaded bodyweight training is to not rely on the weight itself to become bigger and stronger. Using external weight is just like any other form of training. Your results don't come from using certain equipment or even doing an individual exercise. Success depends on the skills and knowledge you bring *to* that weight or that exercise. Weight doesn't produce or control muscle tension, only your mind can do that. Instead, weight contributes to resistance which is a big influence to your muscle tension, but it isn't everything. Chasing solely after weight and reps instead of skill and tension can leave you vulnerable to poor quality training.

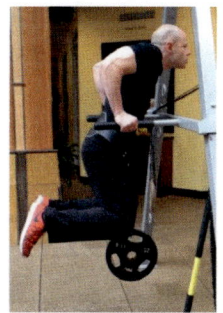

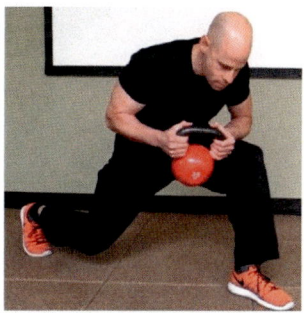

I used to depend on weights and equipment rather than skill to get results. I used to "shrug" my dips because my back wasn't strong enough. I also used to do shallow lunges and lean forward to lunge with heavy weight.

Let's take weighted pull-ups for example. Let's say that on any given day you can do close grip pull-ups with a large range of motion and a pause at the top and bottom of each rep. You're also proficient at keeping your legs from moving throughout each rep. You can do 15 reps in a row with relative ease.

Since your goal is to keep getting stronger, you decide to experiment with adding some extra weight. You strap on a dip belt with 20 pounds and get to work. You get a good eight reps in and pat yourself on the back for stepping up your routine. Over the next few weeks, you add reps and weight until you're doing pull-ups with a solid 45 pounds.

Now the real question isn't if you're actually stronger or not. Obviously, if you added weight and reps to some degree, you're gaining some measure of strength. The more important question is if you are regressing your technique to progress the amount of weight you can lift. Are you bringing your elbows and shoulders through the same range of motion? Are you still driving your chest into your hands at the top? Are you still pausing at the top and bottom of each rep? Is your muscle tension evenly distributed throughout your pull chain? How is your breathing and body position compared to when you did pull-ups without the weight?

These are the things to ponder when doing weighted calisthenics. The purpose of your training is to manipulate muscle tension, not just to lift stuff up. You are not a crane on a construction site.

Lift harder, not just heavier

Don't make the mistake of letting your technique erode for the sake of lifting more weight. I used to make excuses why I couldn't squat as deep with heavy weight or needed to change my body position under a heavy load. It was all an effort to protect my ego so I could lift more weight. It didn't make me much stronger, and my joints suffered for it.

When I got into calisthenics, my mindset shifted from using an easier technique to lift more weight, to using a harder technique to create more tension with just my bodyweight. I started to use technical details like range of tension, timing, and proactive tension to make my muscles work harder.

When you have this mindset, you'll probably find you don't need nearly as much weight to make your muscles work very hard. Even adding an extra 10-20 pounds can be a significant increase in many exercises. You'll also find you won't need much extra weight with a more advanced technique. You can lift a lot more weight when doing push-ups with your arms wide apart. Keeping your hands close together will be much more difficult, and you won't need as much load.

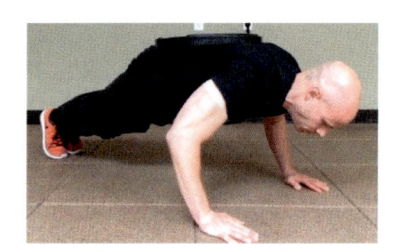

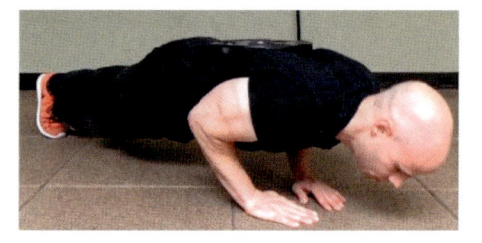

You can combine progressive technique with weighted calisthenics. The picture on the left shows me doing wide push-ups with a 45-pound plate on my back. On the left, I'm using a more difficult close push-up but with only 25 pounds on my back.

Building muscle and strength doesn't come from weight or a fancy routine. It comes from using basic exercises to create progressive tension in your muscles. It doesn't do you much good to lift a lot of weight while using an easy technique. You're just regressing one aspect of your training while progressing in another. If you want to get stronger, stop doing your exercises the easy way. The bulk of your resistance should still come from using an advanced technique, and the weight is used to supplement the resistance your body produces against gravity.

Most other forms of strength training use weight as an asset, something that's vital to your progress and performance. Over the years, I've come to perceive weight as more of a liability. While it is true that a heavy load can influence the amount of tension in your muscles, that influence can come at a cost. Weight doesn't just place stress on your muscles, but it also creates stress on your joints, nervous system and tissues. When you learn to create a lot of tension with less weight you essentially make your training more effective with less cost to your body.

To sum up, weighted calisthenics is perfectly fine and even safe as long as you approach them with the right attitude and skill set. Use them as another tool in your toolbox. Just don't make the mistake of believing one tool is the supreme way to achieve the results you want.

Points To Ponder

1. Start light and go easy on the weight. There's always time to add more weight later on, but let your body get used to a given load for a week or two before adding more weight.
2. Always emphasize your range of tension. Reducing your range for the sake of weight is usually a sign that the weight is too heavy.

3. Be sure to warm up without any load for a set or two. Strive to make your technique as perfect as possible during that warm-up set and try to do the weighted reps the exact same way.
4. If doing a weighted exercise is part of your usual routine, plan to do a non-weighted version of that exercise at some point in the week. This will help improve technique and give your joints a break.

Chapter 14 Calisthenics Cardio

I used to be a big-time cardio junkie before I discovered the power of strength training. Back in college, I spent more time on an elliptical than in class. As a bike racer, I used to take 2-hour Spinning classes and put countless miles on my exercise bike almost every day.

These days, you have a better chance of spotting Sasquatch than catching me on an exercise bike. It's been over ten years since I've done much gym-style cardio and I haven't missed it one bit. I would even say I'm much better off without it. It's not because I think gym-style cardio is bad, it's just that it's so darn expensive.

The High Cost of Cardio

Gym-style cardio can come with a pretty hefty price tag. First, there's the cost of the equipment which you either need to purchase yourself or pay a monthly fee to use at a gym. If you buy it yourself, you're also responsible for its maintenance plus it takes up valuable space in your home. A gym membership requires the additional cost in time and money to travel to and from the gym for each workout.

In addition to the expense of the equipment, you also need to spend the time and energy required to use it. Cardio is usually done for relatively extended periods of time to expend a lot of energy. I was personally spending 2-3 hours every day doing cardio at the peak of my racing career.

It's not just the physical energy, but also the mental energy you need to spend in order to push yourself on a stationary exercise machine. It takes a lot of discipline to run in place as you anxiously wait for the clock to tick down. This mental drudgery is why modern cardio machines come with digital distractions like TV and even the internet to occupy your mind.

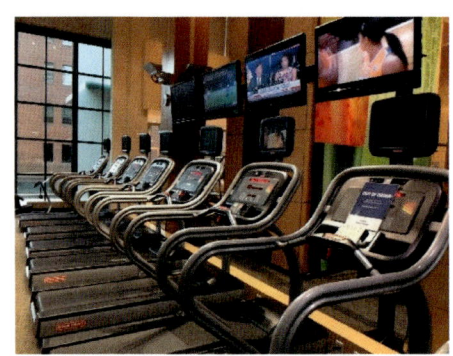

More screens mean more distraction which can be good or bad depending on how you look at it.

It costs a lot to make equipment based cardio a big part of your exercise routine, and that's fine. Results in fitness aren't free, so the costs are entirely justifiable, provided they produce a substantial benefit.

The Limited Benefits Of Cardio

When I first got into fitness, cardiovascular exercise was all the rage as it promised three benefits. These included improving endurance, burning fat, and general health. Let's explore these benefits and the potential influence cardio can have on them.

Cardio for fat loss

Make no mistake, cardio can be an influence on your weight. It doesn't directly cause weight loss or control your weight, but it can certainly be effective for burning hundreds, even thousands of calories in a single workout.

When you practice cardio, you increase how many calories you burn through physical activity. Your physical activity is an influence on your total calorie expenditure with your base metabolic rate and the thermic effect of food making up the other influences.

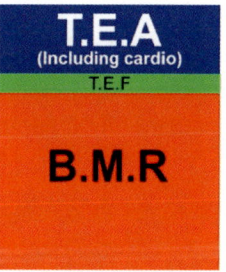

All physical activity and cardio increase your thermic effect of activity which influences your total calorie expenditure. Your base metabolic rate (BMR) and thermic effect of food (TEF) make up the rest of your total calorie expenditure.

While increasing your total calorie expenditure is important, it's not everything. You still have to account for how your total calorie expenditure is related to your total calorie intake. It's the *balance* between the speed you consume and the speed you expend calories that control the amount of fat you have.

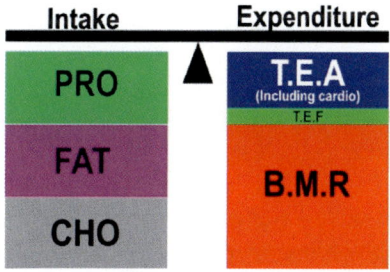

While cardio is an influence toward your thermic effect of activity and your total calorie expenditure, it doesn't directly control your calorie balance which is what's responsible for your body fat level.

While cardio is a perfectly legitimate way to increase your total calorie expenditure it's not everything and other influences, like diet, may be a more important influence depending on your personal circumstances.

Cardio for endurance

Any activity that challenges your stamina will improve your endurance. The question is if the type of exercise you're practicing is developing the endurance you want.

Like strength training, your endurance is specific to the functional demands of the activity you practice. The type of endurance you develop will have limited carryover to activities that require different types of endurance.

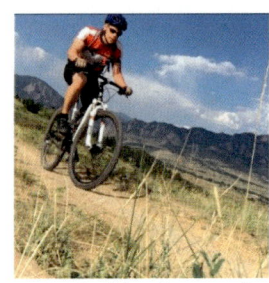

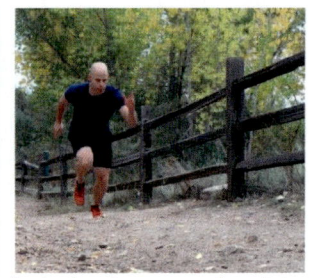

Both cycling and running build endurance, but the body adapts to each activity in a specific way.

A good example of this is the functional demands of running a 10K vs sparring in a ring. In Taekwon-Do, students would sometimes be surprised they had trouble lasting a few rounds of free-sparring despite practicing a regular running routine. The functional demand of running is different than sparring, so there's minimal functional carry over between the two. So while all forms of cardio can improve your endurance, be sure you're building the type of endurance you want.

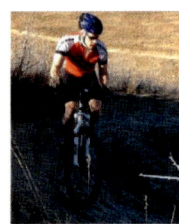

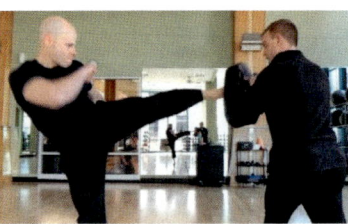

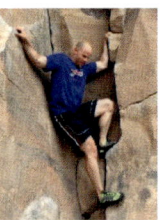

All three of these activities require their own unique endurance. Cycling is more repetitive, kickboxing is more random and rock climbing requires more stamina in the upper body.

Cardio For Health

I thank cardio for a lot of the health benefits I've enjoyed in my life. I've enjoyed good blood work and a robust cardiovascular system. Cardio has also been a source of mental therapy during times of stress. At the same time, I blame it for many of the problems I've had to deal with. Cardio has made many of my muscles stiff and tight despite copious amounts of stretching. I'm still discovering muscle weaknesses and imbalances that were born from long hours on the bike. I've suffered joint pain, fragmented muscle tension, and mental stress over missed workouts. Cardio has truly been a mixed blessing.

Like all fitness habits, cardio can both hurt or heal. It largely depends on understanding how to use it in a healthy way rather than an unhealthy way. Use it, don't abuse it as I like to say.

3 Tips For Smart Cardio

As with many things in fitness, I see cardio as a tool. It's neither good nor bad, and any positive or negative results depend on how well you use it in a smart way. To help you figure out the smartest way to use cardio for your goals I've drafted up the following guidelines.

#1 Use cardio as part of a weight loss/ control plan

Weight control is a lot easier to achieve through a multi-faceted approach. By all means, engage in some regular physical activity to burn more calories, but don't depend on that alone. Keep your diet in check, so you don't end up using cardio to compensate for chronic overeating.

Also, try to be active outside of your workout. All calories burned through physical activity count. Burning 100 calories while mowing the lawn is the same influence on your total calorie expenditure as burning 100 calories on a treadmill. In some cases, the calories you spend through non-exercise physical activity can be more than the calories you burn in a workout.

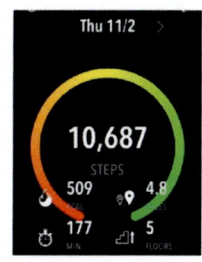

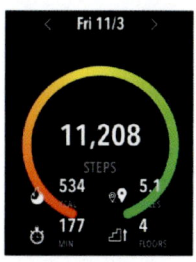

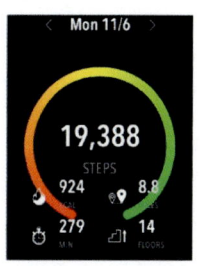

These are sample screenshots of the step counter on my smartphone. I like to track my daily steps because it's loosely correlated to my non-exercise physical activity which can add and burn a lot of calories.

#2 Program your cardio to fulfill the functional demands of your performance goals

Don't make the mistake of training for overall endurance when you need to develop stamina for a particular activity. Using an elliptical for an hour may not help you much if you're preparing to try out for the high school football team. In that case, field sprints with short rest periods might be more applicable since they resemble the functional demand of a football game.

#3 Use cardio as part of a healthy lifestyle

Just like with weight loss, don't over-rely on cardio for your health and well-being. Take other lifestyle factors into account like diet, recreation, and how you handle stress. It also pays to adjust the volume and intensity of your cardio, so it doesn't become an abusive habit. Look out for signs of overdoing it like chronic fatigue and mental burn out along with aches and pains.

The Calisthenics Cardio Advantage

Using an elliptical is fine, but the best cardio equipment by far is your own body. Nothing else comes close especially when you consider the natural advantages calisthenics bring to your performance, health, and even fat loss.

Bodyweight cardio has an incredible amount of functional carry over toward the performance requirements of any sport. Sprinting, running, jumping and even kicking have a lot of functional carryover to sports that require those movements. Sure, you can run on a treadmill, but it's hard to practice agility drills where you have to stop and turn quickly. Even riding a stationary bike doesn't have as much functional carry over as riding a real bike over rocks and dirt.

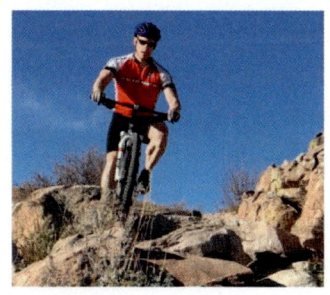

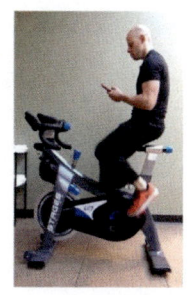

It's a lot easier to check your email on a stationary bike than while riding over a rocky trail. Even though both stationary and real cycling may look similar they are quite different in application.

Another advantage of bodyweight cardio is natural resistance. Fancy cardio machines have adjustable settings so you can dial in a comfortable level of difficulty. Mother Nature doesn't have a resistance control. You're forced to work hard while walking up a hill no matter how motivated or fatigued you feel. However, while the natural world will force you to step up, it will also scale back the difficulty as well. The natural landscape provides a variety of surfaces and levels of difficulty ensuring you won't get stuck always using your body the same way.

Calisthenics based cardio uses the body in a more dynamic way which requires you to use your body in a wider range of ability. For example, running on a treadmill usually involves running at the same pace, with the same stride and the same gait. It creates a particular movement pattern, and you develop a narrow range of physical abilities within that pattern. Now compare that to trail running where the terrain is constantly changing and forcing you to adjust how you move. This variety not only gives you a broader foundation of ability, but it also helps prevent weaknesses and imbalances.

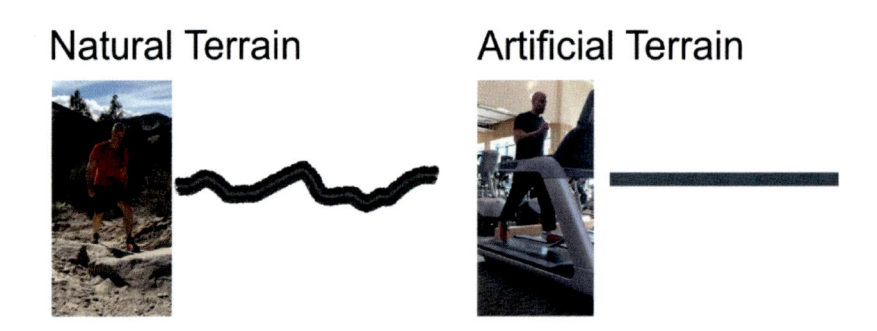

Lastly, let's not forget the calisthenics advantage for fat loss. Moving your body through space forces you to deal with your strength to weight ratio. Carrying around extra fat makes you naturally work harder as you move around.

I've also heard a theory that calisthenics cardio can subliminally help you lose weight since it requires you to be both stronger and lighter. The basic idea is that if you struggle to move around excess weight your body will adapt by shedding that weight to make the exercise more efficient. I don't know if that's true or not, but I have noticed that people who do stationary cardio all winter tend to become leaner when the weather warms up, and they move around outside.

My explanation of this is it's just a lot easier to exercise a lot longer and harder with calisthenics cardio. Just this past weekend I went on a 2-hour hike on Saturday and then a 4-hour bike ride on Sunday. Granted, that's a lot even for me, but that adds up to 6 hours of calorie-torching activity within 48 hours! You couldn't pay me to do 6 hours of gym-based cardio, but I'll gladly do it hiking up a mountain or on a bike.

Not that gym-based cardio is at all bad. It does have its advantages such as convenience. Sometimes it makes sense to take refuge on a treadmill when the weather is nasty outside. It's also a lot better to sit on an exercise bike than on the couch while watching a sports game. But, when you step back and compare the two, calisthenics cardio can bring you a lot of benefit with relatively little cost making it a potent way to improve performance, health, and weight control.

Calisthenics Cardio Ideas

Nearly all forms of natural locomotion are a type of calisthenics exercise. If an activity involves moving around it fits the bill. Certain kinds of training can be up for debate, such as cycling and cross-country skiing because you're using equipment that makes you move in an unnatural way. I don't see much point in getting dogmatic about it though. As long as you're moving around and enjoying yourself, that's what matters most.

Walking

Walking is one of the best forms of exercise bar none. It's so natural and simple that even sedentary people do it a little bit each day. You don't need any special equipment or special skills to do it. You just place one foot in front of the other.

Despite its simple nature, you can progress or regress it to accommodate any fitness level. Adding distance or elevation will challenge even the most hard-core athlete. It can be both relaxing and rejuvenating while helping you strip off the stress of the day.

I find walking can be one of the best ways to escape and take a break from daily stress. Getting out for a walk helps you escape the screens and electronics that continuously bid for your attention and mental energy. It's one of the best ways for your mind to finally relax and sort through the mental noise you've been trying to process all day long.

Even though walking might not always be the most strenuous activity, I have found it to be an effective way to burn a lot of calories. In fact, some of the most notable weight loss stories I've heard involve a lot of walking.

The reason walking can contribute to weight loss is simple. It's not terribly exhausting or hard on the body which means you can do it at a much higher frequency than other high-intensity activities. You can burn a lot more calories running for 45 minutes than walking for the same amount of time, but you can walk every day whereas you might only run 2-3 times a week.

The key to getting a lot of benefit from walking is to treat it as a serious form of training. Plan your route and how long you plan to walk. Don't just wander around the mall and window shop. You don't need to speed walk, but do try to move at a brisk pace. Also, be sure to be mindful of how you're using your squat chain with each step. Pay attention to how you're using your glutes and hamstrings to propel yourself forward with each step. Notice if there's any difference between how you use one leg or the other. Check in with your breathing, posture and even where you're eyes are directed. Walking with your head up and looking ahead is different than being hunched over and looking at the ground.

Jogging/ running/ sprinting

Running variations are the next most popular means of locomotion after walking. Even if you're not a runner you've probably engaged in some form of running in sport or when you're in a rush to go somewhere.

Some people may debate the definitions of jogging, running and sprinting but I find they are similar activities that exist along a spectrum.

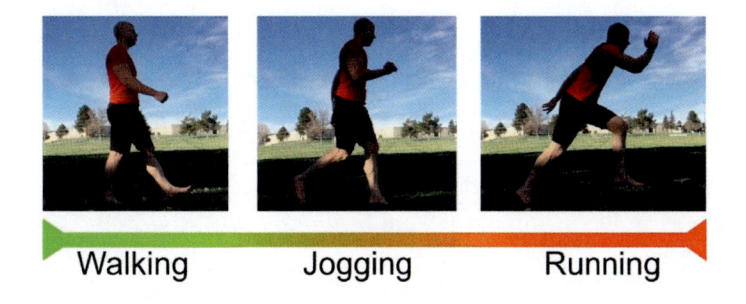

Generally speaking, jogging is a slower and more relaxed pace compared to running. I've always considered going for a jog as something I can do for more than 30 minutes, and it's not fatiguing me to the point where I can't talk. Running is done at a faster pace where it's difficult to talk, and you feel more fatigued afterward. Sprinting is a more short-term and typically doesn't last more than 15-20 seconds.

Each activity alters the relationship between intensity and volume. Jogging uses a lower amount of tension for longer periods of time. Running uses a moderate amount of tension and a moderate amount of time. Sprinting requires high levels of tension and short periods of time.

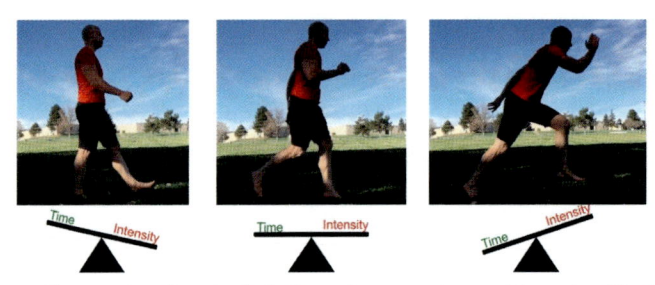

Walking and running are both forms of locomotion that tip the balance between time and intensity. The lower the intensity the more time you can do the activity like a leisurely walk. High-intensity activities like running at high speed are things you can only do for short periods of time.

While these activities are pretty safe, they do carry a much higher risk of injury compared to walking. Injury, burnout, and chronic fatigue are all things you want to be careful to avoid. Be sure to give yourself adequate recovery between workouts and practicing them only a couple of times a week.

I also highly recommend investing in some coaching when getting involved in either jogging, running or sprinting. Seeking the advice of a coach can help minimize risk while maximizing results.

Hiking

Hiking is another one of my favorite activities. It's nothing more than just walking along nature trails, but it's one of the best ways to get out and enjoy nature.

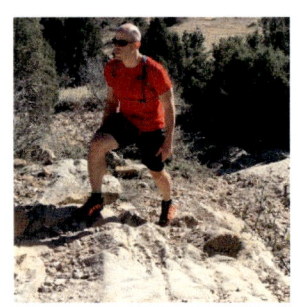

Nothing beats going for a hike in the Rocky Mountains!

Even though hiking is just walking, it is a different experience from walking along a street or walk path in an urban environment. The biggest difference is how hiking usually involves walking along a trail with uneven terrain. Walking on dirt and rocks can help build balance, coordination, and strength unlike using a treadmill or paved surface.

Hiking also often means going up a mountain or a series of inclines which create some unique challenges. This is not only true for going up but also coming down. Walking, or even running, down a mountain will condition you for benefits you won't gain from working out in a gym. The most notable benefit is learning how to use your muscles to absorb stress and control momentum so it doesn't wear out your joints.

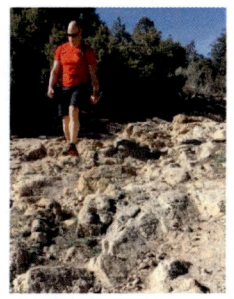

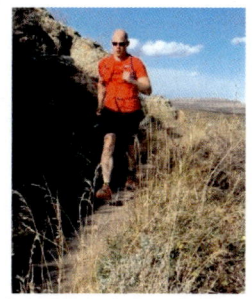

Walking down a rocky trail and running along a dirt path provides benefits you can't gain on a stationary piece of gym equipment.

You can also jog and run on any trail to make things more intense. Just be aware that the risk of tripping and falling increases on uneven terrain so start slow and be sure to keep your eyes open for hazards.

Some people like to hike with trekking poles. Using poles can work your upper body more which both increases muscle activation and improves stability.

Swimming

I'm not much of a swimmer. To me, swimming is something I do to keep from drowning when I'm in deep water. I do have to admit though that swimming is one heck of a workout. Even swimming across a pool once is enough to send my heart rate sky high.

Swimming offers several benefits over land-based cardio. It makes you use a lot of muscle so it can significantly increase your rate of calorie expenditure. There's minimal impact on your body which makes it ideal for people with joint issues. It's also great for cross training and helps you break you out of out of a neurological rut.

Like with running, I highly recommend looking into some coaching to help you avoid potential issues while increasing the quality of your workout.

Cycling

Like swimming, riding a bike is a low impact activity, while the frame of the bike supports your weight instead of your legs. Using a bike with a range of gears gives you the freedom to adjust the resistance of the exercise sort of like a weight machine.

There are many types of bicycles available ranging from basic and inexpensive to some costing as much as a decent used car. Even though there are many styles available, your neural code will be pretty much the same from one bike to the next. It's not the bike that matters, it's what you do with it.

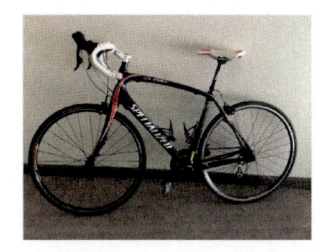

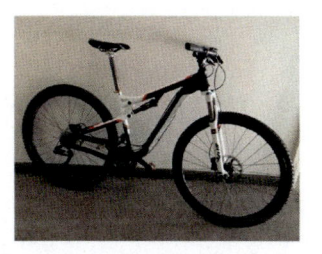

My road bike on the left may look different than my mountain bike on the right, but they both produce very similar neural codes since they make my body move in similar ways.

Something that can make a big difference is the type of terrain you plan on riding. Many prefer to stick to pavement and bike paths as these environments are usually more available.

Mountain biking is a fun way to ride closer to nature but typically involves more technical skills and varied terrain. Both options will burn calories and build strength just fine. It's more a question of which options appeal most to you.

If you're in the market for a new ride, don't worry too much about choosing the perfect bike. The most important considerations are fit, comfort and reliability. You want to make sure you're using a bike that's safe and comfortable. If you already have a bike, it's well worth the investment to get it tuned up and keep it running well.

Kicking and punching

Calisthenics cardio doesn't have to be limited to highly repetitive locomotion exercises. Boxing or kickboxing type exercises are a fun way to learn a new skill while unleashing your inner action star.

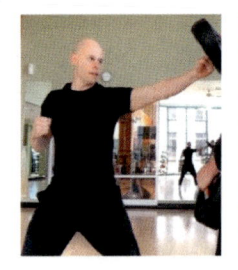

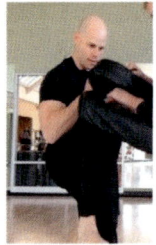

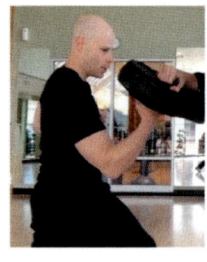

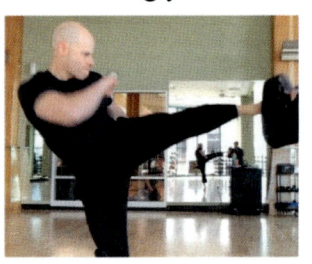

There is a bigger learning curve with kicking and punching based cardio, so it pays to take a class and get some professional instruction.

Jumping rope

Skipping rope is one those traditional exercises that don't require much time or equipment, yet pays massive dividends. It's also a challenging game of skill that requires mental focus, so it doesn't feel like drudgery when you do it.

I recommend mixing in a little jump rope in with your circuit training to change up the pace and tempo of a workout.

Circuit training

Circuit training is an excellent way to mix strength and cardio to gain multiple benefits in one time-efficient workout.

Setting up a circuit is simple. You just select some exercises and string them together, so you move from one exercise to another with little rest in between. While circuit training is about moving between tasks quickly, don't make it a race against the clock. There's a difference between moving quickly and rushing through each set. Be sure to maintain the quality of your technique even if that means moving a little slower through the workout.

There are plenty of ways you can set up a circuit. I like to think of each exercise as a building block, and you put them together to assemble your workout.

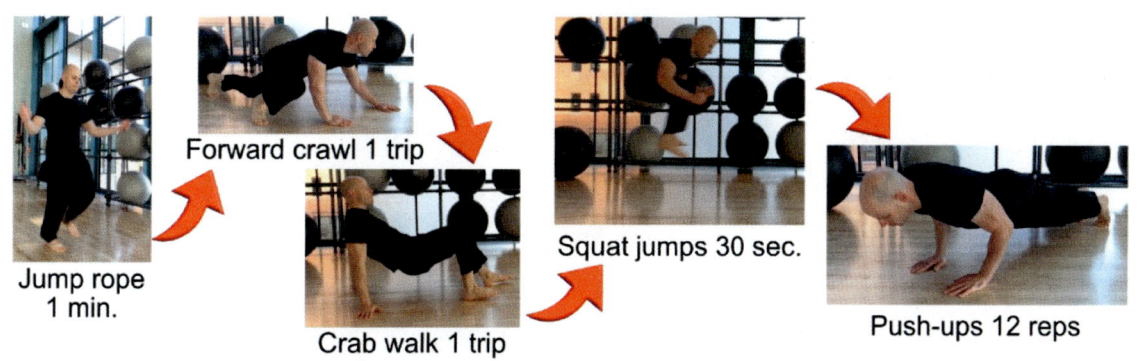

A sample circuit workout combining exercises for strength, mobility, endurance, and power. You can also see how you can mix different program methods such as time, distance and reps for various exercises.

While circuit training is a mix of cardio and strength, you can emphasize various levels of each depending on your exercise selection. For example, a strength circuit might involve a lot of strength calisthenics like push-ups, squats, and rows. A cardio circuit might include activities like jumping, kicking, sprinting and crawling. You can also go 50/50 by alternating between strength and cardio exercises.

You can set up your circuit a few ways. One way is to do each exercise for a given amount of time. You just set a timer and do your first exercise for that amount of time. When the timer beeps you move onto the next task. The timer is sort of like a personal trainer telling you to change what you're doing and keeps you on track.

The other option is to do each exercise for a given amount of work, like 30 push-ups, and you move to the next exercise once you complete that set. This method is useful for working without a timer or when you want to pace yourself and change exercises when you wish.

A lot of people like to create different circuits for each workout; others prefer to stick to a handful of workouts and repeat them over time. Either way can help you get a great cardiovascular workout.

Field or court sports

Sports are an attractive option for those who suffer from a lack of motivation. Playing field or court sports can motivate you to both show up to play and push yourself to higher levels of performance. You'll have a lot more incentive to show up when you have a partner or teammates counting on you. You'll also find yourself pushing your physical abilities as you sprint and chase points in a competitive setting.

There are plenty of sports from basketball and ultimate Frisbee to tennis and racquetball. You can find plenty of local clubs and organizations online and through Meetup.com. Just pick something you enjoy and have fun.

Winter cardio calisthenics

You don't have to shackle yourself to a cardio machine if you live in a place that gets cold and snowy each winter. Some of the most fun and enjoyable forms of cardio are things you can do in the snow.

Cross-country skiing/ backcountry skiing

I like to think of X-C skiing as hiking with a gliding motion. It's a fantastic calorie burner because it uses a lot of muscle mass, plus it's a low impact activity which can be easy on the joints.

Backcountry skiing is essentially hiking up a mountain with special equipment that allows you to use your skis like snowshoes. Like cross country skiing you trek up in a gliding motion and ski back down. It's a full body workout that burns loads of calories while helping you escape the crowded resorts and long lift lines.

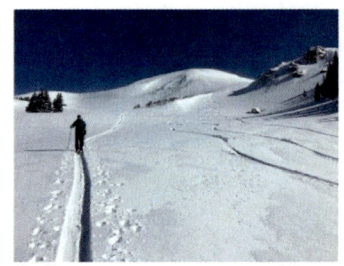

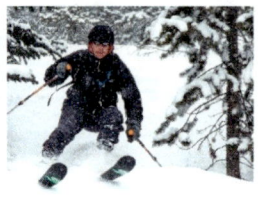

Hike up and ski down, it's a simple and effective way to get out and burn a bunch of calories. While it is not for the novice skier, it can be a fun way to make skiing more exciting if you're getting bored with the same old runs at the resort.

Cross-country skiing is easier to start off with since backcountry skiing does require you to be a pretty good skier to ski through woods and over the ungroomed terrain. There is also a higher risk of encountering avalanches in the backcountry. These are just a few of the reasons why skiing in the backcountry can be a more costly and risky form of recreation. X-C skiing is a lot easier to pick up and you can get started with an afternoon lesson and some rental equipment at your local ski resort.

Sledding

Sledding is traditionally seen as a childhood activity, but it's actually a high-quality cardio workout. It's easy to see why this is the case since you spend most of your time trekking up a   hill and much less time zipping down on a plastic sled. It's actually not that different from backcountry skiing which is pretty much the same thing only you're sledding down rather than skiing.

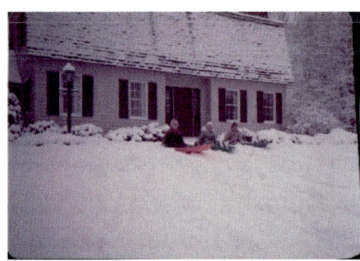

I'm the one on the far right along with my sister in the middle and my childhood friend Matt. We didn't have video games or cable TV back then but a decent sledding hill and a foot of snow were enough to keep us active and having fun all day long.

Even though sledding might seem like child's play, it is one of the riskiest winter activities you can do. Most of this is because you're rocketing down a natural slope, with trees and other hazards on a device with minimal control.

I'm not saying you need to wear motorcycle armor when sledding, just be a little cautious and be aware of your surroundings. Be sure to have plenty of run out room and stay clear of hazards like trees and rocks.

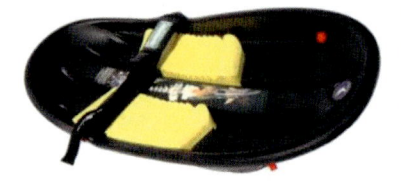

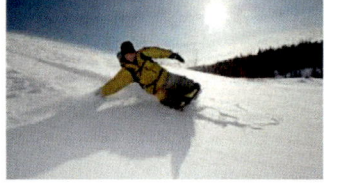

The Mad River Rocket is a fun knee sled some of my friends had back in Vermont. You could carry it on your back as you trekked up a hillside or mountain and you would knee surf down in pillow-soft powder. Photos: madriverrocket.com

Snowshoeing

Snowshoeing is primarily hiking in the wintertime which is a lot of fun and a great workout. It's amazing how a blanket of snow can transform a trail and how you move.

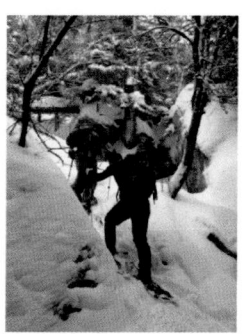

Some friends and I explore the snow-covered trails of Mt. Mansfield on a cold February morning. It's amazing how this trail looks and feels completely different from when we hike it in the summer.

I recommend using a couple of poles when snowshoeing as it improves balance and stability over soft terrain. It also involves more muscle and creates more tension throughout your body.

All of these winter activities require some investment in equipment. You may be able to find local resorts or shops that will rent you the equipment you need. Test drive the activity and see if it's something you want to invest your time and energy in. Once you find something you enjoy doing, you'll be able to stay in shape all winter long and avoid cabin fever.

Points To Ponder

1. Always be conscious of your use of muscle tension during any cardio activity. Try to avoid mentally zoning out too much and allowing your body to work on autopilot.
2. Plan your workouts in advance to prevent yourself from wandering aimlessly during a run or get lost on a hike. This helps quantify your training and helps you avoid being active longer than you should.
3. Be sure to wear appropriate clothing and equipment for your activity to increase comfort, performance, and safety.
4. Do your homework before picking up any new activity. Enlist the help of a friend or colleague who has experience in the activity you're looking to start.
5. Remember that any of these activities are supposed to be fun and enjoyable. Reevaluate your approach if an activity starts to feel like a tedious chore or starts to wear you down.
6. None of these cardio activities are essential. Even the very practice of "cardio" may not be all that important depending on your goals. Feel free to discard any of the above activities, or even cardio in general, if it's not a good fit for you.

Chapter 15 Principles of Programming

This chapter is where you'll start to take all of the exercise bits and pieces you've learned thus far and learn how to put them together into a plan that's best for you. After all, the power to build muscle or burn fat doesn't rest on any particular exercise, but in how you practice your training over time. One of the most important factors in successful training is to follow a planned out workout routine.

Building a solid workout routine isn't rocket science, but some experts like to treat it as such. The internet has loads of formulas and programs that approach exercise as if it's more complex than landing a man on the moon.

There is a time and place for elite level routines, especially when you need elite level performance. The best athletes in the world require programs that dial in every detail to gain a competitive edge. That's great if you're an Olympic athlete, but if you don't need to shave .10 seconds off a lap around a track, such complexity is not only unnecessary, it can distract you from what's most important for your goals. The simpler you make your workout plan, the more you put the odds in your favor. That's why this chapter is not just about smart programming, but how you can make your routines as simple as possible.

What A Routine Really Does

One of the biggest misconceptions in fitness is that getting results depends on dialing in the perfect workout routine. Once you figure out the perfect formula of sets and reps you'll achieve the body of your dreams. Some people spend years trying one routine after another in their search for that magic workout plan that will make their dreams come true.

Your results don't come from following the perfect routine. They come from using a basic routine to progress muscle tension. It doesn't matter what your routine looks like, if you don't improve how well you use tension you'll struggle to make progress. The purpose of a good routine is to help you train better, but it won't make your training more effective just because you follow a special formula.

Prepare for launch!

A good routine is like a launch pad for a rocket. While that launch pad is necessary, it's not what physically makes the rocket launch into space. Your workout routine is just like that launch pad. It's an important part of your success, but it's not wholly responsible for the results you want. Instead, your workout routine provides the same characteristics as that launch pad provides for a rocket.

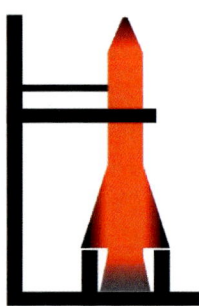

A good routine is just like the launchpad for this rocket. It provides structure and stability while pointing the rocket in the right direction. It plays an important role in getting it into orbit but it's not what physically makes the rocket launch into space.

The Three Elements Of A Good Workout Routine

An effective routine provides three essential structural elements that create the foundation for effective training.

#1 Structure

The biggest asset a routine provides comes from just having a plan in the first place. Writing down what you're going to do and when you'll do it provides structural integrity in your training. If your routine calls for squats on Tuesday and lunges on Friday, then you'll have the structure to ensure you're going to practice those moves on a regular basis. You're not going to be doing 100 squats every day for a week, then hardly any leg exercises for the next month.

#2 Balance

A good routine helps to keep your training balanced, so you avoid overtraining some muscle groups while neglecting others. Balance is of particular importance when it comes to your bodyweight training. It's easy to focus on big exercises like push-ups and pull-ups while neglecting bridges and legwork. Through using a structured routine, you'll have a plan that ensures you spend an equal amount of time on everything without falling victim to personal bias.

#3 Direction

While your routine isn't entirely responsible for your results but it does point you in the right direction. Building a routine that makes you aim for progressions in S.A.I.D, T.U.T or I.C.E. helps keep your eye on the ball, so you don't waste your time and energy on workouts that move you in the wrong direction.

Why You Should Build Your Own Routine

An effective routine has to do more than just require the neural code to progress S.A.I.D, T.U.T or I.C.E. It also needs to integrate with your lifestyle resources, preferances, and influences as easily as possible. The effectiveness of any routine must first and foremost depend on your ability to do that routine on a consistent basis for weeks at a time. It doesn't matter if a particular method has been proven to work for a lot of people. It won't help you achieve your goals if you have trouble sticking to it.

Building your plan around your circumstances is why I'm a big believer in creating your routine yourself. Only you understand your unique resources and limitations. Giving you a cookie-cutter workout would be like handing you a random pair of shoes and expecting you to run a marathon. Chances are, it won't be a good fit and would cause some issues sooner or later. When this happens, most people either quit or search out another random routine hoping for a good fit by sheer luck. Even if they do find a good fit, it won't stay that way forever. Your life, body, and goals change over time, so your routine should follow suit.

Creating your routine gives you the flexibility to customize your workout to fit your needs and preferences. It ensures you don't waste time on unneeded exercises, so your workouts are efficient and effective. It also allows you to make changes when you need to do so.

What Goes Into An Effective Routine?

Building a routine isn't complicated. It's just like building a spaceship out of Legos. You just collect the pieces and put them together according to your needs and preferences. You might ask yourself "how do

I know how everything goes together?" That's where S.A.I.D, T.U.T, and I.C.E. comes in. They are like compass needles pointing you in the direction you want to go. Just contemplate how any choice you make will influence the specific performance you need, the time under tension or your calorie expenditure.

So let's start by digging into the toy box for the pieces you need.

Piece 1 Exercises

Be sure to select exercises that require you to create a neural code that can satisfy S.A.I.D, T.U.T or I.C.E. There's not much sense in doing 100 push-ups every day when you want to become a fast sprinter or run every day when you want to build your upper body. Select exercises that can help you increase calorie expenditure, put tension in your muscles or challenge the functional abilities you want.

Piece 2 The volume to intensity ratio

This is actually 2 pieces, but they come super glued together because they are used in balance to one another. The more you do an exercise the less intensity you can use and vice versa. Think of running a marathon or running a sprint. You can't sprint a marathon nor would you get much from doing a marathon pace for 200 meters.

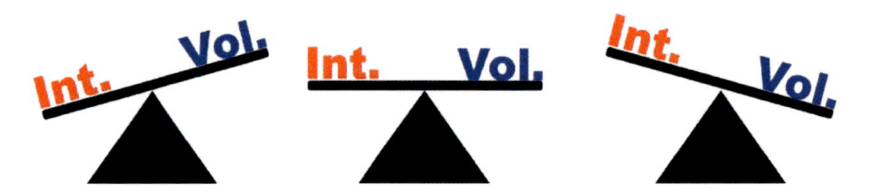

A good routine will balance volume and intensity according to your personal needs and goals. The more intensity you need the less volume you'll use and vice versa.

Piece 3 Frequency

Frequency usually refers to how many times you train in a week, but it can also refer to how often you train each year, month, or day as well.

So there's not too much to it, you just have a given exercise, a ratio of intensity and volume and the frequency. Pretty much all routine variations will adjust one or all three of those variables. The trick is figuring out the best combination for your goals and lifestyle. To help get you started, here are some routine guidelines for building workouts focused on S.A.I.D, T.U.T, and I.C.E.

Building A Routine For Muscle Growth (Progression Of T.U.T)

Exercise selection

Use basic compound exercises that require a moderate to high degree of tension along your muscle chains. The exercises listed in the chapters on how to work your muscle chains are all good examples.

Volume / intensity ratio

Muscle building routines use a range of both intensity and volume. Some workouts use hard exercises with relatively low volume while others use easier exercises and more volume. Most muscle building routines involve using enough resistance to fatigue your muscles within 15-90 seconds.

Frequency

Train each muscle group 1-3 times a week.

Routine objective

The purpose of a muscle building routine is to bring your muscles to a high level of fatigue and then to let them recover over several days. This type of training uses the natural cycle of eliciting a stress-inducing stimulus followed by super-compensation when your muscles come back a little bigger and stronger than before.

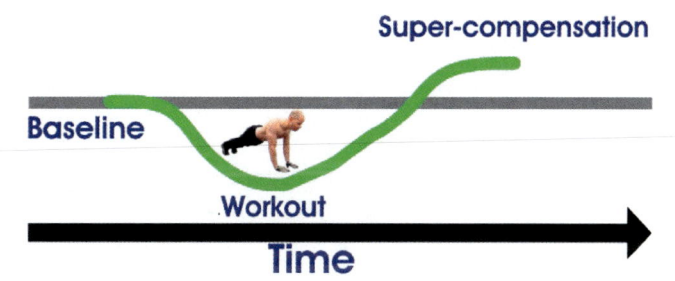

Muscle building workouts use up a lot of muscle energy which creates a lot of fatigue. The body then super compensates when it recovers by building up slightly more capability in the muscle than it had before. Repeating this cycle over time is how you build muscle.

Routine progression

Progression involves see-sawing the volume and intensity ratio to increase the work capacity of the muscles you're training. Athletes practice this by selecting an exercise that places a given amount of tension in the muscle, which typically allowing for 5-12 or more reps.

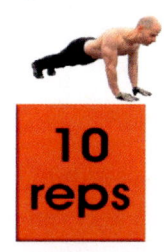

From there you progress the volume of the exercise by adding reps or the amount of time you can perform that exercise.

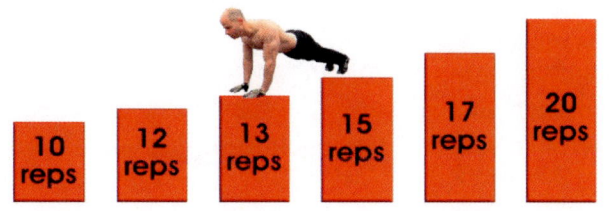

Adding volume to the same amount of intensity helps you build the work capacity of the muscle which in this case is a standard military style push-up.

Once you have added a significant amount of volume, you add more resistance which will drop the amount of time you can do the exercise, and the process starts over again.

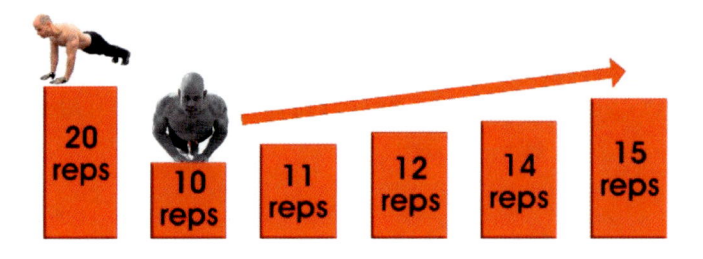

Once you've built up some stamina with a given technique, you progress to a more advanced variation (in this case close push-ups) which will drop your reps. You then build your reps back up with the harder exercise and repeat the process.

Other considerations

This routine is all about creating and controlling muscle fatigue. Both exercise time and rest time are variables you can manipulate to progress fatigue. You can progress muscle fatigue by shortening the rest time between sets even if the resistance and time under tension are the same.

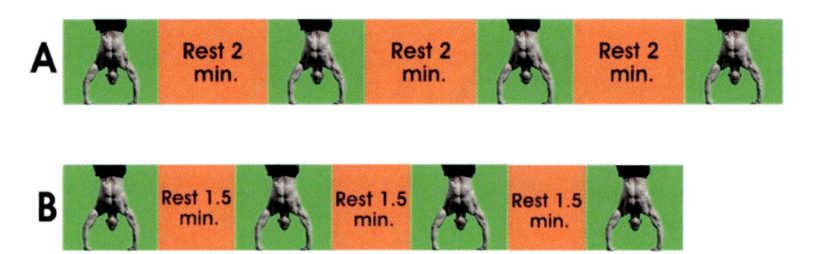

Both handstand workout A and B use the same exercise for the same amount of time, but workout B uses a shorter rest period between each set. This creates more total fatigue and potential muscle building stimulus even though the actual workload is the same.

Resting between 45-90 seconds works well in most cases, but start off with a rest period that feels right for you and shorten it if you want. The most important thing is to keep your rest periods consistent. Keeping a regular rest period prevents inconsistent levels of fatigue from one workout to the next which can compromise long-term results.

The number of sets is a bit of a topic of debate. Some experts, whom I call sprinters, swear by hitting the muscle fast and hard with 1-2 intense sets. Others, who are like marathon runners, claim volume is the way to go and endorse as many as ten sets.

Both strategies use different extremes of the volume and intensity balance. Sprinters use intensity to bring the muscles to a high level of fatigue very quickly while marathoners use volume to reach a high state of fatigue but at a slower pace.

I find the best strategy for you may depend on your attitude and the mentality you bring to training. It takes a different type of mental discipline to emphasize either intensity or volume. People tend to do better with an emphasis on either volume or intensity and seldom do as well if they change to the other method. When a sprinter attempts volume training, they burn themselves out very quickly. They might not even be able to complete the workout. If a marathoner attempts a low volume routine, they lack the ability to use the required intensity to get much from just one or two sets. Pay attention to what feels best for you.

In either case, neither high volume nor intensity will produce results if you don't progress your training over time. You'll need to progress both volume and intensity to some degree either way.

Full body or split training?

There are benefits to both split training and full body workouts. Split training allows you to focus a lot of energy toward working a few select muscle chains. For example, a squat chain workout can involve doing lunges, squats, calf raises and hill sprints. All of those exercises can take a lot of time and energy making it impractical to do that much work for all muscle groups in a full body workout.

A full body routine can help you maintain a consistent amount of work on a muscle group, especially if your schedule is unpredictable. I like to give full body routines to my clients who travel a lot and find they can't reliably train 4-5 times a week. Giving them a full body routine ensures they work all of their muscle chains 2-3 times a week even when their schedule is hectic.

My experience is that both full body and split routines can work very well so it's best to use whichever method works best for you. Your results depend more on the amount of work you do over weeks, months and years. 10 pull chain workouts a month will produce the same basic results regardless of if you do them in a split routine or full body workouts.

Should you train to failure?

Training to muscular failure is a topic of debate among muscle building athletes. Some claim you need to push yourself until you can't do one more rep while others claim doing so is unnecessary and even dangerous.

My experience is that what people tend to call "failure" is more about the mind failing rather than the body. Training to true muscular failure is incredibly difficult to do. I've pushed my legs to muscular failure no more than twice in my entire training career. In both cases, I had to lay down for a while because my leg muscles refused to do anything I asked of them. I couldn't even stand up!

Sometimes training to failure refers to "technical failure" where you do an exercise until you can't continue to do it anymore with good form. This is a lot easier to do, but it's still mostly a mental limitation than a physical one. There are countless examples of athletes going beyond their perceived limitations once they change their mental state.

So pushing yourself as hard as you can is something you can only do once in a great while, and a mental illusion the rest of the time. This is why I'm not a big believer in the idea of training to failure. Most of the time, it only reinforces your current mental limits. The more you hit a perceived limitation the more you reinforce that limit. When someone says "I can only do 4 pull-ups, how can I do more?" I first tell them to stop saying they can only do 4 pull-ups!

Leaving a little left in the tank may help your body recover faster, but more importantly, it prevents you from getting mentally stuck. Thinking "I could have pushed a little harder" sets you up for more progress in your next workout because you know you can go beyond what you did before.

Lastly, you don't have to push your muscles until they are completely drained to stimulate muscle growth. If you finish a leg workout, and can still walk and climb stairs, then you still left some energy in your leg muscles. Don't worry though, because I promise you'll still build muscle even though you can walk around afterward. Bringing your muscles to a state of "high fatigue" means exactly that. They aren't completely trashed, they are just pretty tired and that's enough to stimulate the growth you want.

Building A Routine for Performance And Capability (Progressions Of S.A.I.D)

Exercise selection

Use exercises and drills that challenge the specific performance you want to improve. For example, do hill sprints if you want to run faster, or do slow sidekicks if you want to improve hip control and stability.

Volume / intensity ratio

Training for functional capability can span a wide range of volume and intensity. Some capabilities, like strength, speed, and power, can require a lot of intensity and don't use a lot of volume. Other capabilities, like stability, balance, and mobility are not very physically demanding and often require much more volume. The general rule of thumb is the more fatigue the training creates the less volume you use and vice versa.

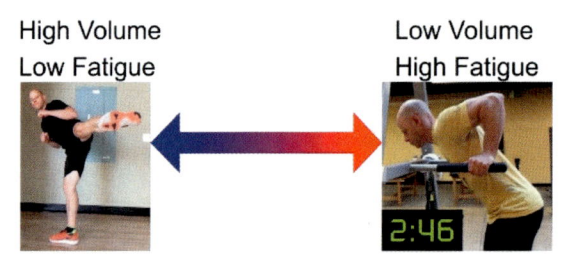

Low fatigue training, like holding a sidekick for 5 seconds is something you can practice every day. High fatigue training, like doing dips for 3 minutes is something you only practice once or twice a week to allow for more recovery.

Frequency

Frequency depends on the amount of fatigue your training produces. Methods that produce a lot of fatigue should be done for low-frequency like around 1-2 times a week. Exercises that do not produce a lot of fatigue can be practiced every day, or even multiple times a day.

Routine objective

The purpose of a S.A.I.D focused routine is to practice producing the neural code that creates the functional ability you want. Each training session is where you try to make your body do something better. It could be trying to jump higher, squat deeper or holding a handstand without shaking.

Routine progression

Progression happens when you become more proficient in your ability to do what you're trying to do. Sometimes, this can be obvious through quantifiable measurements like time, speed or reps. Other times, an improvement in performance is self-evident as it becomes easier to accomplish what used to be more difficult.

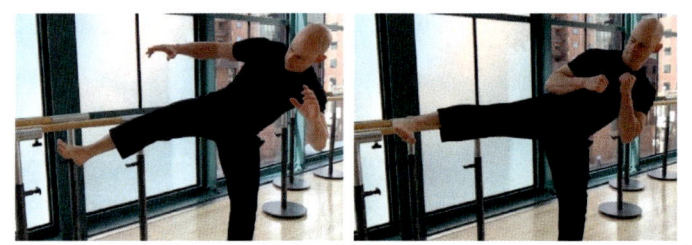

Performance improvements are usually self-evident. It doesn't take a trained eye to notice how my sidekick is better in the image on the right compared to the sloppy kick on the left.

Other considerations

Don't fall for the myth that practice makes perfect and progress will come if you put in enough time and effort. While improvement does require hard work, it's always possible to be no faster, stronger or capable than before despite even years of training.

Any improvement in your ability to do something comes from concentrating on how you're training and constantly trying to improve. In other words, consistently trying to improve your neural code, so you use your body to produce a better performance.

Performance training can become confusing which is why hiring a coach can be extremely helpful. A trained expert can observe what you do and advise you on how to progress your technique.

A good coach will tell you how to use your body in a smarter way. They'll show you how to use your hips to jump higher, or where to look when dribbling down the court. They will not only ask you to perform better but tell you exactly what to do to make that happen.

While a coach or trainer can be a powerful asset, you may not always have access to someone who can help you. In this case, you'll have to be your own coach. While this may not always be ideal, it's not an impossible situation either.

I recommend using what I call comparative training. Comparative training is when you observe the differences between times when you perform better, and times you perform worse. For example, say you're working on your handstands. In one workout you feel stable and strong while holding a handstand. A few days later you feel sloppy and unstable. Your mission is to figure out why there was a difference between the two workouts. Maybe you didn't have enough tension in your back. Perhaps you forgot to keep your hands clenched into the floor. Once you find that difference, you'll know what you need to work on to improve.

Building A Routine For Fat Loss (Progression Of I.C.E)

Exercise selection

Use exercises that work a lot of muscle to speed up your caloric expenditure. Most calorie burning exercises make extensive use of the lower body for this reason. You'll also probably use a lot of exercises that involve fast repetitive motions like stepping or pedaling to be able to do them for relatively long periods of time.

Volume / intensity ratio

Both volume and intensity can increase the rate at which you burn calories. You'll burn a greater total number of calories through either training longer or harder. Many fat burning routines will involve a variety of activities that use a range of both intensity and volume.

Frequency

Like with performance workouts, calorie burning workouts can produce various levels of fatigue. The frequency of a workout depends on the amount of fatigue you experience from your workout. A bout of exercise that creates a lot of fatigue, like a hard run, is something you'll only do 1-2 times a week. However, something like a short walk after dinner is something you can do daily.

Routine objective

The aim of an I.C.E routine is to accelerate the rate at which you burn calories to increase your total calorie expenditure. In other words, burn those calories by the truckload!

Routine progression

Like with a T.U.T routine, you can progress your I.C.E routine by adding either tension (intensity) or time (volume) to your routine. Adding either will increase the rate at which you burn calories and result in a greater total calorie expenditure. You might have a high-intensity activity, like that 5K race once a week, but you can always add a moderate to low intensity activity, like a casual hiking, throughout the week. In short, doing more helps you burn more.

With that said, your I.C.E routine isn't something you typically progress over time like you would a S.A.I.D or T.U.T routine. You'll probably find yourself settling on a consistent activity, like a bi-weekly 3-mile run, and maintain that without any major progressions after the first few months. You don't always have to progress your I.C.E routine to keep seeing results. Since the objective is to burn calories, you'll be successful simply by being more active. You don't always have to add more exercise and effort to your routine. You can also seek to progress the T.U.T or S.A.I.D qualities of your I.C.E routine. You might work to smooth out your stride during your run or seek to decrease your 5K run time. You can also progress the tension control in your muscles as you exercise or add a little resistance by pedaling in a higher gear.

Don't forget you can also progress weight loss through making changes in your diet and lifestyle habits as well.

Other considerations

An I.C.E routine is one of the simplest and most basic forms of training you can do. It doesn't usually require much skill, but it may help to get some coaching to prevent injury from your exercise of choice.

The most important thing is not to become too dependent upon your calorie expending workouts to control your weight. Adjust both diet and activity levels to help manage your weight. That way, you won't fall into the trap of using exercise to compensate for a poor diet, or a super strict diet to make up for a lack of physical activity.

How To Create Your Own Workout Routine

As the saying goes, if you're not planning to succeed you're planning to fail. A lot of your success will come, not from getting every detail right, but from having a weekly plan in the first place. Once you have a plan in place, you'll be in a much better position to succeed. Follow these simple steps to establish your basic game plan.

Step 1 Establish the objective of your training

The first step is to decide what you want to accomplish with your training. Do you want to build muscle, improve performance or burn fat? Remember, you're going to be working on all 3 to some degree no matter what you do. You're just selecting the area you want to emphasize your results.

You can also pursue multiple goals at once. You can practice hitting a punching bag to work on your punching technique while improving endurance and burning calories at the same time. You don't have to always select one goal at the expense of the other two, but it does help to prioritize what's most important to you.

Step 2 Build your weekly plan

I find most people like to work off of a seven-day plan so pull out a calendar and plan out what you're going to do every day of the week. If you're planning on taking a rest day, then make sure you plan those as well.

If your goal is to improve performance, plan what days you're going to practice your skills. Include what days you'll meet with your coach and which days you'll rest. If you're practicing something that requires more recovery plan what days you'll work harder and which days you'll go easier.

Weekly Workout Plan for Karate

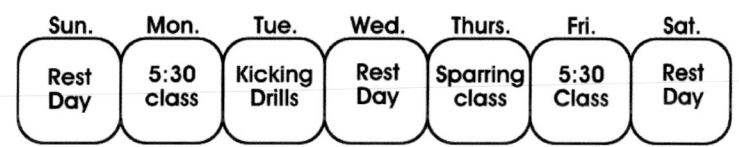

Sun.	Mon.	Tue.	Wed.	Thurs.	Fri.	Sat.
Rest Day	5:30 class	Kicking Drills	Rest Day	Sparring class	5:30 Class	Rest Day

This sample weekly training plan shows what you might practice on each day to prepare for a Karate tournament. This plan keeps your training structured and consistent while ensuring you're working on what is most important to you.

If building muscle or strength is your goal, plan which days you'll work each muscle chain.

Weekly Workout Plan for Building Muscle

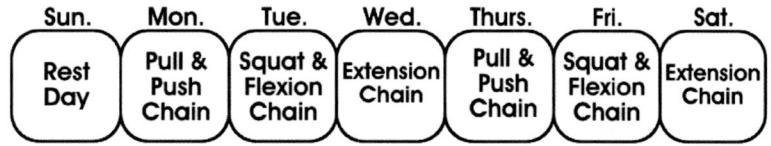

Sun.	Mon.	Tue.	Wed.	Thurs.	Fri.	Sat.
Rest Day	Pull & Push Chain	Squat & Flexion Chain	Extension Chain	Pull & Push Chain	Squat & Flexion Chain	Extension Chain

This sample workout plan details what muscle chains you might work throughout the week. It's a classic 3-way split which repeats twice while giving you one full rest day on Sunday. This example also gives you 3-4 days to recover from each workout.

If you want to pursue multiple goals plan which days you'll train toward each objective.

Weekly Workout Plan for Karate & Building Muscle

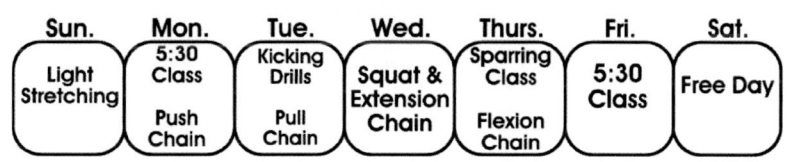

Sun.	Mon.	Tue.	Wed.	Thurs.	Fri.	Sat.
Light Stretching	5:30 Class / Push Chain	Kicking Drills / Pull Chain	Squat & Extension Chain	Sparring Class / Flexion Chain	5:30 Class	Free Day

A hypothetical weekly plan for training in Karate and building muscle. This plan works the major muscle chains once a week alongside martial arts training. It also uses a free day for freestyle and playful activity.

Step 3 Plan each training session

Once you have your weekly routine, it's time to plan what you'll do during each session. What activities are you going to do? What muscle chains are you going to work? What skills are you going to practice? How long are you going to walk for? How many sets are you going to do? Don't worry too much about getting everything perfect. This step isn't about figuring out what will get you results. It's just about figuring out what will get you started.

Monday Plan

```
Mon.
5:30
Class      - Take class & stay after to
             work on forms.
Push       - 3 sets of close push-ups.
Chain      - Isometric handstand hold
             for time. 2 sets.
```

This sample plan for Monday outlines what you might work on for the day. The Karate class would be mostly up to the instructor but you've made a note to work on some additional skills. The strength training routine is a simple workout of push-ups and isometric handstand work.

Step 4 Test out your plan and establish a baseline of performance

At this point, your plan isn't 100% perfect, but it doesn't have to be. All you need is a general idea of what to do each day of the week and what you'll do in each training session.

I recommend easing into your training plan and not pushing yourself as hard as possible. Keep in mind that your results don't depend on always pushing yourself to your limit. They depend on progressing your muscle tension over time. Holding back a little can make it easier to progress compared to rushing forward. If you feel you might be able to do 50 push-ups, do 35. If you think you might be able to run 3 miles 3x a week, just run 2 miles twice a week. There's plenty of time to ramp things up later, and you're playing the long game here.

Now is also the ideal time to start keeping a log of what you're doing. Your workout journal doesn't need to be anything fancy. Just write down what you do and how you do it. Doing so will help you remember what you've done and remind you how to progress in your next workout.

Step 5 Progress, modify and adjust

This is the step that will make or break most of your success. Your results won't be from some special routine or plan; they come from the progressions and modifications you make to the plan you practice.

Start each session by checking your workout log to remind yourself what you're working on to improve. Are you adding a few reps to those push-ups? Are you focusing on keeping your shoulders square while shooting free-throws? Maybe you're just trying to relax your shoulders when running.

Go through your workout while taking notes (mental or physical) about your experience. At the end of your workout contemplate how it went and what you can do to improve. Write down anything you discover or think might be helpful for the next time. This simple habit of thinking about what you're doing and contemplating how to improve is the essence of smart training.

Trust your experience

Your experience is the most valuable asset in your training. It gives you accurate neural feedback about what is happening. Only you can feel how you're doing an exercise. You're the only person on earth who can receive the honest negative and positive feedback from every moment in your workout.

Pay attention to your hunches and ideas. If you're thinking about moving your leg workout from Friday to Wednesday, there's probably a good reason for that. An effective workout involves a degree of trial and error so don't be afraid to experiment.

How Often Should You Change Your Routine?

I'm not a big believer in the idea that you should change your routine as a matter of habit. When you overhaul your program, you run the risk of potentially losing some of the progress you've built. Change is always a gamble, and there's no promise that you'll stimulate progress just because you're doing something different.

Sometimes it's good to make changes, but it's better to change out of necessity rather than novelty. Some good reasons to make a change include fitting your training around a change in your schedule or adjusting your workouts to address weaknesses. If you think making a change might improve some aspect of your training, then go right ahead and make the change. Don't wait four weeks, just give it a shot. If your routine is feeling a little stale, by all means, change it up a bit, just make sure you're still focusing on appropriately using tension for your goals. Always keep your mind looking for better ways to train rather than just different ways to train.

Tips For A Smart Warm Up

Warming up is important, but it's easy to overcomplicate it. I've even met some people whose warm-up is longer than their actual workout. Just as with your workouts, you want your warm-up to be simple, efficient and smart. You can make this happen the following ways.

#1 Be specific to the activity you want to do

Most of your warm-up should involve doing lighter versions of the very movements you plan on doing. Do some light jogging or marching in place if you're going for a run. Do incline push-ups before close push-ups. Gently swing your golf club before crushing the ball off the first tee.

Too many people waste time and energy with warm-up activities that are metabolically and neurologically different than their actual workout. Running on a treadmill is both metabolically and neurologically different than doing pull-ups. While it might get your heart rate up, it won't do a lot to prepare you for hanging from a bar.

#2 Address personal issues

A good warm-up should also address any physical issues you may have. This might include some tight or sore areas of your body or performance challenges like balance or tension control.

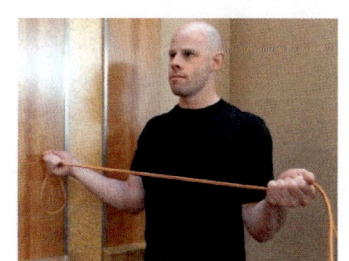

I suffered multiple shoulder issues due to chronic internal rotation. Using a band to strengthen my external shoulder rotation became a regular part of my warm-up for several months.

Issues like tightness or soreness often originate from your neural code. No one has a sore lower back from a lack of foam rolling or not enough time on a stretching machine. Most of the time, these passive warm-up exercises do very little to address the true issue which is how you're using muscle tension. Maybe your lower back is tight because of weak hips. Your shoulders could be sore because you lack scapular control. Whatever the issue is, stiff and sore areas of your body are usually the result of how you use your body on a daily basis rather than a lack of a proper warm up. Consult with a coach or therapist who can diagnose what's going on so you can target the real issue that's holding you back.

#3 Move and loosen up every day

A lot of people feel they can't exercise without a long warm-up because they feel stiff and cold before every workout. They go through a long routine and finally feel like they are ready to train. The fact is, they probably don't need a long warm up to get ready to exercise. They need a long warm up to recover from extended periods of being sedentary.

It's no secret that modern living has made even moderately active people more sedentary. I'm a personal trainer who works in a gym, and even I find myself sitting for hours at a stretch. This lack of activity causes even the most active people to grow stiff and weak between workouts thus requiring more preparation before moving.

The solution isn't to make your warm up more costly and complicated; it's to be more active every day so you don't need a long warm up in the first place.

You don't need to work out for hours every day to be more action ready from one workout to the next. Habitually engaging in small activities throughout the day can do wonders. For example, I make a habit of squatting down to pick things up off the floor. Doing this helps keep my legs pretty lumber and ready to go at any time. I can take off for a jog at the drop of a hat and hard leg workouts only take a minute or two to prepare for.

My muscles and joints were always stiff and tight which required an extensive warm up before every workout. Now, I can kick, run and jump without any warm-up because I squat down every day like when cleaning equipment at the gym.

Other examples can include joint circles and light stretching throughout the day for a few moments. Standing tall and rolling your shoulders might not seem like a lot, but it doesn't take much to combat the effects of sitting at a desk for hours at a time.

Breaking Out Of The Workout Prison

The notion of being active every day might seem a little extreme, but this is actually how your body was designed to be used. These days, people are working out and exercising more than ever, yet daily activity levels are still on the decline.

The idea of being active with a workout is actually an artificial invention. All throughout history, people have been active as a form of labor and utility. Look at manual laborers such as farmers. They don't fit their activity into orderly scheduled bouts of exercise at regular intervals. If they need to load hay they do it for however long it takes to get the job done. They are not worried about optimal sets and reps or overtraining.

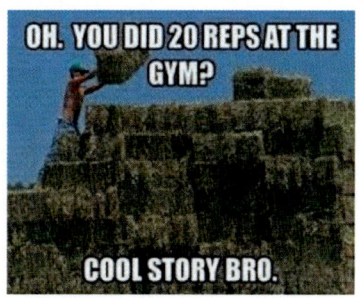

I can relate to this image because I did a lot of manual labor when I was younger. I never worried about overtraining or keeping my physical activity in scheduled chunks. I just worked hard until the job was done which is all your body cares about.

Modern fitness workouts have done the same thing to human activity as zoos do to animals. It takes something natural and organic and confines it into an artificial system that uses imposed schedules and guidelines.

Not that I have anything against working out. I love going to the local playground and just working hard for an hour or so. Doing a workout is a great break from the stress of everyday life, and it helps keep your activity levels consistent.

The issue isn't the artificial construct of a workout. It's the fact that this unnatural use of physical activity is just about the only time people are doing any meaningful activity at all.

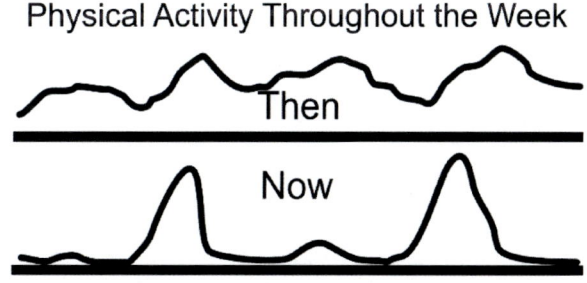

Modern technology has greatly reduced the amount of natural physical activity most people experience on a daily basis. In the past, most people were fairly active throughout the week. Now, most folks are very sedentary with occasional bursts of intense activity that we call "workouts."

The result of this shift is people are working out more than ever, yet are less active overall. The long sessions of sedentary living condition the body to be stiff and weak, and then we expect our body to perform well during high-intensity exercise. It's like taking a car and having it sit in a cold garage for a day or two, and then driving it hard on a race track for an hour 2-3 times a week. Then we act all surprised with things start to break and wear out.

As a human being, you are designed to be active, to some degree, every single day. Sometimes your activity is light and refreshing. Other times it's intense and challenging. The modern approach to exercise fights against this natural tendency. We're either sitting idle or pushing ourselves as hard as possible. It's no wonder people feel stressed and banged up all the time.

Calisthenics helps you escape the artificial workout prison

Using a gym and specific equipment creates the idea that you're only supposed to be active when you're in a specific place at a specific time. The equipment is designed to work the body hard, so we naturally assume that if we're using it we're supposed to be pushing ourselves with very intense exercise.

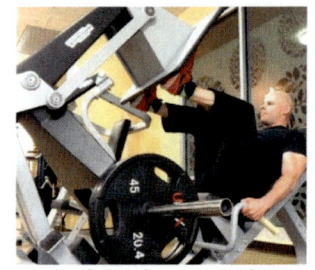

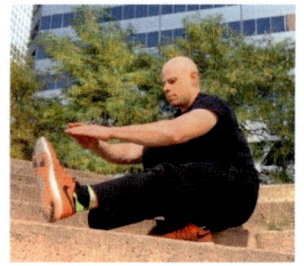

Progressive calisthenics can be done almost anywhere at any time, but a leg press doesn't offer as much flexibility.

Calisthenics helps you break free of the confines of working out because you can do it anywhere at any time. You don't always need to do a workout to use your body; you just need to move. You can squat down to pick up items from the floor. You can hang from a doorway pull-up bar before walking into your room. You can do a set of calf raises while waiting for the bus. You can even stand on one leg while putting on your shoes.

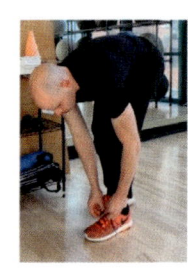

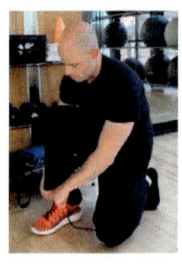

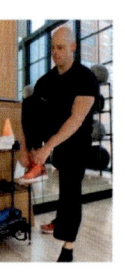

Opportunities to train are everywhere! Even a simple activity, like putting on your shoes, can improve your fitness. You can stretch your hamstrings like in the image on the left, crouch down and work on hip mobility or work on hip stability and strength by standing on one leg.

Sprinkling activity throughout your day will do wonders to increase your activity level outside your workout. It increases your total calorie expenditure, refines your neural code and improves tension control. In other words, it turns the tide against chronic sedentary living without requiring a lot of lifestyle adjustment. Now your training works with your daily routine instead of forcing itself into your schedule while eating up a lot of your limited time and energy.

Points To Ponder

1. Don't worry too much about finding the perfect routine. Remember that success comes from the progression of your training rather than the routine you follow.
2. Feel free to change your routine whenever you feel the need to do so.
3. At the same time, don't make unnecessary changes if they are not called for. Needless changes can jeopardize your consistency and overall progress.
4. If you're struggling to maintain a certain routine scale back and make it shorter so it doesn't require as much time or energy. A shorter routine you can consistently practice will always produce better results than a big routine you struggle to maintain.
5. Stay vigilant against "bloating" your routine by adding exercises that do little for you. Focus on basic moves and be sure anything you add will bring some noticeable value to your fitness. If you're not sure about the effectiveness of an exercise, cut it from your routine for a few weeks and see if you notice any difference.

Chapter 16 Eating For Success

Diet and exercise go together like peas and carrots or as I prefer, chocolate and peanut butter. That's why I thought it made sense to spill a few words about dietary considerations here. Before I get to the meat and potatoes of good dietary habits, let's take a moment to consider if you need to make any changes in your diet in the first place.

Beware of assuming you need to change your diet just because you do something called a workout. Remember, a workout is a theoretical concept people invented to quantify physical activity. Assuming you need to follow certain dietary rules because you do an exercise routine can be a bit risky. A workout can mean anything from a few sets of pull-ups to a 5-hour trail run. Following general dietary rules just because you exercise can be very hit or miss depending on how much influence your training has over your nutritional needs.

Your workout also isn't the only thing that influences your nutritional requirements. It may not even be a big influence on your nutritional needs compared to the rest of your lifestyle. Some workouts don't involve that much activity. Have you ever measured the actual amount of time you're active during a strength workout? I've known some guys who spend hours in the gym, but once you subtract the time they spend talking, watching TV or playing on their phone, they've only been active for around twenty minutes. Afterward, they scarf down a high-calorie protein shake in the belief their body needs it after such a long workout. A few months go by, and they wonder why their pants are tight in the waist, and the scale keeps climbing even though they've been "eating right."

All physical activity can influence your nutritional demand, and sometimes your general physical activity can be more important than your workouts. When I was in school, I used to take on physically active summer jobs that had me moving and lifting stuff for hours every day. I always found myself getting super hungry and tired because I wasn't eating enough. I didn't think washing cars or carrying crates of soda counted because it wasn't a "workout." Looking back, I should have packed a couple of extra sandwiches in my lunch each morning.

I'm telling you this story to illustrate the point that your workouts may or may not require you to make any changes to your diet. Your nutritional requirements depend on a lot of factors, and your workouts are just a few of them. It's for this reason this chapter will be more about general healthy eating for the active individual instead of specific rules that may or may not be required by your workout.

Two Limited Theories About Exercise Nutrition

Throughout the years, I've found most dietary advice for athletes falls into one of two camps. On the one hand, you have the "eat big" strategy. This philosophy is built on the idea that you need to eat a lot to build muscle and fuel your grueling workouts. This approach also champions the notion that you need to be in a calorie surplus to build muscle and fuel your training. It commonly uses strategies that involve eating many times a day while ingesting large quantities of protein. It's also a method that tends to favor quantity over quality while being a little more liberal when it comes to food choices. You're a little more free to eat a bit more calorie-laden "junk foods" to get enough calories and protein.

On the other hand, you have the "eat right" camp. This philosophy is more about food quality over food quantity and tends to be about following a set of dietary rules that claim to be the "correct" way to eat. These rules are often just as much about what you shouldn't eat as much as what you should. Theories range from claims that you shouldn't eat sugar, carbs, processed food, fat, grain, milk, animal products or even food that's cooked.

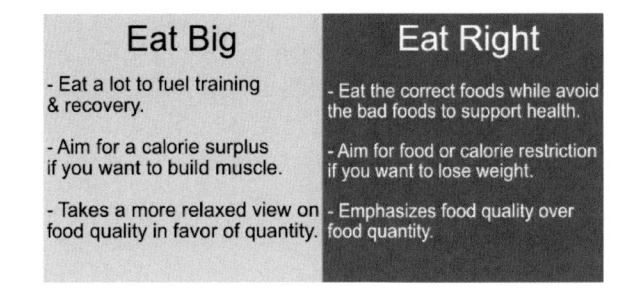

Eat Big	Eat Right
- Eat a lot to fuel training & recovery.	- Eat the correct foods while avoid the bad foods to support health.
- Aim for a calorie surplus if you want to build muscle.	- Aim for food or calorie restriction if you want to lose weight.
- Takes a more relaxed view on food quality in favor of quantity.	- Emphasizes food quality over food quantity.

Both ideologies bring something to the table. The eat big method is great for ensuring you're eating plenty of food to recover and fuel your training. The eat right method is great for ensuring you're not overeating junk food and getting enough nutrients to support recovery.

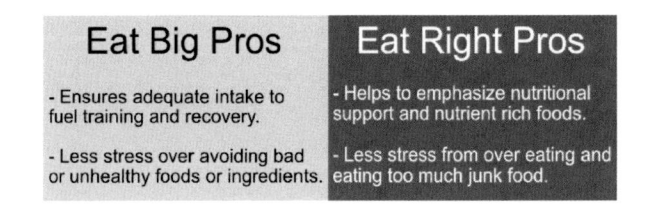

Eat Big Pros	Eat Right Pros
- Ensures adequate intake to fuel training and recovery.	- Helps to emphasize nutritional support and nutrient rich foods.
- Less stress over avoiding bad or unhealthy foods or ingredients.	- Less stress from over eating and eating too much junk food.

Both sides have their drawbacks as well. The eat big idea can potentially cause overeating which is not only stressful on your body but can result in excess body fat. Not only is gaining fat typically undesirable from a health and aesthetic perspective, but it also compromises your strength to weight ratio which is vital to calisthenics training. Meanwhile, eating right might seem ideal on paper, but basing your diet on restriction can cause stressful deprivation, hunger, and cravings.

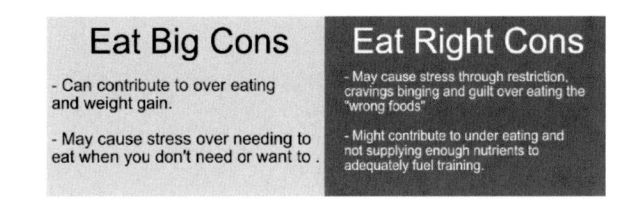

Eat Big Cons	Eat Right Cons
- Can contribute to over eating and weight gain.	- May cause stress through restriction, cravings binging and guilt over eating the "wrong foods"
- May cause stress over needing to eat when you don't need or want to.	- Might contribute to under eating and not supplying enough nutrients to adequately fuel training.

Sadly, both dietary methods portray these negatives as a necessary price to pay for success. I've met people who take pride in suffering such consequences and perceive them as a sign that they are "being good" and following the rules of their dietary theories. They believe gaining some flab is a sure sign they are packing on muscle from that calorie surplus. Fighting cravings just means they're exercising self-control and enduring the noble fight against their "addiction" to whatever evils lurk within the foods a dietary dogma deems to be bad.

I used to bounce between these two schools of thought for years until I started to question what a healthy diet was supposed to do. Was it about losing weight and improving blood work? Was it about trying to live to be 120? Where did the quality of life fit into a healthy diet? Did it make sense to pattern a lifestyle around eating right even if it comprises other aspects of my life?

I decided to do what I do best and dig deep to figure out the real purpose of a healthy diet for all athletes, but especially those who practice calisthenics. It wasn't hard to find once I considered how food related to training.

The True Role Of A Healthy Diet

Basic training theory states you achieve results through controlling a cycle of stress and recovery. You create physical change through a stress-inducing stimulus (training) followed by stress reducing recovery (sleep, R&R, Diet, etc.)

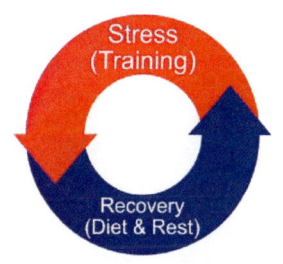

Effective training uses both a stress-inducing stimulus and a period of recovery in a repeating cycle.

Observing this fundamental principle of exercise science brought me to a profound realization. Diet and nutrition played a significant role in *recovery*. It's supposed to help you recover from stress; not cause it.

The idea that a healthy diet removes stress sparked a bit of disruption in how I perceived the two popular dietary theories. Both ideas can potentially relieve stress, but each method can also induce stress when taken to an extreme. Eating big can put you at risk of overeating while restrictive diets carry the risk of under eating. This stress isn't just physical hunger or deprivation. Mentally stressing out over the struggle to eat according to a set of rules can slow your recovery too.

Like many things in life, what's best for you is probably somewhere between the two extremes. Your Goldilocks zone probably resides where you have a mix of both methods. That way, you eat enough to avoid the stress of deprivation but not too much and avoid the stress of overeating.

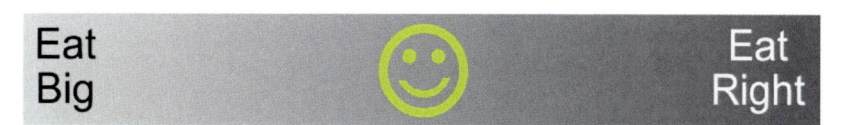

Eating Big and Eating Right are on opposite ends of an infinitely adjustable spectrum. You don't need to fully adhere to, or reject, either school of thought. Your best diet will probably use a mix of both approaches.

The question is, where do you fit along the spectrum with the right amount of each for your personal needs. Everyone brings a different set of circumstances to the table including lifestyle, genetics, and resources. You might lean slightly toward the eat big mentality and need to emphasize a hearty diet without worrying too much about eating "clean" all the time. You may trend toward the eating right side where you do need to be more careful of what you eat and shouldn't be too carefree at the Chinese Buffet.

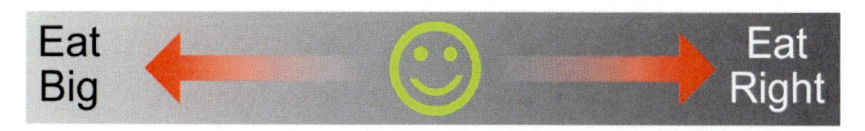

Everyone's dietary needs are unique. You may find you're better off eating more toward one side or the other depending on several lifestyle influences. The important thing is to give yourself permission to do what's best for you.

Keep in mind that your dietary needs can change over time. You may have been more on the eat big side when you were playing rugby in college. Now you're a 60-hour a week desk jockey and you need to be a little more selective about what foods you eat.

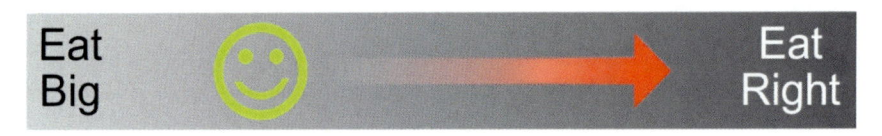

Your dietary needs can change over time. Being flexible in your dietary habits helps prevent the stress that comes from forcing yourself to eat in a way that no longer works for you.

Finding, and maintaining your ideal dietary habits is a skill you hone with practice. It may seem tricky at first, but the long-term payoff is maintaining a healthy diet will become easier and more beneficial over time. On the other hand, the rules of the dietary extremes are straightforward and easy to learn at first, but harder to apply in the long run.

Your best course of action will depend on how you respond to a variety of constantly changing variables that are unique to you. While the rules of a dietary dogma use a one-size-fits-all approach, real healthy eating relies on experience and learning to figure out what's best for you.

These tips can help you create a general plan that works best for you, and you can adjust or modify them as you wish.

#1 Maintain a consistent diet based on wholesome meals

Sitting down to enjoy a balanced meal is becoming less frequent and random as on-the-go snacking has become the normal way to eat in the modern age. Snacking usually involves grabbing whatever cheap and processed foods are readily available which means food quality and satisfaction are compromised.

There are many disadvantages to basing your diet on snack-style foods instead of substantial meals but here are just a few of the biggest reasons.

Meals require planning

A meal requires more forethought and consideration compared to snacking which usually involves making random and impulsive choices. A diet based on 2-3 meals a day puts you in control of your diet while frequent and inconsistent snacking leaves the quality of your diet to random chance and luck.

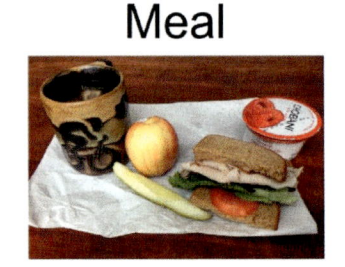

Both snacks and meals have their place in a healthy diet, but it's a lot harder to eat healthy when the bulk of your diet is made out of snack-style foods rather than wholesome meals.

Snacks are often lower quality foods

A meal typically involves more whole foods and ingredients than any snack type food which is often mostly processed ingredients. Such processed ingredients are usually less nutritious and less satisfying.

Meals include more variety

A snack is usually just one or two things like a chocolate bar or a piece of fruit. A meal involves a plethora of ingredients which satisfy both your pallet and nutritional needs a lot better.

Meals create consistency

Meals tend to be something you eat at consistent times, with consistent foods in consistent portions. Keeping to such dietary habits makes it much easier to maintain and improve a healthy diet. In comparison, snacks are much more random and inconsistent which makes it harder to maintain healthy eating habits.

There's nothing wrong with a snack or two each day. The issue isn't snacking itself. The problem is when you look back on the day and realize you never had an actual meal but instead just grazed on snack foods.

#2 Eat plants at each meal

There's more to building muscle and being healthy than just an optimal macronutrient profile. There are vitamins, minerals, antioxidants, phytochemicals and a host of other nutrients that have a role to play. Many of these nutrients can be found primarily in plant-based foods.

Like whole meals, consumption of plant-based foods is diminishing. This decrease might be related to the rise of snacking. Plant-based foods, especially vegetables, seldom satisfy when eaten on their own. A head of lettuce or fistful of green beans isn't a very satisfying snack, but they are enjoyable parts of a wholesome meal. This is why it's important to round out each meal with a healthy amount of plant-based foods.

#3 Include a source of protein at each meal

Protein is a big topic of debate in nutrition. Some say you need a lot; others claim you don't need very much. I say, include some protein in each meal, and you'll probably be fine.

Keep in mind that protein doesn't have to always come from meat or animal products. It can be from nuts, soy and complementary protein sources like beans and rice.

#4 Adjust portions

What you eat is important, but it isn't the only consideration in a healthy diet. Portion size is also critical and can make all the difference in the world.

Consider the portion size of a snack or meal as a whole as well as the various foods in each meal. You may not need to make drastic changes to your diet or adopt any extreme dietary ideas. Adjusting the portion size of what you already eat may be more than enough to improve the health of your diet.

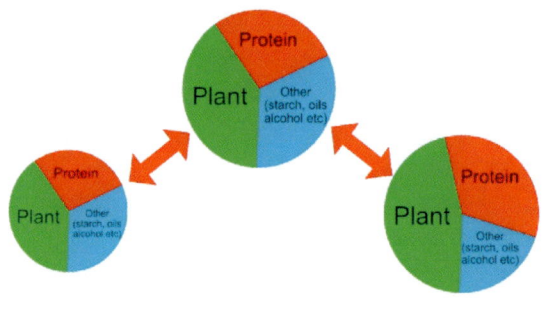

Most athletes don't need to make radical changes to their diet. It's often best to adjust portion sizes to your personal needs. You can change the size of a meal overall like in the example on the left or you can change the amount of each food type like in the example on the right.

#5 Pay attention to your desire and satisfaction curve

A healthy diet requires listening to and respecting the signals your body is sending you. Every day your own body is giving you accurate feedback based on how your diet is influencing your performance and health. This information is far more precise and applicable to you than anything you will read in a book or read on a blog.

Unfortunately, there are a lot of messages in our fitness culture telling you that your body is the root of your problems and such signals are to be ignored or even directly opposed. Such advice is cutting you off from the best available information regarding your health and wellbeing. If you're hungry and feel better eating a certain way, then do that. If following someone's advice increase your stress levels then make a change.

Your mental and physical energy is one of the biggest indicators of a healthy diet. Something probably needs to change if you feel tired or sluggish after eating a meal. You can also become tired if you're not eating enough or getting enough nutrient-dense foods. You're probably on the right track if you make a change and your energy level improves throughout the day.

Appetite and satisfaction are also important considerations. Ideally, you should want something, consume it in a reasonable quantity and then be satisfied. When you follow this cycle, you restore a balance between what you want and what you consume which results in the reduction of stress.

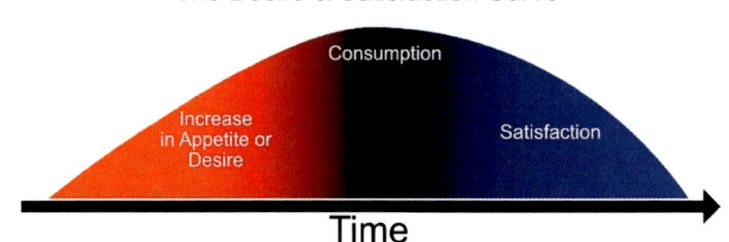

A healthy diet respects the natural bell curve between appetite and satisfaction. Your hunger and desire to eat something increases in time. You then honor your appetite by consuming what you want and satisfaction should quickly follow.

Several influences can disrupt the desire and satisfaction curve. Diets based on restriction and deprivation preach how you should fight, ignore or even hate on your appetites. Many dogmatic theories claim your appetites are the problem and you should seek to eliminate or control them. These messages can cause you to turn your back on the very impulses that tell you what is best for you. Ignoring them causes your appetites to build until you eventually "crack" due to the excess stress that's built up.

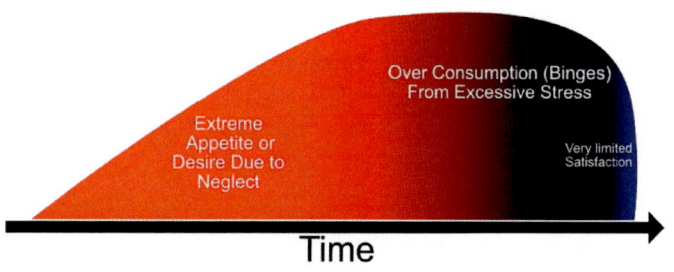

Fighting, or ignoring, your appetites can produce excessive amounts of both physical and mental stress which often results in over-consumption and guilt.

You can also fail to reach a state of satisfaction by not eating what you want or need. A classic example is when you're hungry and ready for a meal but instead, opt for a candy bar and soda from the vending machine on the way to a meeting.

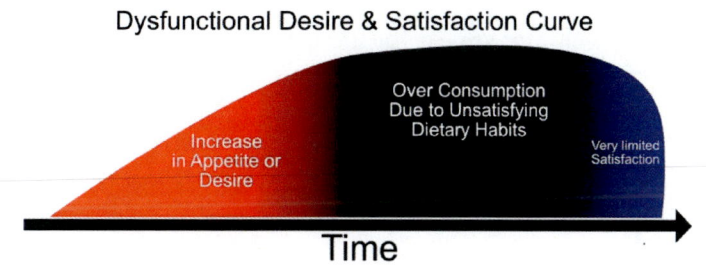

Failing to honor your appetites can result in over-consuming food or drink because it doesn't do a good job at satisfying your true desires. This results in less satisfaction and the over-consumption adds to the stress of your unsatisfied desires.

Mistakenly consuming what you don't want can happen through misinterpreting your appetites. A common instance is when people mistake thirst for hunger and eat something when they really just want a glass of water.

Sometimes, you can miss the mark and feel like you have a hard time becoming satisfied because you don't know what you want or are not getting it. This sort of thing can happen a lot when people try to satisfy emotional appetites with food. They may be bored or lonely and use food as a pacifier. While that food may provide some enjoyment, it fails to satisfy the true emotional desire and leaves you feeling unsatisfied no matter how much you eat.

Like hunger, people can be taught to ignore or fight their feelings of satisfaction and satiety. A common example is a rule that you should always clean your plate or finish your meal. This rule can cause you to continue eating even though your body has told you that it's had enough.

Distraction can also play a role in overshooting your satisfaction target. It's a lot easier to overeat while your attention is on a screen or other form of distraction.

#6 Limit calorie-laden beverages

What you eat is one thing but what you drink can be quite another. It's much easier to consume massive quantities of calories, sugar and artificial substances when those things are in liquid form. Eating three candy bars at once may seem like a lot, but it's pretty easy to drink the equivalent amount of sugar or calories from a single cup.

While it's easy to ingest a lot of calories and sugar through beverages, it's also relatively easy to reduce calories by drinking less juice or soda. Some people drop quite a bit of weight just by drinking less even though they maintain the same food intake.

This can also apply to so-called healthy beverages like protein shakes and smoothies. A meal-in-a-cup isn't always a healthy option just because it has protein or wheatgrass in it.

#7 Emphasize quality and satisfaction when making food choices

There's an old myth that eating healthy means denying yourself the pleasures of food, but the opposite is the case. The more pleasure and satisfaction you gain from food the easier it will be to reduce stress and tame your appetites.

One of the best ways to do this is to emphasize the quality of the foods you select. Choosing fresh whole foods will ensure you gain more value from every bite. This approach also applies to treats and snacks. Why settle for generic sweets that only taste pretty good, when you can spring for a freshly prepared desert that tastes amazing?

So the next time you're shopping, spring for the good stuff and you'll find you won't need nearly as much to satisfy your appetites

I know these ideas aren't very sexy or cutting edge, but that's the point. Like with calisthenics training, a healthy diet shouldn't impose a lot of restrictive rules upon your life. The more you can satisfy your needs without having to stress over every detail the better you'll recover and you'll gain more benefit from your training.

Points To Ponder

1. Don't beat yourself up over making a supposedly "bad" food choice. It probably won't matter very much and adding emotional stress to your dietary choices won't make your diet any healthier.
2. A healthy diet has just as much to do with how you emotionally feel about food as what food physically does to your body. If you want to make big changes to your diet, first pay attention to how you feel about certain foods and contemplate how your choices are influenced by those feelings.
3. There's no need to get caught up in the hype surrounding diet fads and trends. Diet trends come and go because they make inflated promises and are difficult to maintain. The ideal diet for you is one that probably doesn't come with a label attached to it or a celebrity endorsement.
4. Just as your best training comes from basic exercises, the best foods focus on basic ingredients.
5. Invest a little time to learn how to prepare your own favorite dishes so you always look forward to your own home cooking. Usually, the best meals come from simple recipes.
6. Cook in bulk and save food in ready-to-eat portions to save time and money.
7. In general, the more wholesome ingredients you include in a meal, the more satisfying and nutritious it will be.
8. Improve the flavor profile of any dish by adjusting the amount of salt, sweet, fat and acid in the dish. If something doesn't taste quite right, chances are it's missing one of those four things.
9. Refine your palate by giving your food a "kiss" of flavoring. Gradually reduce sauces, spices and other flavor enhancers so you don't need to overload the dish and saturate it with too much salt, sugar or fat.

Bonus Chapter: DIY Tools Of The Trade

One of the best things about bodyweight training is you don't need any fancy equipment to practice it. While it's minimalist nature is appealing, you may want to include a few pieces of equipment to add variety and novelty to your training. Some equipment can also make it easier to progress or regress basic exercises.

Standard pieces of equipment like rings and parallettes can be a great addition to your training. While commercial equipment is effective and reliable, I've always enjoyed making my own calisthenics equipment to suit my personal needs. I'm an inventor at heart and building my equipment became an obsession when I first started calisthenics training. At first, I did it to save money, but each time I made something I found flaws in the design that motivated me to build another version. After several years, I had spent a great deal more than if I had just purchased a commercial version of what I was trying to build. While I didn't save any money, I had developed some designs I really enjoy using more than their commercial counterparts.

Before I show you what I've built, and how you can make them yourself, there are a few things you need to know.

#1 None of these tools are essential

There isn't a single piece in this chapter that will make or break your success. Your results come down to how well you use your body, not how well you can use stuff. Feel free to adopt and discard these tools as you wish.

#2 Build and use these tools at your own risk

All of these tools are simple in both construction and use, but since you're furnishing your materials I can't promise you a risk-free experience. I don't know if the towel you hang from has a tear that will split, or if a plank of wood will give you a splinter. Use both caution and your own best judgment when building and using this equipment.

#3 Feel free to change and modify

All of these designs are the result of my playful experimentation, and I encourage you to do the same. If you think up a way to make any of this stuff work better for you, then go for it.

So without further ado, let's get into some of these designs.

Suspension Trainers

Suspension trainers are the multi-tool of the calisthenics world. You can do hundreds of exercises with them for almost any goal imaginable while mimicking classic weight machine exercises like chest flys, triceps extensions, and core work. They are also the closest thing you can get to a truly portable gym and come in handy when you need to do pull-ups, rows, and dips while traveling.

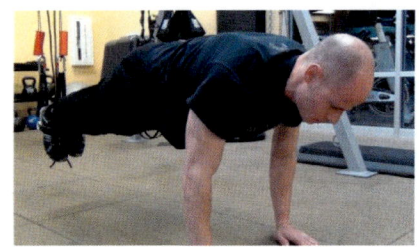

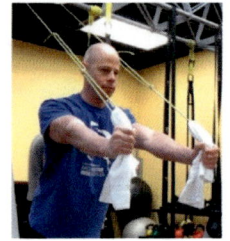

Suspension trainers give you hundreds of exercises that can enhance and supplement your training. Suspending your feet, like in the image on the left, can make planks much more challenging. You can also simulate weight machine exercises, like the triceps extension on the right.

I don't even want to think about the time and money I've spent trying to develop the perfect suspension trainer. With every version I created, I found flaws and drawbacks that prompted me to scrap that design and start all over again. I quickly became obsessively picky with my designs and drew up a list of qualities I wanted. These include:

- Dual anchor points so you can set the straps up to any width to accommodate your unique build and what's best for each exercise.
- Full vertical handle adjustment so the handles can go from an inch above the floor to an overhead reach.
- Small and lightweight, so it's ultra-portable.
- Super easy to set up and take down within a minute.
- Strong, safe and durable enough for weighted dips and pull-ups.
- Ergonomic without any rough edges or elements that impede movement.
- Universal anchoring so you can hang it from above points both inside and outside.
- Quick and easy infinite handle height adjustment so you can place the handles at any height you like.
- Easily accommodate a variety of accessories.
- Made from inexpensive and readily available materials.

I lost a lot of sleep trying to figure out how to make all of these requirements work within one design but I finally got it right with the Prusik Trainer.

Prusik Trainer

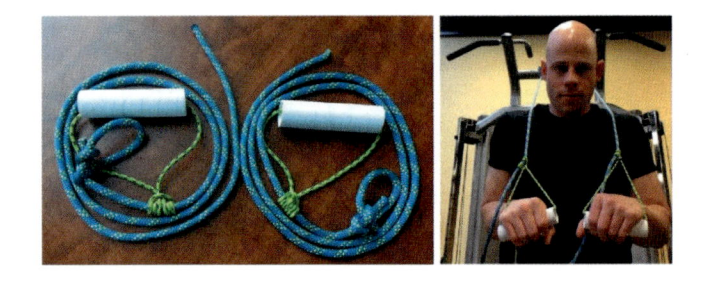

You may notice this trainer uses rope instead of nylon straps like most other trainers. Rope is the ultimate smart device. It's reliable, inexpensive and readily available. You can easily customize every characteristic of the trainer to your specific needs because rope gets its functionality from knots. Nylon suspension straps use metal hardware and stitching which works, but it adds bulk, weight, and cost. It also comprises the trainers' versatility. Once you stitch a loop into a strap you can't make that loop bigger or smaller if need be. Knots gives you all of the functional qualities you need without the weight, bulk, cost, and lack of versatility. Metal hardware can also wear out nylon straps over time whereas knots give you much more longevity.

Materials You'll Need For The Prusik Trainer

- Two lengths of 8mm climbing rope 7-12 feet long
- Two lengths of 4mm climbing rope 3.5 feet long
- Handle material from either PVC or a weight machine handle
- Small razor blade and light grit sandpaper if using PVC handles
- Climbing tape

I get my rope from local outdoor supply stores like REI where they can cut it to the length I need. If possible, have a professional cut your rope there at the shop. Most shops cut the rope with a heated tool that melts the ends and prevents fraying.

Knots you'll need to know

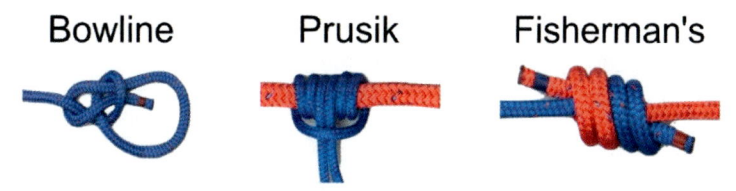

Bowline   Prusik   Fisherman's

www.animatedknots.com

These are cinch knots so the more weight you place on them, the tighter they hold. They are not too complicated, but I do recommend practicing how to tie them correctly before building your first suspension trainer. You can find videos and instructions on how to tie these knots at www.animatedknots.com.

How To Build A Prusik Trainer

Once you understand how to tie your knots building a prusik trainer is quick and easy. First, take your 8mm anchor rope, the one that's long and thick, and tie a bowline knot into one end to create a loop that's about 3 inches in diameter. This loop will serve as your anchor point which you throw over an overhead bar and feed the handle through.

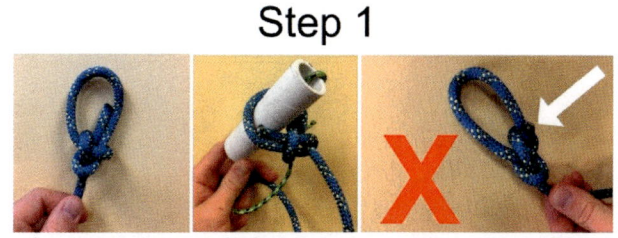

Step 1

Tie a bowline knot into the end of your 8mm rope ensuring the loop is large enough to fit your handle through. This will allow you to set up and take down your trainer without having to remove the handle. Be sure to leave some extra rope on each end of the knot to reduce the risk of it coming undone.

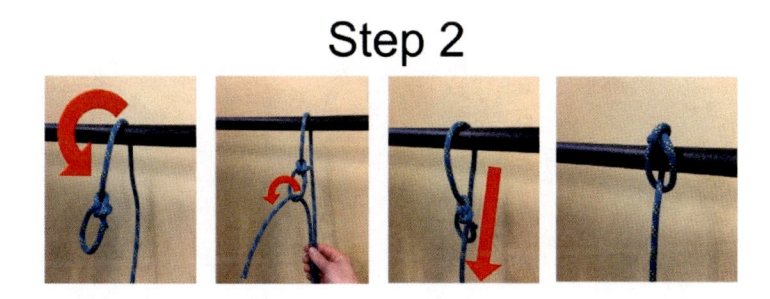

Step 2

Throw the bowline knot over a sturdy overhead support that can easily support your weight. Thread the other end through the loop and pull it down to lock the rope around the support.

Next, take the 4mm handle rope and feed it through your handle and connect the two ends with a fisherman's knot.

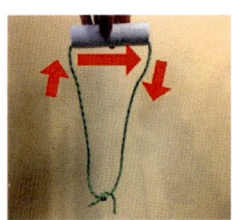

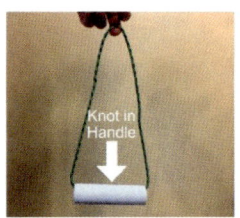

Step 3

Run the 4mm rope through the handle you've selected and tie the ends together with a fisherman's knot. Rotate the rope so the knot is inside the handle.

Lastly, tie the handle rope to your anchor rope with a prusik knot with 3-4 loops. I find it's easier to tie the prusik knot around the anchor rope when it's hanging with some tension pulling down on it. You can stand on the end on the floor or ask someone else to gently pull down on the rope it to keep it tight.

Step 4

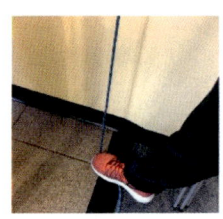

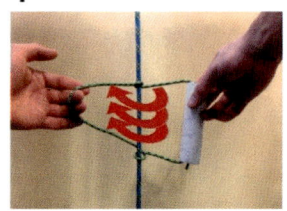

Place some tension on the hanging 8mm rope. Wrap the handle around the 8mm rope 3-4 times. Do this by feeding the handle through the loop on the other side of the handle.

Lastly, smooth out the overlapping handle rope so it hugs the 8mm rope. Be sure your prusik knot loops are flat to securely grip the 8mm rope.

Step 5

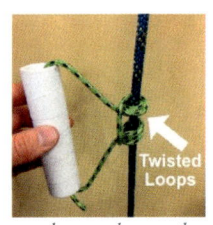

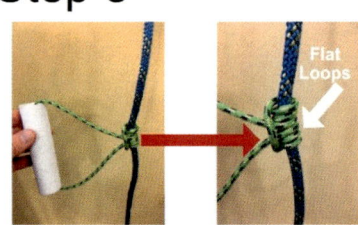

Move the two ends of the prusik knot together and smooth out any overlapping loops so they all lay flat and hug the anchor rope securely.

Be sure the fisherman's knot remains in the handle rather than outside it. One reason is the knot won't rub against your arm while doing push-ups and dips. The other is to prevent the knot from moving to the prusik knot and jamming it. Jamming will compromise the safety of the prusik knot.

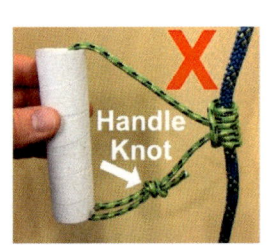

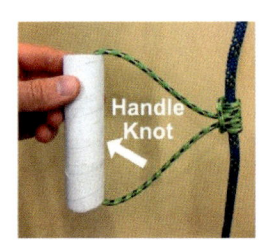

What kind of handle should you use?

You have two options when making your handle for your suspension trainer, PVC pipe or the handle from a commercial weight machine. I've used both and each option has it's pros and cons.

Like with rope, the advantage of using PVC is you can custom build your handle to be the length and diameter you like. People with larger hands prefer a more beefy handle that will be about 1-1.5 inches in diameter and 5.5-6 inches in length. Smaller hands will work best with a 3/4 -1-inch diameter pipe that's about 5 inches in length. PVC is also inexpensive and available in most hardware stores.

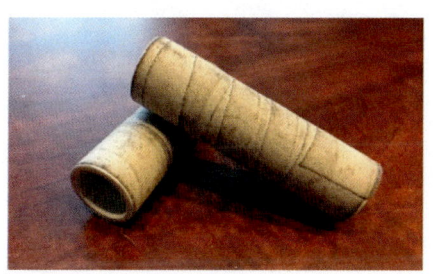

PVC handles are inexpensive and highly customizable, but they do take a little more work to produce a finished handle that works properly.

The disadvantage of PVC is it's a bit tricky to cut and smooth out the edges so they won't wear into the handle rope. If you're going to use PVC, you must make sure to cut each length at a 90-degree angle to avoid angled ends that can make rotating the handle feel uneven. More importantly, you'll need to smooth out the inside and outside edge of the handle edges to minimize wear on your rope. I cannot stress enough how important it is to make sure the rotation of your handle is as smooth as butter under load. If not you'll risk wearing out your rope which can increase the risk of it breaking.

Never use any rope that's worn or frayed!!!!

I've been able to smooth out the ends of PVC with a razor blade and a sand block. Creating a smooth edge takes a little practice to shave off the inside lip without any nicks and bumps. Sanding down the end of the handle takes time and patience, but it's well worth it for a smooth finish.

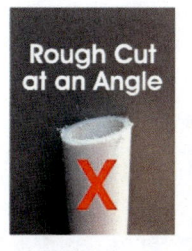

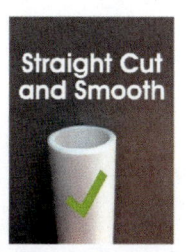

Once you have your handles cut and smoothed, wrap them in climbing tape to give them a grip texture that won't slip. Climbing tape has a similar feel to hockey tape but it holds up better, and the tacky adhesive won't bleed through over time and get on your hands. You can also pick up a roll when buying your rope at the outdoor store.

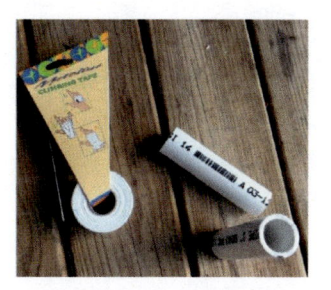

Climbing tape is a useful way to add some grip to the smooth texture of PVC. It's also more durable and doesn't leave a sticky residue like hockey or duct tape.

Your other handle option is to shop for a weight machine handle with a nylon strap. You can find these in many fitness equipment stores or online.

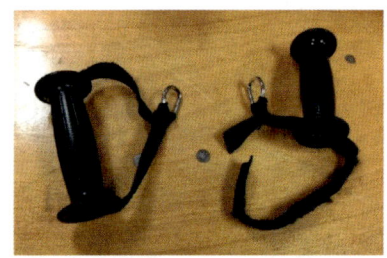

Commercial grade weight machine handles are perfect for building your own suspension trainer. Just cut off the nylon strap and you're good to go!

These handles are more expensive than PVC, but they are a commercially produced product that's designed for physical training. They are a good fit for most size hands, have smooth edges and provide a sure-grip texture. Most of them will come with a nylon loop attached. You can feed your handle rope through the D-ring on the loop, but I just cut it off to save bulk and weight. The D-rings can also get in the way of your arm or elbow during pushing moves.

Bowline Trainer

The bowline trainer offers the ultimate in portability with its compact and lightweight design. Whereas most other suspension trainers can fit in your gym bag, the Bowline trainer can fit in your pocket.

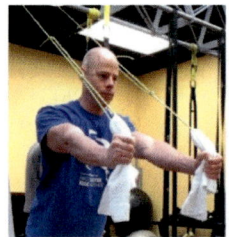

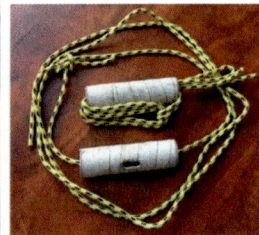

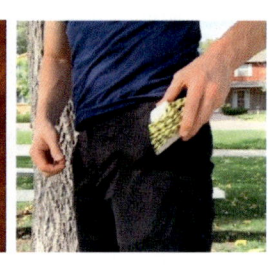

Materials You'll Need For The Bowline Trainer
- Two lengths of 6mm climbing rope 10-15 feet long
- PVC handles or commercial handles
- Small razor blade and light grit sandpaper if using PVC handles
- Climbing tape for PVC handle

Knots you'll need to know
- Bowline knot

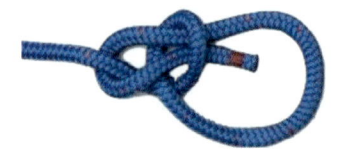

The bowline knot is the only knot you'll need to use for your bowline trainer. Photo: animatedknots.com

The bowline trainer is the simplest and easiest to build and set up. Start off tying a bowline loop for the anchor point just like with the prusik trainer. You don't need to pass a handle through this loop so feel free to make it about 1-2 inches in diameter. Attach to an overhead anchor the same way you would with the prussic trainer.

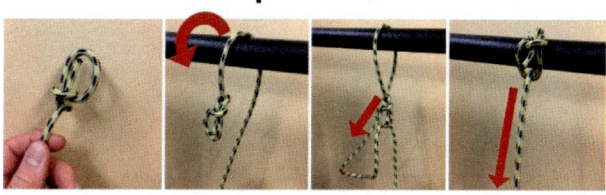

Steps 1 & 2

Make a bowline knot leaving about an inch of line on each end of the knot just as with the prusik trainer. Sling the knot over a sturdy support and feed the other end of the rope through the loop of the bowline knot and pull it tight to the support.

Feed the other end of the rope through your handle and tie a bowline knot above it, so the handle is at the height you wish.

Steps 3 & 4

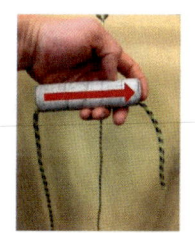

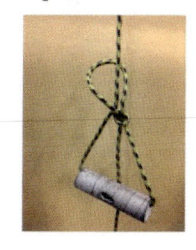

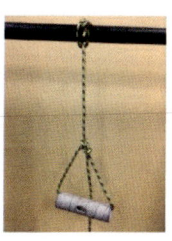

Feed the end of the rope through your handle or attachment of choice and tie another bowline knot.

Complete the same process for the other handle, and you're finished.

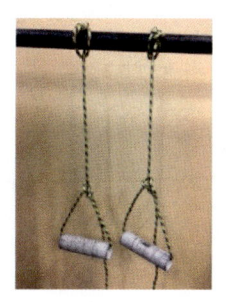

Adjusting the height of the handle is a little more cumbersome than with the prussic trainer. You can make small adjustments by loosening the bowline knot near the handle to make the handle loop bigger or smaller. To make larger changes in height, you'll have to undo the handle knot and retie it at a different level. This type of adjustment is why the bowline trainer is best suited for workouts where you'll only need one or two handle heights.

Suspension Trainer Accessories

Suspension trainers are like cable-style weight machines where you can attach all kinds of accessories to them. Once again, none of them are necessary, but they can add some fun and variety to your training.

Foot slings

Foot slings give you the ability to suspend your feet off the ground just like your hands do with handles. They can help with exercises like the hamstring curls and planks I mentioned earlier in the book. There are a few different ways you can build your slings with various pros and cons.

Note: The nylon straps in this chapter can be found at www.strapworks.com.

The first and possibly easiest way to to make a foot sling is to run a 1-inch wide by 2-foot long nylon strap through your handle with a cam buckle to attach and adjust the length.

Materials you'll need for foot slings
- Two lengths of 1-inch x 2-foot nylon straps with attached steel cam buckles

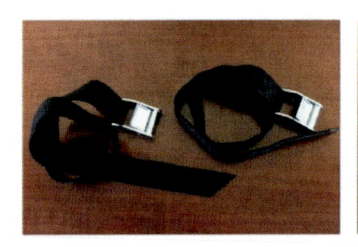

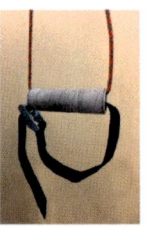

Simply feed the strap through the handle of your suspension trainer and into the cam-buckle on the other end. You then adjust the size of the loop for a perfect fit for you. This design also gives you the ability to remove the straps, so they don't get in the way when you're not using them.

The next option is a foot sling with a quick-adjust foot support. This design is bigger and heavier, so it's probably not something you'll travel with, but it's a great accessory for training at home or in the gym.

Materials you'll need for quick-adjust foot slings
- Two lengths of 1-inch x 3-foot long "simple slings" with 2-inch loops each end
- Two 1-inch PVC T joint
- Two climbing quality carabiners

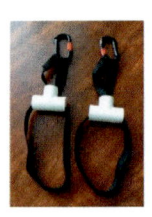

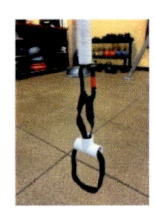

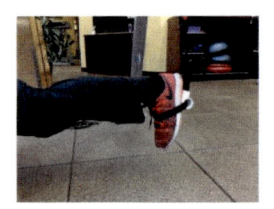

These clip-on foot slings instantly adjust to the perfect size no matter what size foot you have or what type of footwear you have on. They're even a perfect fit if you're barefoot.

The advantage of this foot sling is you can adjust the size of the foot loop by sliding the PVC foot support up and down. The foot support will lock in place once you place weight on the loop. You can quickly bring your foot in and out of a big loop and then pull the support down to fit your foot perfectly. After all, everyone has different size feet and shoes so why should everyone be expected to use the same size foot sling?

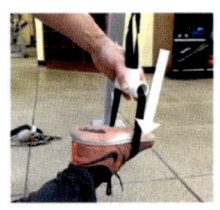

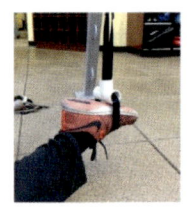

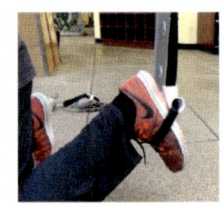

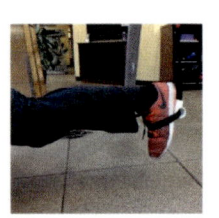

Place your foot in the loop. Slide the PVC foot support down to the bottom of your foot. The support will not slide if you're placing weight on the strap. Next, press your heel against the support and lift your knee off the floor while the foot sling securely suspends your foot.

The adjustable loop provides support for dorsiflexion in a prone position. I've used far too many foot slings that were too big for me to press my heel against the handle to pull my toes forward. While this isn't bad, it can compromise your stability and tension along your flexion chain.

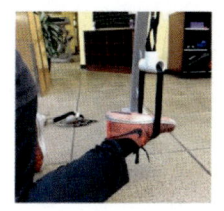

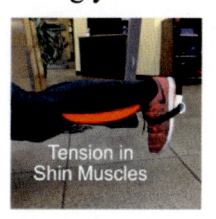

Being able to confidently push your heel against a foot support locks your foot in place and allows much greater tension along your shin muscles.

There's also a minimalist foot sling option for the Bowline Trainer that mimics the adjustable foot sling without any additional hardware. All you need to do is cut a small 1"x1/3" inch hole in the middle of each handle.

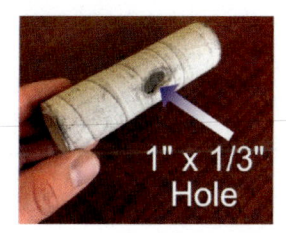

I find the easiest way to create this hole is to drill a few holes with a drill bit that's slightly wider than the rope you're using and make it about 1-inch long. Be sure to smooth out any rough edges.

From there, you feed the rope through the hole in the top, around the bottom of the handle and back up through the hole. Tie it with a bowline knot at the top making sure you have enough room to slide the handle/ foot support up and down to fit your foot through.

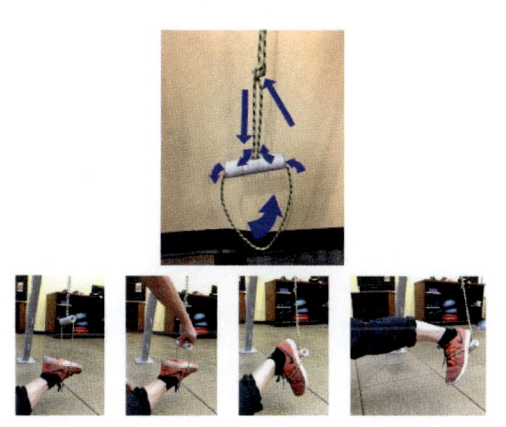

The bowline foot sling works by feeding the end of the rope through the hole in the top, around the bottom and back up through the hole where you tie it off with a bowline knot. It works the same way as the clip-on adjustable foot slings.

Press and ROM Blocks

Push-up handles are a popular piece of DIY calisthenics equipment, and it was one of the first tools I built. After using them for a year or two, a mentor suggested I give them up and keep my hands flat on the floor. After following his advice, I had to admit he was right. The discomfort I felt in my wrists and hands disappeared as my lower arm became stronger and more flexible. I thought I had been using those handles because my wrists were tight and stiff, but it turned out they were a crutch that was contributing to the problem.

Not that I jumped right into full flat-palm training right away. That would be like insisting everyone should jump into full depth squats without any gradual progression. Instead, I used a pair of what I call press blocks as a progressive step between using handles and a flat palm.

Materials You'll Need For ROM Blocks

- Two blocks of 2x4 6 inches in length
- Sandpaper

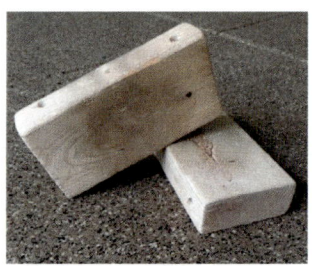

They may look like ordinary blocks of wood, but they are a truly versatile training aid.

These press blocks allow you to work with a flat palm and bent wrist, but your fingers can curl over the edge. This position gives you some of the control and support of a flat palm without requiring quite as much flexibility in your wrists. You can progress the exercise by adjusting how much your fingers are off the edge until you're hands are ready for a full flat palm on the floor.

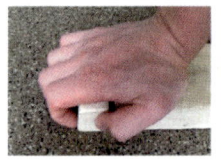

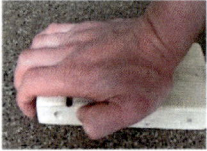

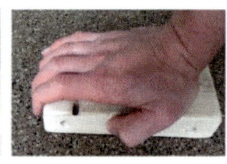

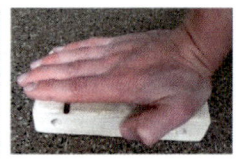

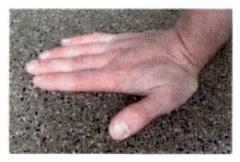

Many calisthenics exercises are best done with a flat hand on the ground. This can be difficult for those who have stiff and weak wrists. Progressively placing more of your hand on the top of a block allows your hand and wrist to develop the strength needed for flat hand exercises.

Making press blocks is simple. You just cut two 6-inch lengths of a 2x4 which you can get at any hardware store. Sand down any rough surfaces and edges. You can also apply paint or varnish to give them a finished look.

Press blocks also work as range of motion blocks. You can stack them up to quantify exercises like push-ups and leg raises.

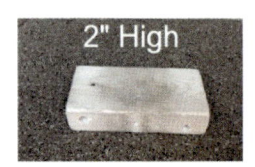

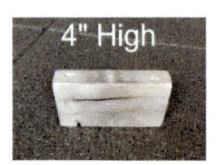

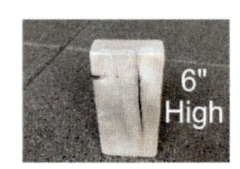

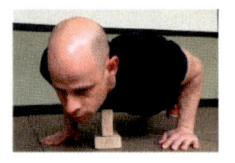

A 6-inch length of 2x4 can be set at 3 different heights which makes them ideal for stacking and quantifying your range of motion in many exercises.

Suspension Press Blocks

Once I experienced the value of pressing with a flat palm on the floor, I wondered how to bring the same benefits to suspension trainers. It took me a lot of failed designs before I finally figured out how to make suspension press blocks.

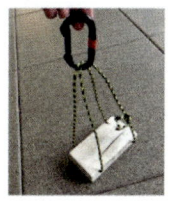

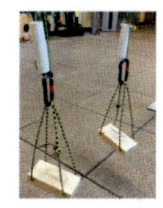

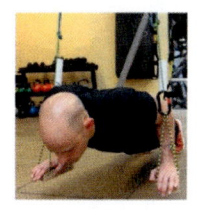

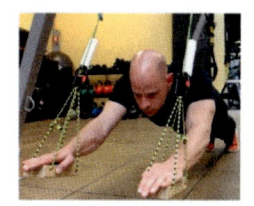

Materials You'll Need For Suspension Press Blocks

- Two 6-inch lengths of wooden 2x4
- Sandpaper
- Two 2-foot lengths of 6mm climbing rope
- Drill with 3/8" drill bit
- 2 carabiners

These are easy to make, and you can use the press blocks you already have on hand. All you need to do is drill two holes widthwise into the sides of two press blocks. Be sure to drill each hole about 3/4 of an inch from each end. Then take a 2-foot length of 6mm rope and feed it through the holes. Connect the two with a double fisherman's knot.

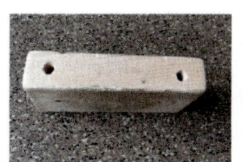

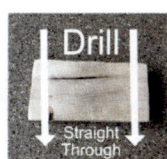

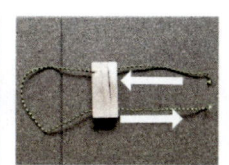

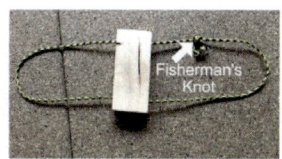

Connect the two loops with a carabiner or through the rope on your bowline trainer.

Be aware these blocks can twist and pivot when you place weight on them. They provide a little more challenge to your hand and wrist stability which can make your joints stronger and more resilient.

Towel Grips

Towels are a simple and versatile accessory you can add to your suspension trainer. You don't even need to build or assemble anything. Just loop a towel over your handle rope, and you're ready to go. These are perfect for pull-ups, rows, rear flies, triceps extensions, and curls. You can also use towels for grip training with hanging exercises.

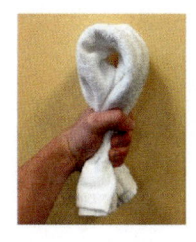

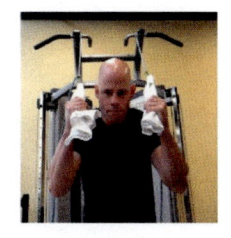

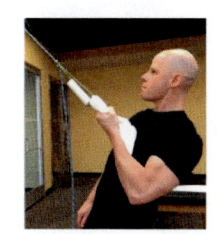

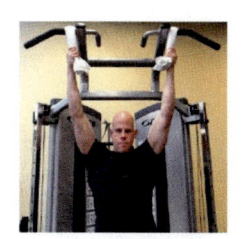

Towels are an economical way to improve grip strength and build up the forearms. They also allow you to work some unique angles with rows and triceps extensions.

The grip used with towels does a great job of strengthening the whole hand and the muscles in the forearm. It's important to grab the towel with both the palm and the fingers. I like to grip with the palm first and then wrap the fingers around the towel.

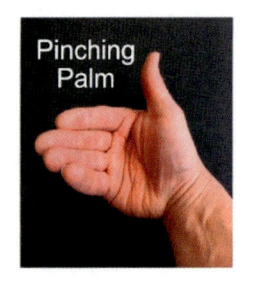

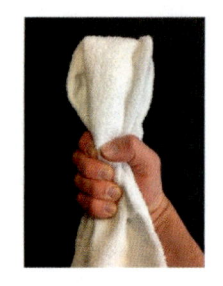

Towel work can be hard on the fingers so I make sure to pinch the towel first with the palm and then wrap the fingers around towards the wrist.

Small hand towels are a perfect size and you can find them in most home goods stores.

Grip Grenades

These are another fun toy to challenge your grip and add variety to your training.

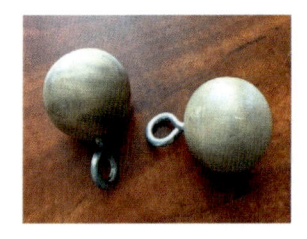

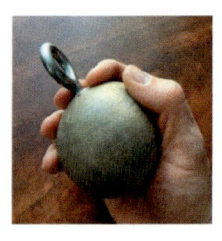

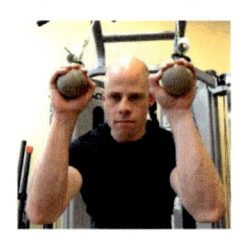

Materials You'll Need For Grip Grenades
- Two wooden craft balls 2.5-3 inches in diameter
- 2 I-bolts with 2 inch long threads
- Drill with a drill bit slightly smaller than the threads of your I-bolts
- Wood glue

The trickiest part about making these is finding a place where you can buy the wood balls. Some craft stores might carry them, but I've always had to purchase them online. The size of the ball you use depends on the size of your hand with larger sizes providing a more challenging grip. I use a 2.5-3 inch diameter size which works well for most people.

Construction is simple. Drill a hole into the very top of each wooden ball that's slightly narrower than the threads of the I-bolt. Squeeze some wood glue into the hole and screw the I-bolt into the top using a wrench for leverage.

You can then attach the grip grenades to a suspension trainer or overhead bar with a carabiner or simple sling.

Straight bar

Using two independent handles or press pads is great, but sometimes you might want to use a straight bar. As you can see in the image, adding a straight bar to your suspension trainer is pretty simple.

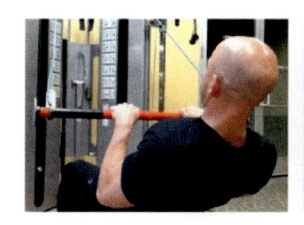

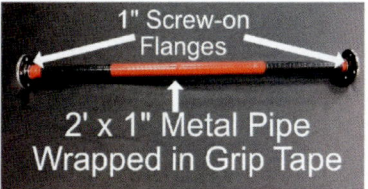

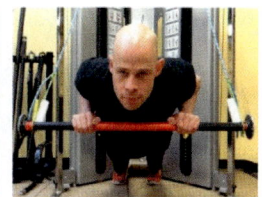

Materials You'll Need For A Straight Suspension Bar

- One 1-inch wide and 2.5-3 foot long metal pipe
- Two metal flanges to screw into each end of the pipe
- Grip tape
- Electrical tape if you want to rotate the bar

All you need is a 2.5-3 foot long metal pipe with a flange screwed onto each end to prevent it from slipping off the rope. You'll want to wrap the bar with climbing tape, but I suggest wrapping the ends in electrical tape to allow the bar to rotate against your suspension trainer for exercises like curls.

Push-Up Lever

The push-up lever adds extra resistance to your push-ups without loading your upper back or spine with a lot of weight. It loads your hips which work not only your pushing strength but also core and hip strength as well. Some people find their abs are sorer than their upper body after using it the first time.

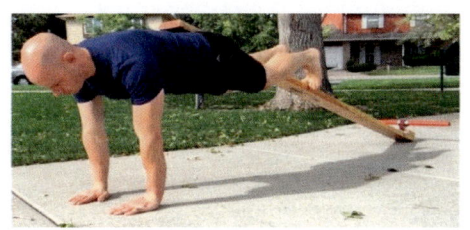

The Push-Up Lever Loads your hips so you don't place any stress directly on your neck or spine like weight vests or placing weight on your back.

A push-up lever can be anything that's over 5 feet long and won't bend or flex. The first version I ever "made" was just a standard pine 2x4. You can also use a length of pipe or a barbell. I like to use a 2x6 because the wider board allows more room for my feet to push into the board.

Using a push-up lever is simple, but not easy. Start by lying on the floor and place the lever on your hips. Wrap your feet around the lever while squeezing the back and inside of your knees against the lever.

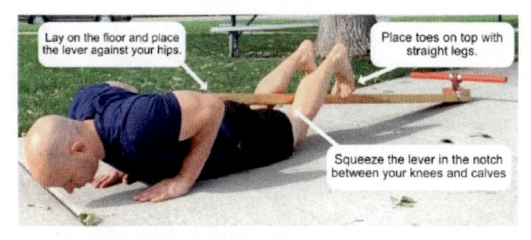

Brace your entire flexion chain by pushing down on the lever with your feet while pushing your hips up. You'll probably find your hips want to sag a bit if your abs aren't tight enough. Unlike with a traditional push-up, you want to push your hips slightly higher than normal, so they are roughly the same height as your shoulders at the top of each rep. Do your best to lower your hips and shoulders at the same speed, so your body stays parallel to the floor through the whole range of motion.

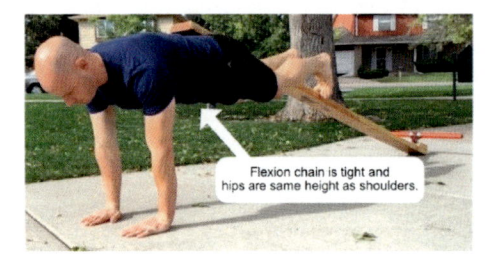

You can slightly adjust the resistance by moving the end of the lever further in or out from your feet.

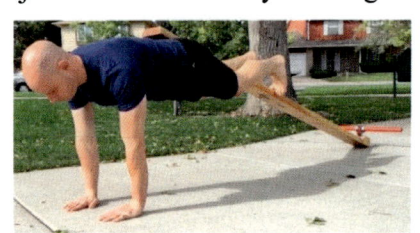

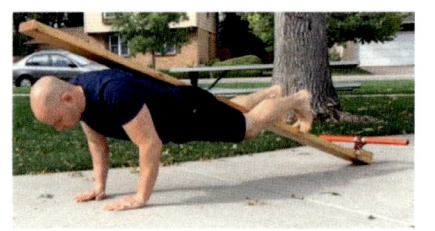

The image on the left shows the end of the lever near my hips which is the most difficult position. On the right, I've moved the lever up which reduces the resistance.

Push-Up Lever 2.0

You can add an insane amount of resistance by adding some weight pins to one end of the board. Just screw on a pipe flange and mounting a T-junction with a 1-inch pipe and two 6 inch pipes.

Materials You'll Need For Push-Up Lever 2.0

- Push-up lever board either 2x4 or 2x6
- 1-inch pipe flange
- 1-inch x 1-inch long metal pipe joiner
- 1-inch metal pipe T junction
- Two 6-inch long 1-inch metal pipes
- 1.5-inch long screws
- Rope or carabiner to attach it to suspension trainer

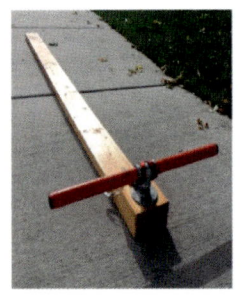

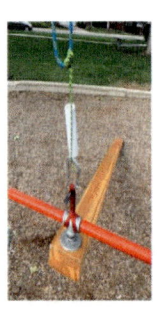

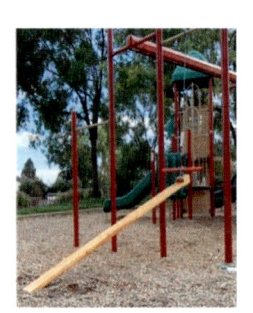

Adding a simple T-bar at one end of the lever allows you to hang that end a few feet off the ground with your suspension trainer.

This version involves extending the end of the lever in front and above you. You can use your suspension trainer to set this up by attaching the weight pins to the rope handle or tying it up with a bowline knot. You'll want to suspend the end of the lever about 1.5-2 feet off the floor depending on how much room you'll need underneath.

Slide yourself under the lever with your feet close to the end on the floor and your hips wedged between the lever and the floor. Press yourself up just as you would using the lever on the floor while lifting the end of the weight pins. Be sure to lift the lever a few times by hand to make sure the rope won't come off the weight pins.

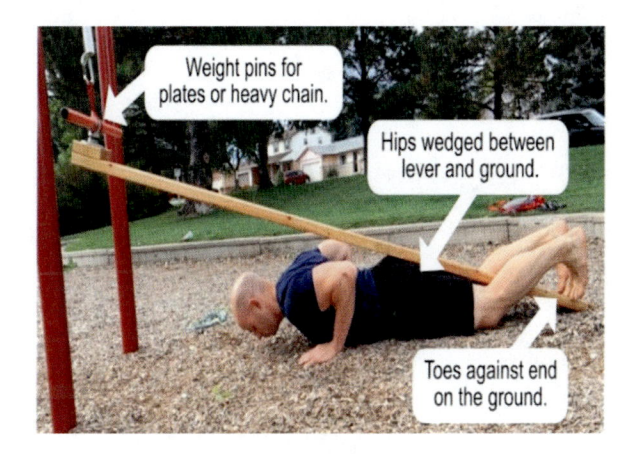

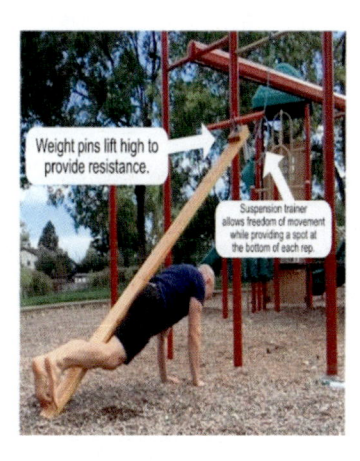

A little weight goes a long way with this method. I've found 10-20 pounds on the weight pins is plenty for most athletes. I've maxed out powerlifters with just 45 pounds. As with all loaded calisthenics listen to your body and go easy at first.

You can also use the lever for rows. All you need to do is set your handles low enough to grab while laying on your back. Rest one end of the lever on your hips and wrap your heels around to the front of the board. From there, reach up and grab the handles and pull yourself up while keeping your extension chain tight.

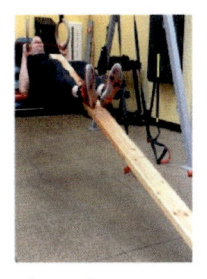

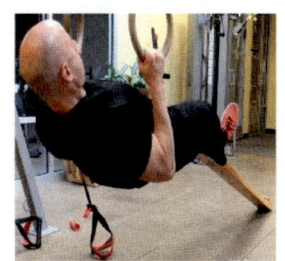

You can make rows harder just as you can make push-ups more difficult. Just lay on the floor, rest the lever on your hips and press in with the back of your heels.

Dip Belt

The dip belt is a staple for those who enjoy weighted calisthenics. Like the ab rollers, you might be better off just purchasing a simple commercial dip belt. With that said, I have invented a unique design you might wish to build for yourself.

The easiest, and crudest way, to make a dip belt is just to use a length of rope or chain around your waist. This style can work, but I've got something better for you.

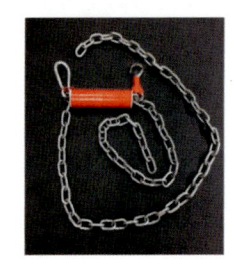

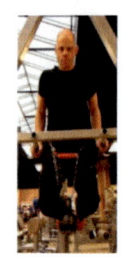

My unique belt has two adjustable loops, one for you and one for the weight. You can custom fit the belt to the size of your waist and the load you're lifting. It also gives you a handle to carry the weight and offers support for your lower abs.

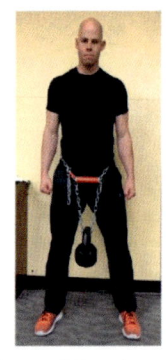

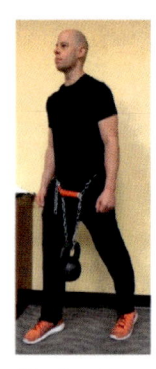

This dip belt offers a custom fit for both the weight you lift and your waist. The handle rests securely against your hips and allows you to move around with the weight attached.

Materials You'll Need For Dip Belt

- One 4-foot length of chain
- One 6-inch length of 1-inch PVC
- One metal S-hook
- One small carabiner
- Climbing tape

Making the dip belt is easy. Just wrap the PCV in grip tape and feed the chain about halfway through. Clip the carabiner on one side of the handle and the S hook on the other. Place some climbing tape on the S-hook so that it won't come off the chain.

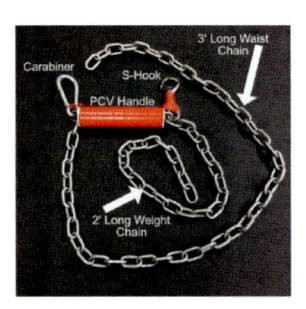

To use it, feed the lower end of the chain through your weight of choice and clip it to the carabiner. Then pick it up by the handle and wrap the other end around your waist to clip it onto the S-hook at your desired length.

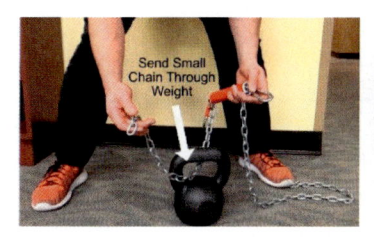

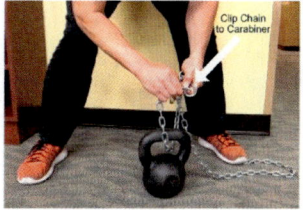

You can also pad this dip belt with a length of foam insulation.

You'll probably find this belt is best suited for relatively light loads. I've seen videos of guys doing dips with hundreds of pounds, so you'll probably want to use a leather belt for such a purpose. I usually do my dips on straps which don't require nearly as much weight as solid bars.

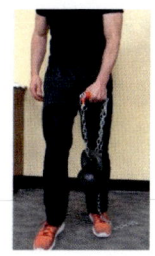

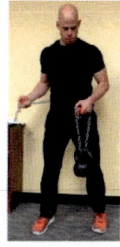

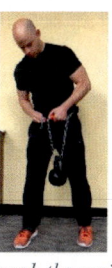

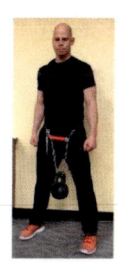

Once you have the weight hooked up, you can lift it up by the handle and hook the waist chain around your hips and hook it to the S-hook.

Squat Stick

It's easy to ignore the small ways you can move your arms and torso to make your squats and lunges easier. The squat stick helps you become more aware of these little movements and provides a way to quantify them for accurate progression.

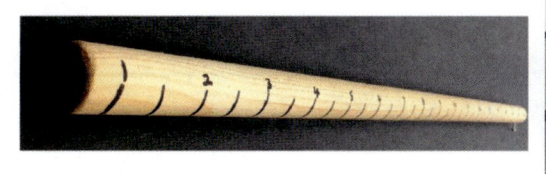

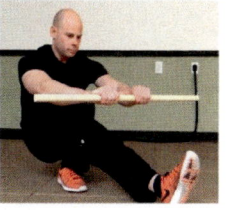

It may look like an ordinary stick but this simple piece of wood can do wonders for your calisthenics training.

Materials You'll Need For A Squat Stick

- One 3-foot long wooden dowel about 1 inch in diameter
- Measuring tape
- Permanent marker

The squat stick serves a couple of purposes. It helps keep your upper body still so you don't move it to make the exercise easier. It also helps point out weaknesses by amplifying any tilting or twisting you might habitually do while squatting.

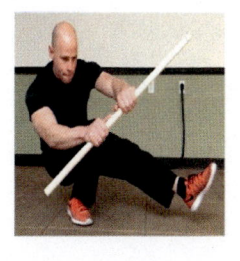

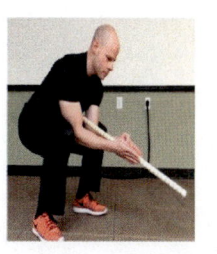

The Squat Stick amplifies any upper body movement that helps you become more aware of important, yet slight, alterations in technique.

You can use the stick two ways. The first is to hold it straight out with the stick horizontal. You can then progress the difficulty of the exercise by how close your hands are together.

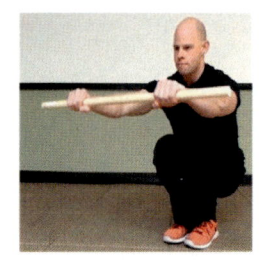

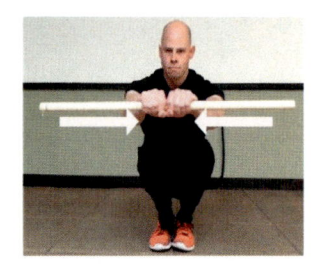

The width of your hands can make a big difference in the difficulty of your squat. The squat stick allows you to both quantify and maintain your hand width while training.

You can also hold the stick straight out from your chest. This position can highlight any excessive twisting and lean forward as you squat. Press your hands together and try to pull the stick into your chest as you do your reps. This position will show you if and when you reach or lean forward to make the exercise easier. You can make the exercise harder by holding your hands the closer to your body.

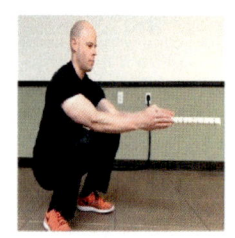

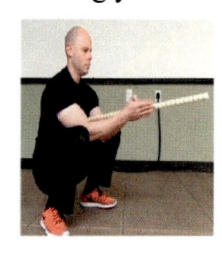

Placing the stick at the bottom of your chest allows you to quantify how far you reach forward during squats.

The squat stick can also be handy for quantifying hand width during push-ups or detecting knee flexion during leg raises.

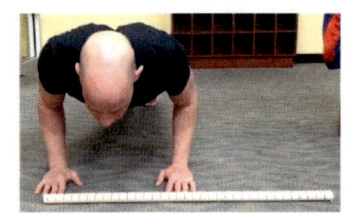

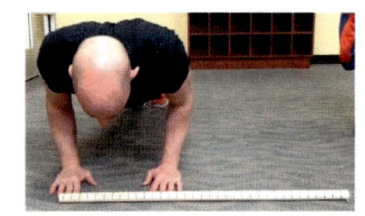

The numbers on the squat stick come in handy for quantifying hand width during push-ups and other floor based exercises.

Playgrounds

Playgrounds are free outdoor 24-hour access calisthenics gyms. They are pet and kid friendly and can be found almost anywhere you travel. The only membership fee you have to pay is just to show up.

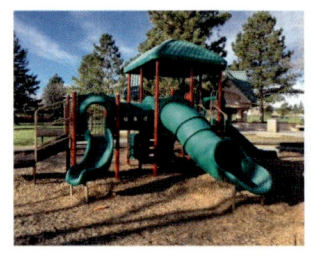

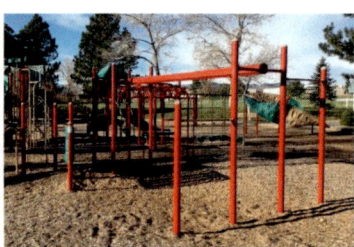

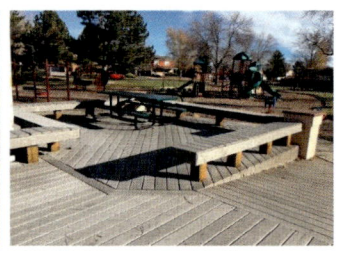

Look for elements that include a lot of metal bars and supports like in the center image. Plastic elements (left) won't offer many opportunities for training. Elements like ledges, benches and finished surfaces (right) are also valuable.

Where to find them and what to look for

You may have a lot of playgrounds near you depending on where you live, but not all of them may be suitable. To find the best options, I recommend starting with playgrounds in public recreation areas like parks or running paths. These areas are typically open at any time and include elements adults can use for calisthenics. You can find these parks with the map app on your phone or do an internet search for parks and recreation areas.

The second best place to look is schools. While these playgrounds can work, the equipment is usually intended for children, and it's best to use them well outside of hours of operation like in the evening or on a Sunday.

Also, be on the lookout for useful calisthenics elements when scoping out playgrounds. The general rule is metal parts are good, while plastic is not as useful. The more bars and metal elements you have, the more exercises you can potentially perform. It also helps to find bars that are high enough for you to reach with a full body hang. Lastly, try to find places with concrete or a surface you're comfortable laying down on for floor work.

What to bring to the playground

A good playground will provide you with a lot of options, but you'll still want to bring a few things to get the most benefit from using it.

Suspension trainer

Packing a suspension trainer with you will give you more variety and versatility. It's also handy to use one to progress or regress any of the moves you're planning to do.

Water and sun protection

A workout on a playground is just like any other outdoor activity. Make sure you bring sun protection, wear appropriate clothing and have plenty of water with you. I prefer to keep everything in a hydration backpack that can hold much more water than a typical water bottle.

Gloves

Playgrounds can involve some environmental risks you might not find in an indoor gym. There can be sharp objects on the ground and surfaces where the paint is chipping or rusty mental edges. I bring a pair of full-finger cycling or work gloves with me to provide protection against these hazards. Gloves also improve comfort when grabbing hot or cold metal bars.

Towel

A beach towel can improve comfort when laying on the ground or hard surfaces. You can also use it to wipe off water from rain or snow so that you won't slip on metal bars. Towels are also great for grip work.

A sense of creativity

Playgrounds offer some unique elements you may not have in an indoor gym. A classic monkey bar and a lot of space to run around are good examples. So feel free to break from your usual routine and get creative. Try crawling across the monkey bars while doing a pull-up at each rung. Do dips and push-ups on the parallel bars. Or just run from one end of the park to the other after each strength set. Use your imagination and think outside of your regular workout to breathe some new life into exercises that may be getting stale.

Well, my friend, you've come to the end of the book, but your journey is just beginning. By now you've learned a lot but I'm sure you may have plenty of questions as well. Calisthenics is a massive discipline and the information in this book is just scratching the surface. There are still many other exercises and approaches I wasn't able to cover so this book is by no means a complete set of instructions. This is just a good starting point and something you can refer to over the years.

Above all, remember that you're the one who's in charge of your training. Be playful and experiment with your approaches while letting the basic principles of S.A.I.D, T.U.T, and I.C.E be your guide. Free free to discard or modify any of the exercises as you see fit. Always listen to your body and have fun.

You can continue to learn more through the Red Delta Project Podcast and the Red Delta Project YouTube channel.

Happy training and as always, be fit & live free!

- Matt Schifferle

Made in the USA
Coppell, TX
04 January 2020